Body Knowledge and Control

Contemporary westernised societies are besotted with the 'body', its size, shape and 'health'. Governments, business and the popular media spend and earn fortunes encouraging populations to get healthy, eat properly, exercise daily and get thin. But how are contemporary social trends and attitudes towards the 'body' reflected in the curriculum of schools, in the teaching of physical education and health? How do teachers and health professionals influence young people's experiences of their own and others' bodies? Is health education liberating or merely another form of regulation and social control?

Drawing together some of the latest research on the body and schooling, *Body Knowledge and Control* offers a sharp and challenging critique of (post) modern day attitudes toward obesity, health, childhood and the mainstream science and business interests that promote narrow body-centred ways of thinking. Includes:

- A critical history of notions of body, identity and health in schools.
- Analysis of the 'obesity epidemic', eating disorders and the influence of nurtured body image in racism, sexism, homophobia and body elitism in schools.

John Evans is Professor of Sociology of Education and Physical Education in the School of Sport and Exercise Sciences, Loughborough University. **Brian Davies** is Professor of Education in the School of Social Sciences, University of Cardiff. **Jan Wright** is an Associate Professor and Associate Dean (Research) in the Graduate School of Education, University of Wollongong, Australia.

Body Knowledge and Control

Studies in the sociology of physical education and health

Edited by John Evans, Brian Davies, Jan Wright

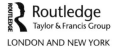
Routledge
Taylor & Francis Group

LONDON AND NEW YORK

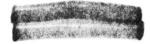

First published 2004
by Routledge
11 New Fetter Lane, London EC4P 4EE

Simultaneously published in the USA and Canada
by Routledge
29 West 35th Street, New York, NY 10001

Routledge is an imprint of the Taylor & Francis Group

© 2004 Selection and editorial matter John Evans, Brian Davies,
Jan Wright; individual chapters, the contributors

Typeset in Times New Roman by
Keystroke, Jacaranda Lodge, Wolverhampton
Printed and bound in Great Britain by
TJ International Ltd, Padstow, Cornwall

British Library Cataloguing in Publication Data
A catalogue record for this book is available from the British Library

Library of Congress Cataloging in Publication Data
A catalog record for this book has been requested

ISBN 0–415–30645–0 (pbk)
ISBN 0–415–30644–2 (hbk)

For Mamgu

Contents

Preface

In recent years 'health' has become a major, multi-million pound industry, a topic of routine everyday conversation, a matter of political concern. So much so that many are inclined to accept the health knowledge and advice that is offered in 'the public interest' and define health issues and agendas as well-meant, ideologically innocent, even incontrovertible matters of fact that should be better reflected in the curriculum of schools. This book arises out of growing misgivings among professionals working internationally in fields of physical education and health regarding such developments. It challenges the core assumption that schools, especially the teaching of physical education and health as currently configured in them, are inherently 'good' for children's and young people's well-being and health. We contend that the insights gained from the sociology of Emile Durkheim, reflected in the work of the British sociologist Basil Bernstein, can further our understandings of the complex relationships between 'society', schools and the 'embodied self'. Part I introduces the contents of this book, highlighting the importance of Bernstein's work in understanding how 'ability', 'health' and corporeality are fashioned in schools. It also illustrates how the influential work of the French sociologist Michel Foucault can inform research methodologies inter-rogating the relationships between social practices and power relations both inside and outside schools. Part II highlights the place of social theory in research and curriculum development. It considers the importance of locating curriculum developments in schools in a 'risk society' and wider socio-historical and political contexts. Questions are raised about the ways in which contemporary discourses around 'obesity', 'childhood' and 'health' are socially constructed, politically regulated and mediated by government policies and school practices. Part III takes us into physical education and health classrooms and sport contexts in schools. Here critical questions are raised about the nature of health education teaching; playground and other behaviour; peer group cultures and relationships; physical culture; 'ability' and 'impairment'; eating disorders; and spatial matters. These are considered in relation to issues of 'healthism', racism, sexism, elitism and homophobia in schools. Part IV clarifies the concepts of 'performance' and 'perfection' and cautiously draws out the implications of the studies reported in this text for future research and curriculum development in physical education and health in initial teacher education and schools.

Contributors

Lisette Burrows is a Senior Lecturer in pedagogy at the School of Physical Education, University of Otago, New Zealand. She has published articles on gender, developmental discourses in physical education and young people's perspectives on health. She is currently co-editing a text on teaching health and physical education in New Zealand and a book on critical problem-solving in physical education. Her research interests are in two areas: sociology of health and the social construction of physical education curriculum.

Gill Clarke is a Senior Lecturer in physical education and biographical studies at Southampton University and Deputy Director of the Centre for Biography and Education. She co-edited *Researching Women and Sport* (Macmillan, 1997) and has published widely on sexuality in physical education and sport. She is on the editorial board of *Sport, Education and Society* and *Auto/Biography*. She is currently writing a book on the war artist Evelyn Dunbar, having received a grant from the Paul Mellon Centre for Studies in British Art to complete this research. Her research interests centre around the narratives of women's lives, be these in the sporting arena or on the home front.

Brian Davies is Professor of Education in the School of Social Sciences, Cardiff University, Wales. Since his *Social Control and Education* (Methuen, 1976) he has taught and written widely on social theory and research, educational policy and pedagogic practice. He is currently editing a second collection of research papers arising from the work of Basil Bernstein, with Joe Muller and Ana Morias.

John Evans is Professor of Sociology of Education and Physical Education at Loughborough University, England. He teaches and writes on issues of equity, education policy, identity and processes of schooling. With Emma Rich and Rachel Holroyd he currently is researching the relationships between formal education and eating disorders. He has authored and edited a number of papers and books in the sociology of education and physical education and co-authored with Dawn Penney, *Politics, Policy and Practice in Physical Education* (E & FN Spon, 1999).

Michael Gard is a Senior Lecturer in dance, physical and health education at Charles Sturt University's Bathurst campus, Australia. He teaches and writes about the human body, gender and sexuality, the shortcomings of biological determinism in all its forms, and the use and misuse of dance within physical education. He is also working on the biography of Robert Helpmann, the famous Australian ballet dancer. He is co-author with Jan Wright from the University of Wollongong of *The Obesity Epidemic: Science and Ideology* (Routledge, 2004), which expands on the arguments raised in his contribution to this volume.

Robyne Garrett is a Lecturer in sociology, physical education and dance at the University of South Australia. Her research interests include gender and physical activity, physical education methodology and alternative movement approaches. Her recently completed Ph.D. thesis entitled 'How Young Women Move' investigates the construction of gender in physical activity contexts for young women. The research employed a storytelling approach, resulting in a series of 'physical stories', which will be further utilised as a strategy for the development of critical reflection in teacher education courses.

Jo Harris is a Senior Lecturer in physical education and Director of teacher education at Loughborough University and is President of the Physical Education Association of the United Kingdom (PEA UK). She has produced numerous teaching resources on health education, presented at national and international conferences and has published many articles in professional and academic journals. She is editor of *Health-Related Exercise in the National Curriculum* (Human Kinetics, 2000) and with Lorraine Cale is currently co-editing a book on young people, physical activity and health. Her research focuses on health within the National Curriculum for Physical Education.

Lyn Harrison is a Senior Lecturer in health and physical education at Deakin University, Australia. Her research interests include: adolescent risk-taking and HIV/AIDS; community and school-based sexuality education; early school-leavers; gender and identity. Her research findings have contributed to policy development in school-based STD/AIDS prevention education at the state and national level and have been presented at national and international conferences and published in both Australian and international journals.

Rachel Holroyd is a Research Associate with the School of Sport and Exercise Sciences, Loughborough University. Her doctoral research examined the areas of young people, embodied identity and physical culture. She has published a number of papers in international journals. Her current research involves an examination of the relationship between formal education and disordered eating among young people, and an evaluation of the use of physical activity programmes with disaffected youth in schools.

David Kirk is Professor of Physical Education and Sport in the School of Sport and Exercise Sciences, Loughborough University. He has published widely on the social construction of physical education from contemporary and historical perspectives, and on the part physical education and sport practices play in the social regulation of the body.

Rosary Lalik is an Associate Professor of literacy studies at Virginia Tech. There she teachers courses in pedagogy and research and has been selected for membership in the Academy of Teaching Excellence. Her research has been published as articles in refereed journals and as chapters in scholarly books. With Kimberly Oliver she has co-authored a book entitled *Bodily Knowledge: Learning about Equity and Justice with Adolescent Girls* (Peter Lang Publishers, 2000).

Deana Leahy is a Lecturer in health and physical education in the Faculty of Education, Deakin University, Australia. Her research interests include post-structuralist and genealogical approaches to health education. She is currently completing a Ph.D. exploring the productive effects of health education discourses in curriculum policy and classroom pedagogies.

Kimberly L. Oliver is an Assistant Professor in physical education at New Mexico State University where she teaches courses in pedagogy and socio-cultural issues in physical education. She is the co-author, with Rosary Lalik, of *Bodily Knowledge: Learning about Equity and Justice with Adolescent Girls* (Peter Lang Publishers, 2000).

Dawn Penney is a Senior Lecturer in the School of Education at Edith Cowan University, Australia. Since 1990 she has been engaged in critical policy research focusing upon contemporary developments in physical education, in both the United Kingdom and Australia. She is co-author with John Evans of *Politics, Policy and Practice in Physical Education* (E&FN Spon, 1999) and editor of *Gender and Physical Education. Contemporary Issues and Future Directions* (Routledge, 2000).

Emma Rich is a Lecturer in gender, identity, health and physical education at Loughborough University, UK. She has published in refereed journals and books in sociology, education and feminist studies, including *International Studies in Sociology of Education and Pedagogy, Culture and Society*. Her research interests include issues of gender, identity, teacher education, eating disorders, cyber-culture, and gender and Olympic governance. Her current research with John Evans and Rachel Holroyd is centred on the relationships between education and the aetiology of eating disorders.

Chris Shilling is Professor of Sociology at the University of Portsmouth. A second edition of his *The Body and Social Theory* was published in 2003 by Sage Press, and other recent studies include *The Sociological Ambition* (Sage, 2001, co-authored with P.A. Mellor), and *Re-forming the Body* (Sage, 1997, co-authored with P.A. Mellor). He teaches mainly in the areas of the body and society, classical and contemporary sociology and social theory, and the emotions and social life, and is currently completing a sole-authored book entitled *The Body in Culture, Technology and Society* (Sage, 2004).

Andrew C. Sparkes is Professor of Social Theory and Director of the Qualitative

Research Unit in the School of Sport and Health Sciences, University of Exeter. His research interests are eclectic and include: interrupted body projects, identity dilemmas, and the narrative (re)construction of self; and the lives and careers of marginalised individuals. These interests are framed by a desire to seek interpretive forms of understanding and an aspiration to represent lived experience using a variety of genres. His most recent book is *Telling Tales in Sport and Physical Activity: A Qualitative Journey* (Human Kinetics Press, 2002).

Richard Tinning is Professor of Pedagogy and Physical Education in the School of Human Movement Studies at the University of Queensland. As a teacher educator he has been involved in major Australian curriculum development projects, worked on large-scale professional development programmes for teachers, and been a consultant to both schools and universities. Richard's research interests are informed by a socially critical perspective and, since the early 1980s when he wrote 'Physical education and the cult of slenderness: a critique', he has been increasingly interested in pedagogical work on/for the body and the role of physical education in the making of the 'healthy' citizen.

Jan Wright is currently Associate Professor and Associate Dean (Research) in the Faculty of Education at the University of Wollongong. She is co-author with Richard Tinning, Doune MacDonald and Chris Hickey of *Becoming a Physical Education Teacher* (Prentice Hall) and, with Doune MacDonald and Lisette Burrows, *Critical Inquiry and Problem Solving in Physical Education* (Routledge, forthcoming). Her most recent research draws on a feminist post-structuralist approach to explore the place and meaning of physical activity in the lives of young people. She has also published in a number of other areas including: media representation of sporting bodies; and the social construction of gendered bodies in physical education. She is currently working with Michael Gard on a book, *The Obesity Epidemic: Science and Ideology* (Routledge, 2004).

Foreword

Educating bodies: schooling and the constitution of society

Chris Shilling

Introduction

Schooling has historically been implicated in 'civilising' the bodies of children: the physical capacities and appearances of each new generation undergo development and disciplining in schools, while teachers have long sought to encourage their charges to exert control over when and how they should translate impulses and affects into actions (Elias 2000 [1939]). These 'civilised' standards are not neutral or universal, but reflect the specific norms and expectations of societies at particular stages in their development. They are also stratified, having long been applied in different ways to young people depending on their social background. Nevertheless, it is on the basis of such standards of physical control and stimulation that the organisation and transmission of educational knowledge is deployed within schools. Knowledge is not dispensed and received by a 'circuit of minds', but flows within a corporeal context that determines its salience and that shapes what particular individuals make of the curriculum on offer to them. Until relatively recently, however, the embodied nature of schooling has constituted something of an 'absent presence' in the sociology of education (Shilling 2003). The physical targets of pedagogical knowledge, be they preschoolers or university students, usually appeared only fleetingly before fading and even disappearing from the analytical landscape.

This relative neglect of the body had serious implications for the sociology of education. Without taking into account the corporeal preconditions and characteristics of social action, and the ways in which structures of power and control impacted on the bodies of those subject to them, its multiplying perspectives were fated to construct partial explanations which misrepresented the mechanisms associated with the organisation, delivery and reception of education. In these cases, it was never properly clear how educational outcomes actually occurred because it was never properly clear how the *physical* habits, senses and dispositions of embodied students responded to and were shaped by the organisation and transmission of knowledge within schools. Judging by many educational studies, indeed, it was possible to conclude that the subject matter of educational studies consisted of a variety of young *minds*. These may have been active minds, enabled differentially by the symbolic codes that structured their family environment (and they were certainly characterised by cognitive dispositions that varied according to social class, gender and 'race', and structured by the unequal distribution of cultural capital within the school system), but the individuals they belonged to were often described in a peculiarly ethereal manner.

This neglect was rooted in the mind/body dualism characteristic of that dominant tradition of Western thought which has marginalised body matters on the assumption that it is the *mind* that makes us distinctively human. As Descartes argued in *The Meditations*, 'I am . . . only a thing that thinks', and 'my mind . . . is entirely and truly distinct from my body and may exist without it' (Descartes 1973: 105, 156). Just as the body was not ignored completely within philosophy, however, neither was it totally absent from the study of education. While the enfleshed subjects of educational knowledge may rarely have been presented to us in their sensory entirety, some of the most insightful commentators on the subject recognised the significance of the organisation of bodies in schools. Basil Bernstein's *et al.*'s (1973 [1966]) paper on ritual in education still provides us with a rich source of ideas on the subject (even if the body remains something of a shadowy presence), while other educational studies usefully highlighted the quite remarkable levels of bodily constraint that children were subject to. Wolfson's and Jackson's (1969) report on ethnographies of nursery school children, for example, demonstrated how educational life was dominated by a series of physical mishaps and constraints. Some children experienced as many as thirty physical constraints on their behaviour in each hour, a figure which translates into thousands of corrections over a single year. It is difficult to overestimate the importance of these bodily engagements: it is through them that children begin, literally, to feel the parameters and demands of the educational environments through which they pass, and to associate the delivery of school knowledge with the cultivation of 'acceptable bodies'.

The dearth of educational studies which took the body as their explicit focus begun to change alongside the general explosion of writings on the body in sociology, and across the humanities and social sciences, that occurred during the 1980s and 1990s. However, this concern to address a novel subject in education was accompanied by a hunger for theoretical novelty which was not entirely productive. The turning away from classical figures in the field was associated with a new enthusiasm for all things Foucauldian, post-structuralist and post-modernist. These perspectives have yielded important insights – and some of the contributors to this volume continue to find them of use – but the writings of more traditional figures can still offer much in helping us to consider the significance of schooling within a democratic state. In this context, I want to use this foreword to examine how the writings of the most significant 'founding father' of the sociological study of education, Emile Durkheim, can productively be employed to analyse the relationship between the body, education and society. The editors of this volume seek to reinstate the significance of Durkheim for the analysis of education, largely through a critical appreciation of the Durkheimian theories of Basil Bernstein, so this is an appropriate point to revisit and re-interpret his general significance for accounts of the schooled body.

There has been a tendency in recent years to neglect the value of Durkheim's writings for the study of educational organisation and knowledge (Davies 1994), yet I want to suggest that his work can help us appreciate the body as a *multi-dimensional medium* for the constitution of society. This broad approach allows us to recognise the creation, sustenance and degeneration of social relationships as an inescapably corporeal process, and to highlight the significance of the embodiment of education. Instead of being a subject of marginal academic import, Durkheim allows us to view physical education (in the broadest sense of that term) as vital to the health of society. In what follows, I first examine Durkheim's analysis of the relationship between the body and society before focusing on his specific understanding of the contribution of schooling to this process.

Durkheim and the body

Social theories have made great strides in combating the view that the body is a wholly natural phenomenon, immune to the influence of society, but have sometimes substituted the biological essentialism they are hostile to with an equally one-sided social essentialism which loses any hold on the material facticity of the body. In contrast, Durkheim's writings highlight how the body is not only a physical *location* on which society inscribes its effects, but a material *source* of social categories and relations, and a sensual *means* by which people are attached to or dislocated from social forms.[1] Durkheim's most detailed explication of this theoretical approach can be found in his *The Elementary Forms of Religious Life*, an analysis he undertook in order to establish the fundamental processes governing the constitution of *all* societies (Durkheim 1995 [1912]). The broad corporeal principles underlying this study can be summarised as follows.

First, Durkheim views the body as a prime *location* for society. Society exists prior to the birth of each new generation, and the dominant patterns of social relations and institutions exert an inevitable effect on the development of embodied subjects. In particular, the common morality that turns a collection of people into a society for Durkheim is expressed through a symbolic order which structures not only the conscience and consciousness of its members, but the exterior of their bodies. This occurs when social values affect the physical size, shape and appearance of a social population. Thus, the body is surrounded by a series of totemic prohibitions and imperatives which seek to consolidate the moral order of society by determining how people relate to the topography and look of their own flesh and the flesh of each new generation (ibid.: 125, 138). Historically speaking, Durkheim argues that the image-imprinted-on-flesh 'is in fact and by far, the most important' mode of representation that exists. It is because bodies 'share in a common life, [that] they are often led, almost instinctively, to paint themselves or to imprint images on their bodies that remind them' of this life (ibid.: 223). Such 'tribal' markings may be less common in the contemporary world, but Durkheim identifies the elementary features of cultural norms which ensure appearance constitutes a strong marker of identity and belonging.

If the exterior of the flesh is a location for the effects of society, so too are the 'interior' dispositions and capacities of the body. These were analysed most effectively by Durkheim's close colleague, Marcel Mauss, who argued that those social techniques which are both traditional and effective to a society become ingrained through apprenticeships into the prime characteristics of the body. For Mauss (1973 [1934]: 71–2) 'there is perhaps no "natural" way for the adult' to manage their body and, therefore, 'each society has', and has to have, 'its own special habits' pertaining to the body.[2] These techniques are transmitted by initiation and education in which the surfaces of the body are penetrated and in which social symbolism enters the heart of the individual's physical self. As Durkheim (1995 [1912]: 211) argued, in order for *any* society to exist the life of the group must become 'organised within' the bodily being of individuals. These body techniques remain vital to modern societies because their transmission involves an 'education in composure' and rationalisation congruent with the needs of a specialised society (Mauss 1973 [1934]: 86).

The second principle recognised by Durkheim as fundamental to the constitution of social life recognises that while society pre-exists each new generation, the embodied capacities of individuals endow them with the ability to act creatively on their environment. In this respect, the body is not only a location for society but is also a *source* of the social space in which moral symbols and norms exist and develop. Indeed, the body possesses a particular importance in Durkheim's work because of his realisation that without the body neither life nor society can be (re)generated (Janssen and Verheggen 1997). Thus, while Durkheim (1982 [1895]) initially defined the social in opposition to the natural, he subsequently associated the creative powers of the body with a capacity for generating a social symbolism. This symbolism was significant because it created a space in which individuals could transcend their self-oriented impulses, and recognise others as common participants in collective life (Durkheim 1995 [1912]: 125, 138, 233). The potency of such symbols was such that they could enable people to reaffirm their commitment to a social order or envisage alternative ways of being.

Third, the body is not just a location on which society inscribes its effects and a source of social space, but also constitutes a *means* through which people are positioned within (attached to, or distanced from) their social milieu. For Durkheim, bodies are 'energised' via the social force of 'collective effervescence' during collective gatherings. When these gatherings are ritualised, they have the capacity to 'fix' individual emotions to common symbols: a process which structures the inner lives of individuals and enables a social group to know and feel itself to be a moral community (ibid.: 221–3, 229, 239). The process of attachment to society is such that it substitutes the world immediately available to an individual's perceptions for another, moral world in which people can interact on the basis of shared understandings (Durkheim 1974 [1914]). By 'drawing us outside ourselves', such attachment also 'puts us precisely in the position of developing our personalities' (Durkheim 1961: 73).

While the body is an indispensable means through which individuals can be attached to society for Durkheim, this attachment is not automatic and remains dependent on a periodic recharging provided by the effervescence of group life.

When group life weakens, the symbolic order of society loses the energy that gave rise to it and the reality it incarnated (Durkheim 1995 [1912]: 217, 342). Individuals can 'fall out' of society and, as Durkheim's (1952 [1897]) study of suicide illustrates, may even lose their thirst for life itself. Egoistic suicide, for example, is associated with a loss of meaning and an 'excessive individualism' in which the individual loses the support of that collective energy that attaches them to society (ibid.: 209–11). Life seems empty and 'the bond attaching man to life relaxes because that attaching him to society is itself slack' (ibid.: 214–15).

This view of the body may appear initially to have little to do with our concern for the education of bodies, yet it actually proposes a normative vision of the relationship between the body and society which has significant implications for the operation and analysis of schooling. For Durkheim, society could either develop the capacities of embodied individuals in ways that helped them fulfil their social potentialities (through, for example a 'normal' division of labour which matched the abilities and interests of individuals to the demands of the occupational structure), or could be structured in ways that left individuals isolated and cut adrift from social relations through which they could pursue realistic ambitions (Durkheim 1974 [1914]). What Durkheim (1961: 77) refers to as 'centrifugal' nationalism, for example, warps the development of people by placing 'national sentiment in conflict with commitments to mankind' and stands in dangerous contrast with the emotions encouraged by a healthy form of patriotism dedicated towards the scientific, artistic and peaceful improvement of society. This improvement of society, which was actually based on principles that worked towards the enhancement of humanity *as a whole*, operated by maximising the bodily capacities of individuals and the opportunities they had for contributing towards the general good (Durkheim 1961).

Schooling the body

Durkheim (1961: 150) recognised that schools played a major role in 'organising' society on and within embodied individuals, and viewed the school class as 'a small society'. He devoted a series of lectures to the subject of how they could instil the 'spirit of discipline' (involving a regularity of conduct and an internally felt obligation to obey) into pupils in order to assist in the reproduction of the moral order of society (Durkheim 1961). Properly executed, the function of schooling should be to foster in children an appreciation of human dignity that would help contribute to the fullest possible development of humanity (ibid., 1977 [1938]). This was a thoroughly physical process which should engage with bodily emotion as well as with the mind: the organisation of school ritual and the principles regulating the delivery of school knowledge should help promote individual and social good by engaging with *desires* as well as with thought (Durkheim 1961: 43). Collective representations must be given 'enough color, form and life' to stimulate moral action (ibid.: 228–9). That is, they should not operate exclusively at an intellectual level, but 'must have something emotional; they must have the characteristic of a sentiment' if they are to shape the personalities of pupils (ibid.: 229). As

Durkheim (ibid.: 229) elaborates 'The point here is not to enrich the mind with some theoretical notion, a speculative conception; but to give it a principle of action'.

Durkheim recognised that schooling was, in one sense, an imposition on pupils: it treated its embodied subjects as a *location* on which social designs could be imprinted However, he also emphasised that the moral order of schooling should simultaneously operate as a means by which individuals could realise their *own* potential (ibid.: 124). This order could only be sustained, furthermore, because, it builds on children's own preference for habitual action and on the ease with which children imitate and get attached to all manner of things outside themselves, including the sentiments of others. The organisation and delivery of educational knowledge did not, then, simply locate itself on the bodies of children. Instead, the bodily capacities of young people – capacities such as the 'aptitude' for sympathy that Durkheim (ibid.: 220) viewed as a first form of an eminently 'altruistic and social tendency' – constituted a *source* for this education and a prerequisite for the *attachment* of individuals to the society of which they were a part.

Durkheim's analysis of schooling had deeply practical implications. He was disturbed by the moral health of the society at the time he was writing, and his books *Suicide* and *The Division of Labour in Society* made it clear that he was concerned that modern society contained a number of tendencies which might frustrate rather than nurture the capacities of humans to revitalise the social environment in which they lived. In this context, he identified the school as the only proper intermediate organisation that existed between the family and the state. For Durkheim (ibid.: 232) 'communal life' had become 'very impoverished and now holds a very secondary place in our consciousness'. The corporeal processes involved in schooling, however, contained the potential to assist in the moral revitalisation of society.

Times have obviously changed since Durkheim was writing, but the Durkheimian scholar Basil Bernstein has expressed similar concerns about the relationship between schooling and the moral order of democracies in the contemporary era. More than that, Bernstein has argued that the organisation of power relations and discourse within education knowledge means that schools have *failed* in their duty to society. Instead of helping people feel they have a genuine stake in society, that they have a right to be included in society, and that they have the right to participate in procedures whereby social order is maintained and changed, Bernstein (1996: 5) associates schools with the production and reproduction of distributive injustices. Such biases are highly damaging to our social system. As Bernstein (ibid.) argues, 'these biases can reach down to drain the very springs of affirmation, motivation and imagination . . . [and] can become, and often are, an economic and cultural threat to democracy'.

Bodies of knowledge

The study of physical education has traditionally been a low-status subject within sociology, yet there is little justification for this as *all* education involves a physical education of the body. Antonio Gramsci (1971), for example, wrote about the importance of people being trained to acquire the stamina necessary to endure long hours of relative physical passivity if they were to study and engage critically with the hegemonic ideals of society, while figures as politically diverse as Adam Smith and Karl Marx recognised the importance of schooling in ensuring the health of young people. *Body Knowledge* seeks to reconnect our appreciation of physical education to such general evaluations of the significance of the body in schooling. Of particular importance in this respect is the editors' analysis of the uneasy coexistence of what they refer to as performance codes (stressing authority, discipline, hierarchy and order) with perfection codes (stressing autonomy, self-responsibility, surveillance and control). This essentially Durkheimian analysis draws on the work of Bernstein but extends it into the explicit analysis of the body in schooling in order to examine the socially stratified and contradictory demands placed on young people today.

The contributors to this volume explore a range of related phenomenon and while they do not all draw on the Durkheimian concerns of Bernstein in framing their discussions about the physical education of young people's bodies, they range widely across the several ways in which the body constitutes a medium for the constitution of society. Most examine how societies locate themselves on the bodies of students, but some of the contributions here also provide us with the potential of appreciating how corporeal creativity and change is possible, and highlight how educational practices emotionally stimulate the attachment and repulsion of different groups of students to different forms of physical education. In doing this, they draw on a range of authors and theories but all contribute to the invaluable task set out by Durkheim for the sociology of education. That is, to analyse how education becomes embodied in subjects, to explore the conse-quences of this embodiment for the moral health of society, and to recognise that embodied beings are not simply a location for society, but possess creative capacities which can also revitalise and begin to change the social space in which they exist. The enduring relevance of Durkheim for this task, I would argue, lies in his recognition that embodied subjects are a source of, as well as a location for, schooling and society, and that it is the complex interaction between bodies, educational knowledge, and wider social conditions, that determines how different groups of people are positioned within the education system. The value of this collection lies in its contribution to this task.

Notes

1 For a detailed discussion of these points, see Shilling 2004a and 2004b.
2 Even techniques of breathing are not immune from social intervention. In the West we tend to breath 'into' and 'out from' our chest, yet various Eastern forms of med-itation and exercise cultivate the use of the lower abdomen as a means of assisting the passage of breath into the body.

References

Bernstein, B. (1996) *Pedagogy, Symbolic Control and Identity*, London: Taylor & Francis.

Bernstein, B., Peters, R. and Elvin, L. (1973 [1966]) 'Ritual in education', reprinted in B. Bernstein *Class, Codes and Control, Vol. 3*, London: Routledge.

Davies, B. (1994) 'Durkheim and the sociology of education in Britain', *British Journal of Sociology of Education* 15(1): 3–25.

Descartes, R. (1973) *The Philosophical Works of Descartes*, Volume 1, trans. E. Haldane and G.R.T. Ross, Cambridge: Cambridge Univeristy Press.

Durkheim, E. (1952 [1897]) *Suicide*, London: Routledge.

Durkheim, E. (1961) *Moral Education. A Study in the Theory and Application of the Sociology of Education*, New York: Free Press.

Durkheim, E. (1974 [1914]) 'The dualism of human nature and its social conditions', in R.N. Bellah (ed.) *Emile Durkheim on Morality and Society*, Chicago: University of Chicago Press.

Durkheim, E. (1977 [1938]) *The Evolution of Educational Thought. Lectures on the Formation and Development of Secondary Education in France*, London: Routledge.

Durkheim, E. (1982 [1895]) *The Rules of Sociological Method*, Houndmills: Macmillan.

Durkheim, E. (1995 [1912]) *The Elementary Forms of Religious Life*, New York: Free Press.

Elias, N. (2000 [1939]) *The Civilizing Process*, Oxford: Blackwell.

Gramsci, A. (1971) *Selections from the Prison Notebooks*, tr. and ed. Q. Hoare and G.N. Smith, London: Lawrence and Wishart.

Janssen, J. and Verheggen, T. (1997) 'The double center of gravity in Durkheim's symbol theory: bringing the symbolism of the body back in', *Sociological Theory* 15(3): 294–306.

Mauss, M. (1973 [1934]) 'Techniques of the Body', *Economy and Society* 2: 70–88.

Shilling, C. (2003 second edition) *The Body and Social Theory*, London: Sage.

Shilling, C. (2004a) 'Embodiment, emotions and the foundations of social order. Durkheim's enduring contribution', in J. Alexander and P. Smith (eds) *The Cambridge Companion to Durkheim*, Cambridge: Cambridge University Press.

Shilling, C. (2004b) *The Body in Culture, Technology and Society*, London: Sage.

Wolfson, B. and Jackson, J. (1969) 'An intensive look at the daily experiences of young children', *Research into Education* 2: 1–12.

Acknowledgements

The editors would like to thank the contributors for agreeing to be part of this project, and for their patience and enthusiasm. It has been a pleasure working with so many colleagues across nations, a hugely rewarding experience throughout. We would also like to thank Samantha Grant and Michelle Bacca at Routledge for their editorial assistance, advice and support in publishing this material, and Emma Rich for her tireless and patient assistance with IT matters. John Evans would especially like to thank Janet, Rhianedd and Ceryn Evans for providing insight and motivation for this project, and for their enduring, grounding sense of perspective, love and fun.

Part I

Introduction

Pedagogy, culture and identity

1 Pedagogy, symbolic control, identity and health

John Evans and Brian Davies

Body knowledge and control

> The greatest enemy of scientific progress is orthodoxy.
>
> (John Brignell 2000: 209)

Book titles, said Basil Bernstein (2000: xxvi), are generally retrospective with reference to their contents. In entitling this book we deliberately draw attention to the title of Michael Young's (1971) complex, edited volume, *Knowledge and Control. New Directions for the Sociology of Education*, a text that set out to frame the relation of the sociology of knowledge and education some thirty years ago. Its disparate contents variously inspired, repelled and reflected a growing international 'community' of sociological researchers in education critical of existing education policy, conservative ideology and conventional forms of curriculum organisation, content and practice in schools.[1] The 'new directions' espoused by Young and some of his contributors raised old questions about the political, social class and cultural origins of school knowledge and processes and their inegalitarian outcomes in new and exciting, phenomenologically inspired, ways (see Evans and Davies 1986, 2002). However, they fell some way short of providing the conceptual, methodological and practical pedagogical means to attend to such issues satisfactorily, failing to capitalise on the ideas of Basil Bernstein and Pierre Bourdieu with which they lay, cheek by jowl, in *Knowledge and Control*.[2] Moreover, while raising challenging questions about how school knowledge was organised, transmitted, evaluated and interpreted and influenced the categories used by teachers to select, label and position pupils as 'able', deviant' or otherwise, it had nothing at all directly to say either as to how knowledge is 'embodied', or how 'the body' is schooled (Evans 1988; Shilling 1993a, b).

We will contend that the critical sentiments of *New Directions*, if reconfigured around the past thirty years of Bernsteinian insight on pedagogy, symbolic control and identity along with other recent social theory, can sharpen and guide our attention to ways of looking at how knowledge of 'the body' is implicated in the construction of identity and 'health' and the achievement of social hierarchies, order and control in society and schools. It may also advance our thinking on the policy and practical pedagogical measures to be taken towards the achievement of a curriculum that is both more 'inclusive' and expressive of social democratic ideals. Indeed, it is to show how Bernstein (2001: 364) began the task, inspired by Durkheim, of making 'explicit the social base of the pedagogic relation, its various contingent realisations, the agents and agencies of its enactments', both at the level of the knowledge base of society and the maintenance and change of its modalities of symbolic control, that this and subsequent chapters are dedicated. This required examination of the ideologies and knowledge claims that variously inform, influence and define the configurations of physical education and health curricula (PEH) that are now found in schools internationally, interrogation of the actions of policy-makers, teachers, pupils and others responsible for their enactment and relating these processes to socio-economic trends occurring outside schools. It is also to ask how the pedagogies of PEH help regulate relations within and between social groups, 'impact' the pedagogic consciousness of pupils and, ultimately, are implicated in social and cultural reproduction and the distribution of power and principles of control (Bernstein 2000: 4). In this sense, our title is also prospective, engaging directly with how '*knowledge of the body*' is produced, transmitted, 'received' and embodied through PEH and sport in schools. Its implication in processes of selection, differentiation and the construction of social class and cultural hierarchies, identity and the embodied self have, over the last thirty years, become the business of a vibrant community of critical researchers now variously producing sociological analyses of curriculum and teaching in physical education and sport pedagogy internationally.[3]

Following Bernstein (ibid.: xxvi), *Body Knowledge* is, then, in essence, concerned with understanding the social processes and practices of schooling, especially in PEH 'whereby consciousness and desire are given specific forms, evaluated, distributed, challenged and changed'. It is intended as another step towards understanding the impact that formal education has upon the intellectual, social and emotional development of young people, how practices within PEH and sport in schools are 'en-fleshed' and help in forming individuals' sense of identity and 'embodied' self. This is to suggest that we become as involved in a sociology of the *emotions*, as of the intellect; as concerned, for example, to interrogate the significance of pleasure in the pursuit of healthy *and* un-healthy behaviour, as to understand the role of formal education in defining how we are to think and feel about these matters. In the spirit of doing 'critical sociology' each chapter is intended to ask awkward and difficult and, hopefully, challenging questions about the new orthodoxies being established in schools, particularly those relating to the body and health that reflect wider economic interests, cultural tendencies and themes. These, we claim, are nurtured, rationalised and derive their authority from knowledge/s largely produced by the disciplines of the biological, behavioural and health sciences (see Pronger 2002) and which now constitute largely taken for granted 'regimes of truth' (for example, about 'health' and 'ability') among teachers and others in society, initial teacher education (ITE) and schools. On the surface these might seem to be more socially disinterested, objective and value-free than those of sociology but, as we shall see in the chapters of this book, they are not. They feed and frame policy and practice, influence and give structure and form to interactions and social relations and potentially impact upon the attitudes, emotions, selves and identities of teachers and pupils in schools and ITE. Orthodoxy relating to the place and importance of sport in the PE curriculum, reflecting a wider endeavour to restore 'tradition' and certainty in social worlds characterised by rapid social and technological change, has been well documented critically elsewhere (e.g. Penney and Evans 1999). The focus of this reader, therefore, will be essentially but not exclusively on the new discursive 'truths' relating to 'health' and its nature, place, purpose and position in the curriculum in general and PEH and sport in particular, that have found their way into schools, and into many other sites of cultural practice (e.g. family, work, leisure) that influence young lives. These 'truths', we suggest, express relatively new body-centred *perfection* codes (stressing autonomy, self-responsibility, self-surveillance and control), which happily commingle with those of *performance* (stressing authority, discipline, hierarchy and order) long established in education and the curriculum of PE (see Chapters 7, 11 and 14).[4]

Defining 'ability' 'health' and identity in PEH

Any discussion of 'health' issues within and/or beyond schools, in our view, would of necessity embrace analyses of the relationships between individuals' sense of value, status and embodied self and the ways in which success, failure, achievement and 'ability' are socially constructed (produced, reproduced and defined) by teachers and pupils in schools. It would also explore how parents and guardians are implicated in these processes, investing in, working upon and endorsing particular versions of corporeal 'ability' and 'health'. Amongst other things, this requires that we look afresh at how educational (including 'health') knowledge is selected, organised, differently valued, transmitted and defined.

From the early 1950s the predominant concern of politicians and education policy-makers in Britain and the USA was expressed in the rhetoric of whether educational systems met individual needs in a changing and expanding industrial society (Halsey *et al.* 1961; Karabel and Halsey 1977). Schools were pictured as functioning to socialise children into the values and norms necessary for the effective performance of their roles in society, differentiating their academic achievements and allocating them by 'intelligence' as human resources to the adult occupational system. Deviance or failure to succeed either in gaining academic credentials or, in PE, good *performance* in sport, fitness and health, tended to be explicated in terms of individual lack of 'intelligence', familial or sectional pathology. Pupils, parents or teachers, rather than curriculum structures, content, resources, system failure or government policies on education, were the loci for blame and shame.

This deeply conservative view of schooling has become integral to the policies of successive Conservative and Labour governments in the UK since the 1980s and, elsewhere (see Mills 2002; Apple 2002). For example, the 'abnormal' academic underachievement of boys has been held variously to be the responsibility of 'progressive' pedagogy, weak labour markets or an excess of female teacher role models (see Lingard and Douglas 1999; Mills 2000, 2002; Apple, 2002 for critiques of this discourse). Only recently in the UK has New Labour begun to acknowledge that the conventional status and configuration of the secondary school curriculum may not, for many children, be desirable, let alone ideal. Its claims to have eroded educational inequality, however, are backed by little evidence of change in terms of the educational opportunities available to different social categories of student in UK schools. Rising overall achievement in schools, as measured by the General Certificate of Secondary Education (GCSE) examination success at age 16, has been accompanied by a consistent increase in relative inequalities of attainment in school, especially in relation to social class and ethnic origin (Gillborn and Youdell 2001) and in terms of higher education entry. What is important here, however, is that in these conditions of schooling, 'ability' has now come to be understood by policy-makers, politicians and teachers as 'proxy for common sense notions of "intelligence"' (Demain 2001: 2). The discourse of 'ability' that underlies the multiple and complex selections that separate out the 'able' and the 'less able' within schools provides the opportunity for teachers and senior managers 'to identify the winners and losers at the earliest possible stages, allowing continual checks to ensure that those predicted for success "fulfil" their potential' (Gillborn and Youdell 2001: 97). Increasingly, stratification is operating at an institutional level (through ability-grouping policies) and at an interpersonal level within classes in terms of the time and attention given to different types of students in the UK and elsewhere (see Lynch and Lodge 2002). The significance of these developments for classroom processes, especially for the social re/production of achievement, underachievement, educational aspirations, 'ability' and identity and their intersections with gender, ethnicity and social class (see Francis 2000; Connolly and Neill 2001) has yet to be fully explored, especially in contexts of PEH.

With few notable exceptions (Burrows and Wright 2001; Hill 2003; Brittain 2004; Sparkes, Chapter 11 of this volume) we have little research that enables us to do more than speculate as to whether similarly reductionist conceptions of 'ability' apply across subject cultures. With fashionable search for the 'athletic gene' endorsing the belief that 'ability' is given at birth and differentially 'fixed' in both quality and form in the identities of women and men, we can only be on our guard against such policy developments and tendencies in physical education, sport and health practices in schools and initial teacher education PE (ITEPE) and in the biological, behavioural and health sciences. We might reasonably ask: what potential damage is done to pupils' sense of confidence, competence and embodied self when subjected to pedagogical and discursive practices which consider 'health' to be an individual responsibility while regarding the 'ability' to achieve it by engaging in appropriate health-promoting physical activities as both fixed and unevenly distributed amongst individuals and social groups? How are definitions of 'ability' constructed within contemporary, 'obesity discourses' by the pervasive and potentially perverse desire to make children and young people 'fit' and thin? (see Gard, Chapter 5; Rich *et al.*, Chapter 12). How is 'ability' embodied, displayed, recognised and valued by pupils, peers, teachers and significant others in and outside schools? Are parents and guardians differently positioned by virtue of their social class and culture to invest in, nurture (e.g. through out-of-school leisure activity, personal coaching, etc.) and endorse the forms of 'physical capital' (see Bourdieu 1984) required of children if they are to display 'ability' in schools? How is 'disability' and 'impairment' socially constructed and dealt with in pedagogical contexts driven by performance and perfection codes? (see Sparkes, Chapter 11). And what future is there for inclusive, social democratic comprehensive school ideals when set against government policies and initiatives in the UK driving schools towards elite 'sports college status' and teachers towards 'talent identi-fication' in contexts long governed by performance and perfection rather than competency codes? Will 'ability' and 'talent' be reduced to a commodity simply to be 'spotted,' residing in the few, at the expense of the 'multiple intelligences' and potential immanent in all pupils that all good pedagogues would strive to unfold? Nash (2003: 1) asks whether the 'durable embodied cognitive schemes, acquired by children in classed environments, are the principal cause of observed class variation in educational performances'. Do the thoughts and actions of teachers in contexts of PEH, '*generate* the observed distribution of attainments, as distinct from merely failing to eliminate variance due to the operations of the cognitive' embodied habitus? (ibid: 6). Are the primary effects of socialisation (in the early years, family and home) 'more important than the secondary effects that many sociologists have taken as their proper area of concern?' (ibid: 1). We have barely touched the surface of these issues in research in PEH.

All this compels us to think what some still believe unthinkable: that for a great many young people, particularly those from working-class homes, girls and young women, 'non-mainstream' cultural groups and people with disability, the content and conventional organisation of education and PEH and sport may increasingly be neither worthwhile, nor empowering (Evans and Davies 2002). What passes for education, 'ability' and 'health' and PEH and sport in the school curriculum is neither necessary nor immutable (see Penney and Chandler 2000); they are social constructs laden with values, which may be less than universally desirable. In Bernstein's (1996) terms, they proceed from a number of knowledge bases in the natural and social sciences, the power of whose content is appropriated and selectively privileged by policy-makers and reshaped in both the official recontextualising field (for example, by Central Government Departments of Education and Health) and pedagogic recontextualising fields (such as curriculum agencies and universities). Physical education and sport have more than their fair share of quango-like agencies (for example, in the UK, Sport England and the Youth Sport Trust) that define practice and allocate resources as if they were dispensing largesse. Their reproductive agents, teachers and coaches, tend to be strongly attached to performance, body perfection and product, very often shaped by elite attachment or personal desire for all three.

We need, therefore, to explore the conventions of curricular hierarchies (see Penney and Chandler 2000), deconstructing the ways in which common sense categories, such as the 'good' and 'able' child, 'intelligence', 'physical ability', skill', 'health', 'fitness' and 'educability' are generated and endorsed through the practices of 'science' and academia (see Pronger 2002) and are re/produced and performed in schools and initial teacher education (ITE). We also need to explore how the social ranking of subjects or activities (for example, health-related exercise, games or dance) that are routinely employed within PEH contexts comes to organise and constrain its social reality and to define 'ability' and 'health'. Deconstructing categories largely taken for granted in education and PE helps reveal their socio-cultural and economic origins, enabling us to see more clearly the potential consequences of our curricular and pedagogical actions for the learning opportunities and identities of pupils. At the same time, we need also pursue the relationships between these phenomena and socio-cultural and economic interests, hierarchies and ideologies prevailing both in wider school settings and outside them in society, exploring issues of whose voice and values matter and where lies the locus of power, authority and control. Unsurprisingly these questions may seem nihilistic and damaging to conventional ways of understanding education, especially to those with vested interests in sustaining an inequitable status quo. But all educational realities, categories or subjects stand in need of explanation; the task is to explore through which persons, groups and processes, certain forms of knowledge and organisation, status and identity are sustained in schools and PEH.

Whose body matters in PEH?

We have long held the view that the Durkheimian inspired views of Bernstein (Bernstein 1990, 1996, 2000; Davies 1994), focusing upon educational discourse and pedagogy, appropriately combined with other social theories evident in the chapters of this book, give best purchase on such questions and a way of approaching them in adequate depth. New hierarchies of the body are being nurtured in our primary and secondary schools, relating to size, shape and weight (Evans *et al.* 2003 and Chapter 12). Are such hierarchies congenial to inclusive, egalitarian, comprehensive ideals unlike many aspects of those of gender, race, class, 'ability' and sexuality from which they partly arise and which they may endorse? Paraphrasing Bernstein, we must consider what body shape, form and embodied predisposition is recognised as being of value in schools and PEH. Is there a dominant 'image'[5] of value such that some students are unable to recognise themselves as having a 'body' or 'self' of any value? What body images are excluded by the dominant images of the school? Whose body is seen and heeded? (see Oliver and Lalik, Chapter 8; Rich *et al.*, Chapter 12). In Bernstein's (2000) terms,

> A school metaphorically holds up a mirror in which an image is reflected. There may be several images, positive and negative. A school's ideology may be seen as a construction in a mirror through which images are reflected. The question is: who recognises themselves as of value? What other images are excluded by the dominant image of value so that some students are unable to recognise themselves? In the same way, we can ask about the acoustic of

the school. Whose voice is heard? Who is speaking? Who is hailed by this voice? For whom is it familiar?

(Bernstein 2000: xxi)

In this sense there are visual and temporal features to the images the school reflects and those images are projections of a hierarchy of predominantly class values. These are important issues, reminding us that a distribution of knowledge (for example, of and about 'the body') carries unequal value, power and potential. This matters because the distribution of material, financial and spatial resources (see Clarke Chapter 13), tends to follow the distribution of images such that, for those at the top with the 'right' image or ability to perform, there may be more time, space, opportunity, attention and reward, both emotional and material. As Bernstein goes on to point out, an unequal distribution of images, knowledge, possibilities and resources will also affect the rights of participation, inclusion and individual enhancement of groups of students. In his view, schools disguise and mask power relations external to themselves and produce hierarchies of knowledge, possibility and value. They create 'horizontal solidarities' (allegiances between socio-cultural groups, 'whose object is to contain and ameliorate vertical (hierarchical) cleavages between social groups' (Bernstein 2000: xxiii). To achieve this, he says the school must 'disconnect its own internal hierarchy of success and failure from ineffectiveness of teaching within the school and the external hierarchy of power relations between social groups outside the school' and in such a way that 'failure is attributed to inborn facilities' (cognitive, affective, physical) 'or to the cultural deficits relayed by the family which come to have the force of inborn facilities' (ibid: xxiv). Are teachers of PEH in schools and ITE implicated in processes such as these? How are 'success', 'failure' and achievement produced, defined and rationalised in these contexts, with what effect for pupils' corporeal and intellectual health? What social allegiances are formed amongst pupils in classrooms and playground sub-cultures (see Rich *et al.*, Chapter 12), again, with what consequence for individuals' health? And how are these processes related to contemporary Western discourses of anxiety, uncertainty and 'risk' (see Chapter 3 and Leahy and Harrison, Chapter 9) and to processes of social control? How do parents, guardians, teachers, others, invest in and 'work on' the body, to avoid 'risk' and ensure health and success in schools and beyond? Sociological researchers in Australia, New Zealand, the USA and Europe have gone some way towards illustrating how these social processes feature in and are embodied in curriculum and pedagogy (Macdonald *et al.* 2002).[6] This book seeks to further that goal and contends that the central concerns of the sociology of education with selection, differentiation, identity, equity, the nature of socio-cultural reproduction, order and control, remain as valid now as they were thirty years ago.

Education and health in a social democracy

Schools cannot, of course, compensate for society's social, economic and health ills, any more than they can ever hope to please or touch the interests of every young person in their care, no matter how innovative or progressive they are, or how hard they may try. To think that they could do these things alone, unsupported by the political will and intervention of Central Governments, would be to advocate and pursue illusory ideals. Moreover, schools stand as only one amongst many influences, alongside peers, parents and guardians, popular culture, religion, leisure and employment, acting upon young lives, variously implicated in processes of identity formation, socialisation, cultural reproduction and control (Holroyd 2003). We need to interrogate these processes without at the same time deluding ourselves that schools and PEH teachers are the only, or even the most important, catalysts for progressive social and educational change.

Following Bernstein (2000: xix) however, we are reminded that education 'is central to the knowledge base of society, groups and individuals' and that education, like health, is a 'public institution, central to the production and reproduction of distributive justice'. Biases in its form, content, access and opportunities, therefore, have consequences not only for the economy: they reach down 'to drain the very springs of affirmation, motivation and imagination'. Schools play on, help shape and form the aspirations, the core feelings, emotions and intellect of every individual that passes through them. Education has 'a crucial role in creating tomorrow's optimism in the context of today's pessimism. But if it is to do this then we must have an analysis of the social biases of education' (Bernstein 2000: xix), including how structures and practices within them relate to social practices outside.

It is worth reminding ourselves, especially at a time when teachers and researchers are increasingly steered by the barren managerial mantras of liberal individualism – achievement, assessment and accountability – that higher and worthier principles could drive PEH curricula in their pursuit of educational, social and moral ideals. According to Bernstein (2000), high among the principles that ought to guide our actions and help us assess the merits of what we do to young people in schools, are those that provide for the conditions of an effective social democracy. He claimed the first of these was that people must feel that they have a stake in society, as concerned to receive as to give something. Second, people must have confidence that the political arrangements they create will realise this stake. Translating these conditions in terms of school, parents and students must feel they have a stake in it and confidence that its arrangements will realise or enhance this stake. Is this the case in the PEH curriculum? Recent trends towards centralisation and the elevation of the 'expert' in all knowledge matters (see Chapters 3, 6 and 9) should make us aware of the delicacy of the balance between requiring teachers and pupils to achieve such externally imposed ends and practice and allowing them to feel that they have control and responsibility over what and how they teach and learn. It is made even more difficult by the realisation that many aspects of school allocation policies of diversity and choice are, in operation, illusory, illiberal or in-egalitarian.

Bernstein (2000) is clear that if social democratic conditions are to be realised in schools we will need to have institutionalised three interrelated rights. The first is the right to individual enhancement as 'a condition for experiencing boundaries, be they social, intellectual or personal' (p. xx). In this view, enhancement is not simply 'the right to be *more* personally, *more* intellectually, *more* socially, *more* materially, it is the right to the means of *critical* (our emphasis) understanding and to new possibilities' (ibid.: p. x). In PEH in Britain central government education polices make it nigh impossible for teachers to entertain engagement with forms of pedagogy and curriculum that require them and their pupils to think beyond the ordinary and the conventional, take innovative risks and address socio-cultural and educational issues. This right, however, is the condition for *confidence*, such an important facilitator of behaviour in physical activity and sport, as in all other fields, and it operates at the individual level. The second right is the right to be included, socially, intellectually, culturally and personally, a condition for *communitas* that operates at the level of the social. The third right is the right to participate. This 'is not only about discourse, about discussion, it is about practice, and a practice that must have an outcome', it is 'the right to participate in the procedures by which order is constructed, maintained and changes – it operates at the level of politics' (ibid.: p. xxi). Are such rights – of *enhancement, inclusion and participation* – embedded in the curricula of PEH in schools and ITE? Following Bernstein, we should measure our curriculum and teaching against this model. It presupposes an understanding of our pedagogic practice and a willingness to reshape our institutional structures in a way that challenges existing distributions of power and control. These are not just vulgar matters of 'taking sides' for or against particular forms of pedagogy, social theorising and understanding, or believing that rendering everything problematic puts anything together again. It is to engage pragmatically and reflexively in theoretically informed and socially aware pedagogies of PEH.

It will become clear that the contributors to this book write from a variety of quite different theoretical perspectives, all of which are not intended to fit happily together in an overarching coherent conceptual scheme. But without wishing to sound overly idealistic, or to underestimate the chasms that sometimes exist both between theories and theory and practice and the difficulties of bridging them, we end this section by restating a claim repeated elsewhere (Evans and Davies 2002): that, at its very best, theory is not just the catalytic agent in understanding but also of educational and social change. It is, as we together hope to highlight in subsequent chapters, a vehicle for thinking otherwise, a platform for outrageous hypotheses and for unleashing criticism. It offers a language of challenge and modes of thought other than those articulated by dominant others. Critically, it makes the familiar strange (see Pronger 2002). The purpose of theory, then, whether generated by teachers in schools, or researchers and academics elsewhere, is to de-familiarise present practices and categories, to make them less self-evident and necessary and to open up spaces for the invention of new forms of experience and pedagogy. We erode these elements of our practice, in schools and ITE, at our peril. Policy and practice devoid of empirically informed theory, especially in intensified conditions of school work, is likely to beget ideology, inequity, poetry or fascism rather than 'better education' and social democratic ideals. The message is clear, in physical education and health we should make research and teaching more not less complex, and 'theory', ideas and innovation, not our enemies but friends (Evans and Davies 2002: 31). Science, after all, in whatever form it takes, is, as Giddens (1999: 10) usefully reminds us, 'essentially a critical attitude towards the world in which you are prepared to revise even your most cherished beliefs'. Laying claim to 'orthodoxy' or 'knowledge certainty' as the foundation for policy and practice in PEH in such circumstances may be as misguided as it is inappropriate if the development of 'able', 'healthy', innovative, flexible thinkers for a social democracy is our chosen primary ideal.

Structure and content of the book

Drawing on the recent research of some of the leading figures in the fields of sociology of education and physical culture, *Body Knowledge* attempts to provide both an innovative and critical way of looking at the relationships between education, physical culture, identity and health. Although the text examines the relations between 'the body' and formal education broadly, it has a strong orientation towards issues of health and identity, interrogating in particular how processes of schooling, historically and contemporaneously, have been and continue to be implicated discursively and pedagogically in the social construction and control of 'the body', identity, well-being and health. In so doing it foregrounds and critiques powerful themes within contemporary culture, notably the assumed positive relationship between organised physical activity, sport, schooling and health. It also offers a way of conceptualising education, schooling and physical culture drawing on research that radically challenges not only the practices of professionals concerned with PEH and sport but also the discursive practices of science that guides and informs them. The ambitions of the text are thus both critical and constructive, pointing both to the potency of knowledge and pedagogy as catalysts for agency and change, as well as their potential to restrict and control. In Chapter 2 Jan Wright calls on the work of Michel Foucault to outline key methodological features of post-structuralism, highlighting their possibilities for the analysis of the relations between education, physical culture, identity and health. She argues the merits of discourse analysis as a way of conceptualising and deconstructing relations of power which operate on and within PHE; highlighting 'the body', identity and health, as socially constructed domains. Combined with other means it can be used for the relational analysis of socio-cultural settings and their change.

Part 2 of the book centres on the way in which ideologies, policies and discursive practices outside schools influence thinking and actions within them. Together the authors explore conceptions of childhood, health and identity, illustrating how definitions, agendas and categories employed and often taken for granted by teachers and teacher educators are constructed historically and contemporaneously in changing socio-cultural circumstance and in relation to the policies and practices of science and other economic and political interests outside schools. Chapter 3 sets PEH curricula within a wider social context while outlining how key concepts from the work of Michel Foucault and Basil Bernstein can inform our understandings of the curriculum and pedagogies of schools. We suggest that their work offers a way of conceptualising the connections between the fine detail of classroom life, the coding of embodied consciousness, and the enactment of power and control in societies increasingly characterised by 'risk' (see Chapters 6, 9 and 13). In Chapter 4 David Kirk emphasises that it is not possible to fully grasp the process of socially constructing 'the body' through schooling without the development of a critical history of the relationships between school knowledge and broader public discourses.

With reference to developments in physical activity in Australian schools since the early 1900s, he argues that schools there, as perhaps in other Western societies in the wake of radical socio-cultural change, are currently struggling to maintain their modernist institutional form which has had as a central goal the production of compliant and productive 'modernist' bodies. This, he points out, has a potentially powerful bearing on young people's identities and health. Michael Gard continues this theme in Chapter 5 where he offers a challenging critique of the so called 'obesity epidemic', a discursive resource legitimising a number of academic disciplines, including physical education, industry and public health agendas. Gard's analysis suggests that physical education's alignment with 'the war against obesity' may not only be bad for the development of the subject but also, ironically, for the well-being and health of many children and young people in schools. A curriculum grounded in the interests of business and the health industry, rather than the physical cultures of students and educational aims, is not what young people need. In Chapter 6 Lisette Burrows and Jan Wright further illustrate how cultural categories that are taken for granted, in this case, 'childhood', are constructed in relation to corporeal discourses that define the healthy child. They foreground the influences of the media and other agencies outside schools that define teachers, parents and pupils as culpable in the production of health and illness, documenting how these powerful social forces regulate and constrain the nature of policy and practice not just in schools but also family life. Their arguments resonate with those expressed in Chapter 13 where it is suggested that, in a 'Totally Pedagogised Society' (Bernstein 2001) where health is everyone's concern, almost every disposition and behaviour is amenable to regulation, control and surveillance not just within and by the practices of schools but in the work place, leisure and home. In Chapter 7 Dawn Penney and Jo Harris offer an innovative way of looking at the 'policy process'. They document the 'discursive boundaries' inherent in official policy texts illustrating their impact on the curriculum and teaching of PE and health in schools in the UK, New Zealand and elsewhere. Their analysis, like that of the others, goes beyond critique to speculate on the role of pedagogy in challenging current boundaries of knowledge and extending understandings among teachers and pupils about their bodies, health and physical education.

Part III contains a number of empirically based sociological studies which centre on aspects of schooling and pedagogy in relation to physical culture, the body, identity and health. All raise a variety of critical and challenging questions about the ways in which schools impact upon, regulate and control children's sense of body and self. They also underline the potential that lies in schools for social and cultural production and reform, while recognising the magnitude of the challenge.

Drawing on critical race theory and anti-racist scholarship, in Chapter 9 Kimberley Oliver and Rosary Lalik describe and critique an intervention designed to help 8th grade girls examine 'the Beauty Walk', an annual event in a school in the southeast part of the United States. We learn that the 'white body' is the school enforced ideal for beauty and that, while the girls were able to name and critique this type of institutionalised racism, in many ways they supported its continuation. This chapter raises fundamental questions not only about the nature of racism in schools but also of the limits of research to act as a vehicle for changing deep-seated taken-for-granted attitudes and school practices. Chapter 9 returns to health issues. Here Deana Leahy and Lyn Harrison draw on a case study of a Year 10 health and physical education programme in a metropolitan secondary school in Australia to illustrate how contemporary 'discourses of risk', health and citizenship, reproduced through the curriculum and classroom practices, can operate as mechanism of social regulation and control. They highlight the merits of viewing the classroom as a 'site of governance', where the way in which students and their bodies are positioned within discourses of education, health, citizenship and risk has significant consequences for their developing sense of identity and self. In Chapter 10 Robyne Garrett centres attention on the social construction of gender within contexts of movement, sport and physical culture. Drawing on post-structuralist theory and methodology this chapter directs attention at young women's lived experience and meanings of the body around physical activity and the discursive practices which can either liberate or constrain the development of particular bodies, identities and action. The physical stories of these young women provide a vivid account not only of the opportunities for joy and empowerment for females through physical activity but, equally, the potential for pain and damage to their physical identities. Drawing vividly and innovatively on his 'lived experience' of involvement in top level sport, in Chapter 11 Andrew Sparkes raises a number of critical issues relating to 'impairment' and 'disability' through sport. His narrative analysis prompts us to reflect not only on the nature of male identity but also how we are to deal pedagogically with body malfunction and vulnerability. Nowhere is the potential damage done to young people's sense of well-being and embodied self by the cultures of schooling, physical activity and wider social influences illustrated more clearly than in the study of eating disorders such as anorexia nervosa. In Chapter 12 Emma Rich, Rachael Holroyd and John Evans point to the ways in which formal education may be implicated in the production of eating disorders, as well as in helping young people avoid them. They raise important issues about the merits of analyses that focus overly on 'the cult of slenderness' as the primary factor in the aetiology and development of disorders such as these, suggesting that more relevant and immediate 'toxins', mediated by teachers, pupils and peers, may be found in the taken-for-granted cultural conditions of the school. In Chapter 13 Gill Clarke illustrates one such taken-for-granted factor in the way in which space(s) shape and control pupil and student teachers' bodies and sexual identities in physical education in schools. Clearly, space, that most taken-for-granted element of our lives, is not neutral but laden with power differentials such that bodies are schooled often along narrow, homophobic lines. Schools in England and, we suspect, in many places elsewhere remain largely sites of compulsory heterosexuality, with few students or teachers daring to cross their boundary lines. Together, then, these authors provide a challenging critique of contemporary practices in schools. In Chapter 14 Davies and Evans clarify some of the key concepts of 'performance' and 'perfection' that feature in earlier chapters, pointing to their value for research in PEH. In Chapter 15 Richard Tinning reminds us of the magnitude of the challenges facing teachers and researchers globally. He cautions against idealism, points to the complexity of the influences acting upon young people's and teachers' lives, and highlights the opportunities emerging for progressive practice in research, ITE and schools.

Finally, we are mindful that these pages contain many omissions and silences; certain voices and class cultures are more in evidence than others. They should be read as at best offering only partial insights into social processes of schooling. Much remains to be said about class and cultural diversity and the embodied similarities and differences that make children and young people so special and unique.

Notes

1   Two factors assured it of such a wide range of reception. The first lay in the character of the horizontal knowledge structures of sociology itself (Bernstein 1999). Long on 'commitment' and short on the good research practice that arises from theoretical strength, its elements could be described as embattled or mutually denying, rather than cooperative or cumulative. Indeed, *New Directions* was particularly forthright either in declaring 'old' ones dead, consigning whole approaches to oblivion as tainted with functionalism or ameliorism (e.g. as represented by the classic Halsey, Floud and Anderson collection of 1961 or the mainstream US tradition of a journal such as *Sociology of Education*), or ignoring them as largely unworthy of attention, for example as with the work of Bernstein or Dahloff and Lundgren

2   Changing evaluations of 'new directions' can be traced, among others, through Connell (1983); Apple (1985); Whitty (1985); Wexler (1987); Goodson (1988); Lauder and Brown (1988); Sadovnik (1995); Arnot (2002).

3   We cannot name or do justice to all those internationally who, from very different perspectives, over the last thirty years, have contributed to critical research and curriculum development in PE and sport in schools. The array of work produced, for example, by Bain, Birrell, Crum, Griffin, Hall, Hellison, Jewett, Lawson, Messner, O'Sullivan, Schempp and Siedentop, from Europe, USA, Australia and elsewhere, as well as others too numerous to mention here, featuring in journals such as *Quest*, and *Sport, Education and Society* dedicated to social science research in PEH and sport, continues to define the field. Not all could, or would want to, be classified as 'critical sociologists' though, together, their work has nurtured the reflective development of research and innovation in PE and sport in schools and initial teacher education (ITE) in many countries. (For examples see Evans 1993; Evans and Davies 1986, 1993; Kirk and Tinning 1990; Rovegno and Kirk 1995; Clarke and Humberstone 1997; Fernandez-Balboa 1997; Hickey *et al.* 1998; Macdonald *et al.* 2002; Laker 2002; Pronger 2002).

4   We use the term 'code' following Bernstein (2000: 202) to refer to 'regulative principles which select and integrate relevant meanings (classifications), forms of their realisation (framings) and their evoking contexts. The values (strong/weak) and functions (classifications/framings) carry the code potential. How this potential is actualised is a

function of the struggle to construct and distribute code modalities which regulate pedagogic relations, communication and context management. Conflict is endemic within and between the arenas in the struggle to dominate modalities *and* in the relation between local pedagogic modalities and official modalities'. The making of the National Curriculum PE in the UK provides a good example of such conflict (Penney and Evans 1999). The social class origins and consequences of such coding will be explored in Chapter 14.

5   We use the term 'image' to refer not just to 'body appearance' (how one looks) but the corporeal manifestation of self, the embodied representation of culturally ideal or idealised characteristics and predispositions.

6   The work of Morais, Neves (2001) and their associates provides the best, extended example of the application and development of a Bernsteinian approach to these ideas to the classroom, mainly focused on lower secondary science teaching in Portugal, overviewed in their 2001 article.

References

Anyon, J. (1981) 'Social class and school knowledge', *Curriculum Inquiry* 11(1): 3–42.

Apple, M. (1985) *Education and Power*, London, Boston: ARK Paperbacks.

Apple, M. (2002) *Educating the Right Way. Markets, Standards, God and Inequality*, London: Routledge/Falmer Press.

Arnot, M. (2002) *Reproducing Gender*, London: Routledge/Falmer.

Bernstein, B. (1990) *The Structuring of Pedagogic Discourse*, Volume IV, London: Routledge.

Bernstein, B. (1996) *Pedagogy, Symbolic Control and Identity: Theory, Research and Critique*, London: Taylor & Francis.

Bernstein, B. (1999) 'Vertical and horizontal discourse: an essay', *British Journal of Sociology of Education* 20(2): 157–75.

Bernstein, B. (2000) *Pedagogy, Symbolic Control and Identity: Theory, Research and Critique*, revised edition, London: Rowman & Littlefield.

Bernstein, B. (2001) 'From pedagogies to knowledges', in A. Morais, I. Neves, B. Davies and H. Daniels (eds) *Towards a Sociology of Pedagogy*, New York: Peter Lang.

Bourdieu, P. (1984) *Distinction: A Social Critique of the Judgement of Taste*, London: Routledge.

Brignell, J. (2000) *Sorry, Wrong Number!*, London: Brignell Associates and European Science and Environment Forum.

Brittain, I. (2004) 'The role of schools in constructing self-perceptions regarding sport and physical education in relation to people with disabilities', *Sport, Education and Society*, forthcoming.

Burrows, L. and Wright, J. (2001) 'Developing children in New Zealand school physical education', *Sport, Education and Society* 6(2): 165–83.

Clarke, G. and Humberstone, B. (1997) *Researching Women and Sport*, London: Macmillan Press.

Connell, B. (1983) *Which Way is Up? Essays on Class, Sex and Culture*, London: Allen and Unwin.

Connolly, P. and Neill, J. (2001) 'Boys' underachievement, educational aspirations and constructions of locality: intersections of gender ethnicity and social class', paper presented at the International Sociology of Education Conference: Class, Race, Gender and Disability: Points of commonality and difference, Sheffield, January 2001.

Davies, B. (1994) 'Durkheim and the sociology of education in Britain', *British Journal of Sociology of Education* 15(1): 3–25.

Demain, J. (2001) *Sociology of Education Today*, Basingstoke: Palgrave.

Evans, J. (1988) 'Body matters: towards a socialist physical education', in H. Lauder and P. Brown (eds) (1988) *Education in Search of a Future*, Lewes: Falmer Press.

Evans, J. (1993) *Equality, Education and Physical Education*, Lewes: Falmer Press.

Evans, J. and Davies, B. (1986) 'Sociology, schooling and physical education', in J. Evans (ed.) *Physical Education, Sport and Schooling – Studies in the Sociology of Physical Education*, London: Falmer Press.

Evans, J. and Davies, B. (2002) 'Theoretical background', in A. Laker (ed.) *The Sociology of Sport and Physical Education*, London: Routledge/Falmer.

Evans, J., Evans, B. and Rich, B. (2003) 'Let them eat chips', *Pedagogy, Culture and Society* 11(2).

Fernandez-Balboa, J.-M. (1997) *Critical Postmodernism in Human Movement, Physical Education and Sport*, New York: SUNY.

Francis, B. (2000) *Boys, Girls and Achievement*. London: Routledge.

Giddens, A. (1999) 'The director's lectures. Runaway world', Reith Lectures Revisited, Lecture 2, 17 November 1999, http://www.lse.ac.uk/Giddens/reith_99/week3/week3. htm

Gillborn, D. and Youdell, D. (2001) 'The new IQism: intelligence, ability and the rationing of education', in J. Demain (ed.) *Sociology of Education Today*, Basingstoke: Palgrave.

Goodson, I. (1988) *The Making of the Curriculum*, Lewes: Falmer Press.

Halsey, A.H., Floud, J. and Anderson, C.A. (eds) (1961) *Education, Economy and Society*, New York: Free Press.

Hickey, C., Fitzclarence, L. and Mathews, R. (1998) *Where the Boys Are: Masculinity, Sport and Education*, Deakin: Deakin Centre for Education and Change.

Hill, L.A. (2003) 'Lessons in the gym: an exploration of the relationships between school physical education and the physicality of adolescent girls', unpublished Ph.D. thesis, Leeds: Leeds Metropolitan University.

Karabel, J. and Halsey, A.H. (eds) (1977) *Power and Ideology in Education*, New York: Oxford University Press.

Kirk, D. and Tinning, R. (1990) *Physical Education, Curriculum and Culture*, Lewes: Falmer Press.

Laker, A. (ed.) (2002) *The Sociology of Sport and Physical Education*, London: Falmer/ Routledge.

Lauder, H. and Brown, P. (eds) (1988) *Education in Search of a Future*, Lewes: Falmer Press.

Lingard, B. and Douglas, P. (1999) *Men Engaging Feminism: Pro-feminism, Backlash and Schooling*, Buckingham: Open University Press.

Lynch, K. and Lodge, A. (2002) *Equality and Power in Schools*, London: Routledge/Falmer

Macdonald, D., Kirk, D., Metzler, M., Nilges, L.M., Schempp, P. and Wright, J. (2002) 'It's all very well in theory: theoretical perspectives and their applications in contemporary pedagogical research', *Quest* 54(2): 133–57.

Mills, M. (2000) '"Troubling the failing boys' discourse"', *Discourse: Studies in the Cultural Politics of Education* 21(2): 237–46.

Mills, M. (2002) 'Review symposium of Apple, M. *Educating the Right Way. Markets, Standards, God and Inequality*, London: Routledge/Falmer Press', *British Journal of Sociology of Education* 23(3): 489–94.

Morais, A. and Neves, I. (2001) 'Pedagogic social contexts. Studies for a sociology of learning', in A. Morais, I. Neves, B. Davies and H. Daniels (eds) *Towards a Sociology of Pedagogy*, New York: Peter Lang.

Morais, A., Neves, I., Davies, B. and Daniels, H. (eds) (2001) *Towards a Sociology of Pedagogy. The Contribution of Basil Bernstein to Research*, New York: Peter Lang.

Nash, R. (2003) 'Inequality/difference in New Zealand education: social reproduction and the cognitive habitus', paper presented at the International Sociology of Education Conference 2003, 2–3 January 2003, London.

Penney, D. and Chandler, T. (2000) 'Physical education: what futures?', *Sport, Education and Society* 5(1): 71–89.

Penney, D. and Evans, J. (1999) *Policy, Politics and Practice in Physical Education and Sport*, London: E&FN Spon.

Pronger, B. (2002) *Body Fascism. Salvation in the Technology of Physical Fitness*, London, Ontario: University of Toronto.

Rovegno, I. and Kirk, D. (1995) 'Articulations and silences in socially critical work on physical education: towards a broader agenda', *Quest* 47(4): 475–90.

Sadovnik, A. (1995) 'Basil Bernstein's theory of pedagogic practice: a structuralist approach', in A.R. Sadovnik (ed.) *Knowledge and Pedagogy. The Sociology of Basil Bernstein*, Norwood, New Jersey: Ablex Publishing Co.

Shilling, C. (1993a) 'The body, class and social inequalities', in Evans, J. (1993) *Equality, Education and Physical Education*, Lewes: Falmer Press.

Shilling, C. (1993b) *The Body and Social Theory*, London: Sage.

Wexler, P. (1987) *Social Analysis: After the New Sociology*, London: Routledge & Kegan Paul.

Whitty, G. (1985) *Sociology and School Knowledge: Curriculum Theory, Research and Politics*, London: Methuen.

Young, M.F.D. (ed.) (1971) *Knowledge and Control: New Directions for the Sociology of Education*, London: Collier Macmillan.

2 Post-structural methodologies
The body, schooling and health

Jan Wright

Poststructuralist theory and research

Post-modernism and post-structuralism often appear to be used interchangeably in educational writing and research, with the term post-modernism more likely to be used in North America and post-structuralism more likely to be used by those following a European tradition of philosophy and social analysis (Scheurich 1997). There are arguably, however, differences that go beyond terminology. The latter position tends to draw on the work of Foucault and Derrida, the former on the work of Lyotard. Different questions are raised and considered by each. What they share is 'the need to problematise systems of thought and organisation' (Usher and Edwards 1994: 1) and fixed notions of identity or social relations. In addition, the term post-modernity is also used globally to describe a period which some suggest has already passed and others, has yet to arrive (Giddens 1991; Kirk 1997). This chapter is not so much concerned with the debates about terminology or about post-modernity as a period. It looks at how post-structuralist theory can help to understand the relationship between the self and the social and, specifically for the purposes of this book, how the embodied self is socially constituted in relation to social institutions and discourses associated with health and physical education.

One of the strengths of post-structuralism is that it comes from a tradition that already has an analytic theory and a useful set of analytic techniques with which to undertake research. While not all post-structuralist researchers necessarily interrogate texts as social instantiations, there is thread of post-structuralism which comes directly out of linguistics, that is, after the structuralist linguistics of Saussure and Levi-Strauss (see Silverman 1983). Through the work of Saussure, meaning has come to be understood as not fixed, but as historically and culturally specific. What 'health' means, for instance, has changed, even in the context of the English-speaking world, quite radically over the last century (Lupton 1995) and, as has been argued by those concerned with the health of indigenous peoples, is differently understood by different cultural and socio-economic groups (Wright and Burrows 2003). With the work of Raymond Barthes, structuralism was extended to the study of cultural texts and through his notion of myths to an understanding of how particular meanings came to be more powerful or 'hegemonic' than others, that is, how some meanings took on the status of taken-for-granted truths (Barker and

Galasinski 2001). If we look at the chapters in this book, many challenge the ways in which particular versions of health (e.g. Gard, Chapter 5), childhood (e.g. Burrows and Wright, Chapter 6), the body and physical education are accepted as the dominant ones.

As Hall (1992, cited in Barker and Galasinski 2001) points out, structuralism was important because it allowed for all forms of meaning production, including 'lived experience', to be treated as texts. Thus, ethnographies, interviews, journals, narratives, even physical movements as they are documented by video or in the form of field notes, could now be analysed as texts. This tradition, therefore, provided both the justification and the means – through structural linguistics and semiotics – to systematically interrogate the meanings of texts (written, spoken or visual) as they are constituted in and by specific social and cultural contexts. Institutionally such work often comes under the umbrella of cultural and/or communication studies and/or critical discourse analysis (see, for instance, Fairclough 1989, 1995; Luke *et al.* 1994). In this chapter, and in most of the chapters in the book which use 'discourse' as an analytic technique, a notion of discourse analysis, drawing more or less on the work of Foucault, has been used to conceptualise and deconstruct the relations both within and between physical and health education, the body, identity and health, as socially constructed domains.

Foucault (1972: 49) describes discourse as 'practices that systematically form the objects of which they speak. Discourses are not about objects; they constitute them and in the practice of doing so conceal their own intervention.' It is through discourse that meanings, subjects and subjectivities are formed. Although in this sense discourse is not equivalent to language, choices in language – for instance, choosing to define overweight as an illness – point to those discourses being drawn upon by writers and speakers, and to the ways in which they position themselves and others. Questions can, therefore, be asked about how language works to position speakers (and listeners) in relation to particular discourses and with what effects. Further, post-structuralism, by its very nature, raises questions about how selves are constituted, how power–knowledge relations change across times, places, and in the context of different social, political and cultural contexts. These are the kinds of questions explored in a number of the analyses in this volume. Burrows and Wright in Chapter 6, for instance, look at the social construction of childhood in relation to particular healthism discourses that define the child as a biological entity whose present and future well-being is put at risk through decreasing participation in physical activity and the excessive consumption of 'junk' food.

The notion of discourse provides a means to understand what resources are available to individuals as they make sense of the world and themselves in the world. What it does not provide is an explanation as to why some, rather than others, are taken up by individuals and why different individuals take up the same discourses in different ways. Part of the answer to these questions lies in the relation between power and discourse. Some discourses have more power to persuade than others and are reiterated more often across a wide range of sites and/or by those who are believable and understood to be expert. For Foucault, this is covered by the notion of technologies of power – that is, 'those technologies which determine the conduct of individuals and submit them to certain ends or domination, an objectivising of the subject' (Foucault 1997: 225). In his early work, Foucault was interested in mapping, or constructing a genealogy of, the emergence of particular regimes of truth as they emerged in specific institutional contexts, specifically in relation to the science, medicine and, particularly, in *The Birth of the Clinic*, psychiatry. In doing so Foucault sought to show the 'specificity and materiality' of the interconnections between power and knowledge (Dreyfus and Rabinow 1982: 203). For Foucault, power is not primarily located in structures or in an all-powerful state apparatus, rather institutions act as specific sites where particular techniques of power are channelled and brought to bear on individuals in systematic ways. In this way a school, through its architecture, its organisation, its curriculum and daily practices, becomes a disciplinary site which draws on particular regimes of truth (discourses) to legitimate its existence and to define what it does. Thus, for example, particular pedagogical practices in physical education, such as those associated with assessment, the organisation of classes based on ability, the measuring of bodies for weight, fitness and so on, even the ways in which teams are chosen, can work to produce 'normalising', 'regulating', 'classifying' and 'surveillance' effects.

While in his earlier writing Foucault was more interested in the ways in which individuals are subjected to particular operations of power, his later work was more concerned to understand how individual selves are constituted; how the 'truth games' that he identified through his genealogical analyses of knowledge fields are taken up by individuals and in what circumstances. He used the concept of 'technologies of the self' to describe the ways in which individuals engage in psychic practices which

> permit individuals to effect by their own means, or with the help of others, a certain number of operations on their own bodies and souls, thoughts, conduct, and way of being, so as to transform themselves in order to attain a certain state of happiness, purity, wisdom, perfection, or immortality.
>
> (Foucault 1997: 225)

While he specifically focused on the ways in which this happened in the context of early Greek and Christian writings, his notion of 'technologies of the self' helps us to look more closely at the diverse ways in which individuals take up, resist and challenge the discourses associated with health, the body and physical activity. If we understand that notions of 'perfection', 'happiness', 'purity', 'wisdom' are themselves socially constituted, we can begin to understand why individuals might take up certain discourses rather than others. One example, which will be developed below, is the way in which specific notions of bodily perfection or normality are promoted via a wide range of social institutions including, but not only, schools and the media. Individuals in their desire to attain such perfection avidly consume information that provides instructions on what they must do to achieve this.

In another example, which is particularly relevant to the example of post-structuralist analysis described later in this chapter, namely perfection/happiness in Western societies, is also associated with a coherent sense of self. In this sense the self becomes a project, work has to be done on the self to maintain a sense of coherence and rationality. Such a humanist notion of the self is critiqued by those drawing on post-structuralist theory, which sees selves/subjectivities/identities as multiple and constantly constituted in and through discourse. However, as Edley (2001) points out (writing in the context of discursive psychology), there is a powerful discourse which would want to see individuals as 'unique, self-contained motivational and cognitive universes'. He argues that

> most people in the Western world are invested in a philosophical tradition which values personal integrity and the consistency of identity over time. Westerners are very keen to be seen, by themselves as well as others, as some*one* in particular. This explains why when people are encouraged or forced to see the contradictions in their own identity 'project', they often feel defensive or embarrassed.
>
> (Edley 2001: 195)

In other words individuals have investments in seeing themselves as coherent selves which have continuity over time. In looking at interview texts (which are, after all, dynamic constructions of subjectivities – both the interviewer's and the interviewee's), the work individuals do to maintain this coherence as well as to constitute particular kinds of subjectivities will be recognisable in their choices of language.

Discourse analysis

In this chapter 'discourse' has been discussed as it is used by those working from a post-structuralist perspective. 'Discourse', however, is a widely used term having a range of different technical meanings and uses in social research. In the intro-duction to *Discourse as Data*, Taylor (2001) provides a very helpful description of a range of discourse analytic processes and their underpinning assumptions and consequent ways of working with data. Discourse analysis is a term widely used by those interested in 'looking closely at "language in use" where the analyst is "looking for patterns"' (Taylor 2001: 6). However, how 'language' is interpreted determines the approach to discourse analysis. From a post-structuralist perspective, discourse analysis is the term used to describe the process of capturing regularities of meaning (patterns in language use) as these are 'constitutive of discourses and to show how discourses in turn constitute aspects of society and the people within it' (ibid.: 9).

One of the key assumptions to an analysis of language and other social meaning-making practices is that as people talk, write or construct images, indeed, act in relation to themselves and to others, they are making choices – choices which are limited by the repertoires of meaning-making tools (language, film angles, colours), repertoires of movement and so on, that they have available. Not all individuals have access to the same set of institutional or cultural resources, and the effects of taking up some ways of acting and meaning are not equally valued in all social contexts. Although Edley refers only to language, his point in the following quote makes sense in relation to a whole range of meaning-making practices:

> A language culture may supply a whole range of ways of talking about or constructing an object or event, and speakers are therefore bound to make choices. However the options aren't always equal. Some constructions or formulations will be more available than others. They will be easier to say.
>
> (Edley 2001: 190)

In physical education, for example, there have been several examples of ways in which choices in language contribute to the production of gender (Clarke 1992; Evans *et al*. 1996; Wright 1995, 2000) and of ways of thinking about and making choices about health and physical activity (Wright and Burrows 2003).

Most of the data-based or empirical post-structuralist research in education draws on qualitative methodologies, although it is not unimaginable that numbers might be involved. Researchers tend to use interviews, observations, collect documentation, and take field notes. If specifically interested how language or visual images work to constitute meanings and subjectivities, they may record teacher–student interactions, or collect media texts. In keeping with the theoretical basis of post-structuralism that takes knowledge as socially constructed, researchers do not claim to be capturing truths, rather they are concerned with how individuals, groups, cultures and institutions construct realities and with what effects. In doing so they also recognise that information collected can be only partial, situated in terms of time and place and the context of the specific situation (e.g. the interview or observation).

Investigating the relation between education, physical culture and identity: an empirical example

Moving now from theoretical considerations to the use of post-structuralism for empirical work in physical education, it is useful to consider what questions a researcher might want to ask. Some questions have already been suggested in earlier sections of this chapter and many others are explored in the remaining chapters in this book. Health and physical education provides a rich site for examining specific relations between schooling, the body and identity (or in post-structuralist terms, subjectivity). It provides a context in which to ask questions such as: How are bodies inscribed with meanings? What part does schooling and physical education play in this process and with what effects? What institutional and cultural discourses are brought into play to construct particular identities and social practices associated with health, sport, physical activity in the context of schools? What kinds of selves/bodies are regarded as normal and what not? Who has the power to determine this and on what authority (discursive or structural) do they draw?

Several chapters in the book exemplify how some of these questions might be addressed (e.g. Leahy and Harrison, Chapter 9; Rich, Holroyd and Evans, Chapter 12; Clarke, Chapter 13). To demonstrate in detail what empirical work might look like using a post-structuralist approach, the remainder of this chapter will work through an example which begins by identifying the work of specific discourses as they are constituted in the institutional site of physical and health education textbooks and concludes by demonstrating how these discourses are taken up by young woman Karin, as she talks about herself and describes the choices she makes in relation to physical activity and eating.

The assumption from a post-structuralist perspective is that subjectivities are constituted by drawing on existing discourses or sets of meaning. In the case to be discussed below, an important aspect of recognising and naming the discourses on which Karin draws is to identify the possible ways of making meanings about health currently available to her. Not all meanings about health will have the same salience for all individuals and in all contexts. Part of the empirical task in this case is to identify which discourses have most salience for Karin and with what consequences. One possible first step, then, in this process is to identify institutional and cultural texts that are likely to serve as important sources of the discourses which constitute the field of inquiry. In Karin's case, these are likely to be the popular media, schools and other institutions concerned with health. Texts from these sources will provide indications of how discourses are constituted and how these become invested with personal and cultural desires, needs and so on. For example, popular magazines may provide instructions in how to exercise to become thinner, but thinness only becomes a desirable goal when connected to cultural ideals of attractiveness and/or the moral virtue of the well-disciplined body. In many cases there is a literature which has already begun the work of identifying the discursive field. In addition, as researchers, workers and participants these fields we are also likely to be very familiar with the range of discourses, dominant and otherwise, circulating. It is then a matter of systematically documenting discourses and the work they do.

Another way of working is take a more grounded approach and look for patterns in meaning-making through an analysis of the language of interviews, classroom interaction, school programmes and so on. Since a fundamental assumption of post-structuralism is that individuals in constituting texts draw on discourses (some dominant and others marginal) which are already circulating in particular social and cultural contexts, the task when working from this direction is to determine where these are found, who else is articulating them, with what power do they speak (or write) and with what effects.

In this case there is now a considerable literature which discusses the dominant discourse of health and their means of production and dissemination in Western society (see, for instance, Lupton 1995; Peterson and Bunton 1997). However, for the purposes of this example, the first step to understanding the salience of the particular discourses on which Karin draws will be to investigate specific meanings about health generated in school health education classes. In this case the focus will be on health education textbooks. Another possible or complementary focus could have been the language of the health classroom (see for instance Leahy and Harrison, Chapter 9). This step is concerned, then, to look at a key institutional site in which discourses are constituted as regimes of truth, in this case as ways of thinking about, evaluating and acting on the body in relation to its health.

To illustrate the meanings that are made available in the context of health and physical education I have chosen several texts on the same topic from health and physical education textbooks widely used in both the junior school and for the senior examinable course in New South Wales (Davis *et al.* 1993; Fitzgibbon *et al.* 1992; Parker *et al.* 2000; Rhineberger *et al.* 1994). What could be asked of the textbooks as a whole is: What meanings about health are constructed in these texts? What is the relationship between health and the body/identity/the self? What discourses do writers draw on and with what consequences for how individuals and groups are to be understood and the behaviours evaluated? What messages are produced as to how people are to live their lives? Such a large-scale analysis is not possible within the scope of this chapter but it is certainly important when choosing and using textbooks to recognise that they are productive of social meanings and provide resources for the ways in which individuals come to know themselves and others. For the purpose of this chapter, following the particular theme of the body, physical activity and health, I have chosen the sections of these textbooks that deal with the relationship between energy, food, activity and the body.

These texts all indicate that the way to think about the relationship between food and activity/exercise is one of 'balance' – energy/kilojoules in and energy/kilojoules out. The metaphor of a seesaw is used in each textbook and often made explicit in the diagrams that accompany the text. What is of interest here is how these specific texts are instructive in ways of thinking and evaluating the body and suggestive to the reader of ways of thinking and acting. Each text in very similar ways suggests that individuals/readers should engage in a process of self-monitoring, whereby they calculate what they eat and how that is balanced by the exercise they do. Resources are provided to do this: tables list the energy value of common foods and the energy expenditure of different forms of activity. The message is clear: eat too much and too many of the wrong kinds of foods, and more exercise will be required to work it off. In the following quote, the text directly addresses the reader inviting them to calculate their daily energy balance:

> In order to calculate daily caloric expenditure, add to your BMR the calorie or kilojoule cost of the various activities that make up your day. The energy expenditure of each activity can be calculated by measuring the amount of oxygen used to perform the activity.
>
> (Davis *et al.* 1993: 134)

An example of a record chart is provided to help with the calculations. It is unlikely to be a coincidence that the topic immediately following 'Energy Balance' is 'Overweight and Obesity' – the two are closely linked discursively; that is, if the prescriptions offered in the first chapter are not followed then the consequences are described in the second.

The second step in the analytical task is to look at how these ways of making sense of the relationship between health and the body are taken up by individuals as they work 'to attain a certain mode of being' (Foucault 1997: 225). A section from an interview with Karin is used to exemplify the way in which a discourse analysis can be used to address this question. Karin's texts are derived from the corpus of interviews collected for a project investigating the place and meaning of physical activity and physical culture in young people's lives (see Wright *et al.* 2003 for further details).

The interview begins with a brief exchange about Karin's family's current and past involvement in physical activity and the value they do or don't place on her participation in sport. The interviewer then asks Karin about her definition of health. The kinds of meanings which Karin draws on to construct a response in the first instance respond very closely to the kinds of meanings which seem to be promoted in most health-related classes and in the media (see, for example, Leahy and Burrow, Chapter 9; Burrows and Wright, Chapter 6) and which seem widespread in both this research and other research concerned with the meaning of health. Health is about eating healthy food (and not 'junk' food) and engaging in exercise. How much exercise and for what purposes becomes more evident as the interview progresses, but again like the students in Burrows' and Wright's study (Wright and Burrows 2003; Burrows and Wright, Chapter 6) it is primarily associated with fitness. What is also evident in this first excerpt is the notion of 'balance', a balance between food in and energy out through exercise; a set of meanings which has been already established as reiterated in many physical and health education textbooks. As Karin's choices in language suggest, she takes this construction of health to be common knowledge, the interviewer should be able to fill in the gaps of 'Basically all that stuff'.

As the interview progresses Karin elaborates on her constructions of healthy (and not-healthy food). Again she assumes (and quite rightly in terms of the power of the discourse) that there is a clear distinction between health and junk food – 'pizza' falls into the category of the latter – and that this understanding is shared by the interviewer. As Lupton points out, fast food or food produced away from the home is regarded negatively in the context of the binaries of natural/artificial and unprocessed/processed. As she also points out, these are 'cultural constructs that ignore the realities of food production and distribution in modern societies' (Lupton 1996: 91).

Int: What is your definition of health?

Karin: Um, health. It is trying to be fit. Um, eating healthy food, you know, have a balance of food and all that stuff. Getting enough exercise. Basically all that type of stuff.

Int: Would you say that you're pretty healthy?

Karin: Oh, I don't know about that. I'm not very fit. I try to eat the right foods all the time, accept for the occasional pizza, haha. But I don't know. I think that I get through life, you know, maybe I could try to be a bit healthier. I guess. Try to get fit. In summer I try to do a bit more exercise but winter it's too cold around here, way too cold in the night-time.

In the next section of the interview it becomes clearer that meanings around food and eating are not simply about health, although in talking about her own practices she continues to draw on what she seems to understand as a shared understanding of meanings. Healthy food is 'veggies and fruit and stuff like that' even if they come from the freezer. In this section of the interview, Karin demonstrates how, for her, the most important discursive resources in how she evaluates and makes sense of her body are those associated with the relationship between energy in and energy out through exercise and those which provide instruction as to how she can best engage in personal practices that ensure that the balance is one where she loses weight. In terms of Foucault's notions of 'technologies of the self', Karin's descriptions of what she seeks to do can be understood in terms of a socially constituted notion of perfection – the 'ideal body' defined in terms of contemporary notions of femininity. Her happiness depends on her pursuit and attainment of that body. This becomes quite explicit in the last excerpt from the interview when Karin talks about how happy she was when she was in Years Six and Seven at school, she 'was really skinny then', before she 'shot up'. It seems to be a happiness that she has continued to strive to achieve through a constant monitoring of her weight and her appearance. Perfection is also signified by the comments of others and a lack of 'perfection' in the ways she feels physically in her body – she talks, for instance, about feeling 'terrible', 'lazy' and 'fat and . . . so oily' when she has missed hockey for a week: 'You know you haven't worked off any energy so you feel heavy and, just like you miss the little exercise you need to feel normal.' Normality has become embodied as a material/sensual experience; the feelings that occur when her personal practices move beyond what it takes to be normal are uncomfortable and serve to motivate her to eat less and exercise more. Discourses that link fitness and health with thinness become entangled with fitness as the ability to play hockey well, to be able to cover the field and to be seen to be a 'good player'.

Int: So you mentioned before about health that it involved eating right, what did you mean?

Karin: Oh, like I try to, like it's not a matter of eating veggies and fruit and stuff like that. Like I like it and I'll eat it if it is put down in front of me, but otherwise I couldn't be bothered to go to the freezer and cooking some veggies, like I mean, come on no way, haha. But I mean, like earlier this year I was like fatter that I am now, like really, I had about 15 kilos extra on me. Yeah, and I was really determined to lose the weight. So I started on a diet type thing. Not necessarily a diet but I exercised regularly, 'cause it was summer and I just cut down from eating, . . . Now I have roughly three muffins, the English muffins, I would have three of them a day and that would do me for the whole day. Yep, that's all I would eat, muffins all day. And I loved it. But now after the holidays, because in the holidays

I just eat what I want and now I find that I am eating more again. Not necessarily more, I just find that I eat two meals a day instead of one. Before if would be three muffins a day and I hardly drank anything. I was healthy on that. I felt fine. All my friends at school said 'you're malnutritioned'. But I felt great, you know, losing all this weight and being able to run on to a hockey field. And I mean even people were noticing that I could run more on a hockey field. They were saying 'Jeez, you are fitter than you used to be!' It made me feel great and I was healthy

Int: What were your goals?

Karin: To lose weight, to get fit for hockey, probably to clean up my skin, cause I knew if I didn't eat as much junk food that I wouldn't get as much junk food and stuff. And um I just wanted to look a bit better. You know how you feel? *You know, you feel better if you are what you want to be and I'm still not.* I would like to be skinnier than this, but, you know.

Int: Why?

Karin: Well, I would like to get fitter for hockey and the fitter you are the better you are. And I feel better about myself once you are where you want to be with weight wise and everything, you know. I mean you see obese people, you know, fatter people, at swimming pools and they are wearing shirts over their swimmers and you feel sorry for them. That's why I to get to a point where I am happy with my weight and the way I look and everything like that, you know. So, I'd still like to lose a bit of weight but at the moment it's not happening, haha. No, I'm staying about average at the moment, which is OK, like at least it's better than putting it back on. But in summer I plan to lose at least another 10–15 kilos.

Int: Where did you find out information about this?

Karin: I didn't. I just figured it out. Like, when I was a little kid I was like a chubby kid. I was like fully a fat, chubby kid. And then I was fat until about Year Six and Seven. And then I just grew. I shot up and I was really skinny then and I was happy and then I didn't change my eating style so naturally I just put on the weight, after I'd stopped growing. And then up until this year I have just kept eating normally and now it's just motivated, like I want to stay the way I am or just even better. Like, I mean, I would love to lose more weight, the fitter you are, the better you are, that's for me anyway. The fitter you are the healthier you are, I reckon.

Int: Were you happy during the holidays?

Karin: I was really worried the whole time that I was going to put on weight. I enjoyed eating the food, but every second, like as soon as I saw it, or as soon as picked it up, I thought 'no.' I needed some one to re-sure me that I wasn't going to put on weight straight away. I would say to mum, 'will this hurt me, how much weight will I put on?' And she was going, 'just eat the damn thing!' Anyway, she probably got sick of me asking, but I was really worried that I was going to put on weight 'cause it's so hard to get off and you don't want to put it all back on, especially now. Like you don't want to have done all of this for nothing.

One last indication of the work that Karin does to maintain her sense of self as coherent and appropriate is the ways in which she deals with alternate evaluations of her self and her practices. She reports comments from her parents, her boy-friend and her school friends that suggest that they are all in some way or another concerned with her health, her thinness and/or her eating practices. These are dismissed as misguided – her family and her boyfriend – or as evidence of their own 'slothfulness' and poor lifestyle – her friends. Karin's investments in con-tinuing to follow a set of practices that, from her point of view, will keep her thin and healthy are very powerful. Their power is derived from a number of institutional sources. The popular media and the fashion and advertising industries promote a form of female beauty predicated on a degree of thinness unavailable to most women without extreme regimes of dieting and exercise. School physical and health education syllabuses and textbooks draw on knowledge constituted in the disciplinary fields of epidemiological medicine and nutrition to make the equation between exercise health and body weight/shape. This knowledge becomes recontextualised in the teaching and learning practices of the classroom. The power of these discourses around health is in the way they bring together the 'expertise' of science with desire – the health education textbooks provide the means to realise the ideal, to achieve perfection. Karin in this context is the ideal subject.

Conclusion

A concern with the relationship between the self/identity and society/culture is clearly not specific to post-structuralism, nor would most post-structuralist researchers limit their theoretical resources to Foucault. Most of the authors in the book draw on a range of theoretical and empirical resources, some of which include forms of discourse analysis deriving from Foucauldian work, to formulate their research problems, their mode of inquiry and their interpretations of their data (see for instance Kirk, Chapter 4; Penney and Harris, Chapter 7). What the contributors to the book share is a desire to interrogate, to ask questions about the ways in which institutional and cultural processes work to produce particular forms of identity or selves, particularly as these relate to the social construction and control of the body, well-being and health.

What I have endeavoured to do in this chapter is to demonstrate how researchers might work with a post-structuralist approach to contribute to this project. It is not an approach that is usually described in research method textbooks, although the social construction of knowledge and identity is a fundamental assumption of most contemporary 'qualitative' research. An obvious starting point for those wishing to draw on this perspective are the many books by, and commentaries on, Foucault. Cultural studies and the sociology of pedagogy are useful sources for information on, and models of, textual analysis (see Barker and Galasinski 2001; Lee and Poynton 2000). As described earlier in this chapter there are also now many studies from education and physical education which exemplify this approach.

Research drawing on a post-structuralist perspective offers a powerful means to make visible the relationships between the ways individuals construct their sense of self/their identity and the sets of social meaning and values circulating in society. Moreover this analysis also demonstrates how particular meanings are more powerful than others through their relationship with institutionally privileged discourses, but also through their relationship with personal investments, desires and needs which are themselves culturally constituted. In relation to the specific concerns of this book, such an analysis allows us to understand how the social practices of physical education can contribute to taken-for-granted relationships between health, fitness and body shape and weight that are in the first place not as certain as they are made out to be (see Gard and Wright 2001; Gard, Chapter 5) and in the second, potentially damaging as they promote practices injurious to health and well-being (see Robyne Garrett, Chapter 10).

In other chapters in this book (e.g. Burrows and Wright, Chapter 6; Gard, Chapter 5) the writers take up the post-structuralist challenge of interrogating the relationship between power and knowledge and between discourse and subjectivity to further alert those working in the area of physical education and related fields that our knowledge is neither certain nor neutral in its effect and that the social practices we engage in (knowledge production and reproduction making, pedagogies, classificatory practices and so on) draw on particular technologies of power which in turn provide the resources for the ways selves are constituted.

References

Barker, C. and Galasinski, D. (2001) *Cultural Studies and Discourse Analysis: A Dialogue on Language and Identity*, London: Sage.

Clarke, G. (1992) 'Learning the language: discourse analysis in physical education', in A.C. Sparkes (ed.) *Research in Physical Education and Sport: Exploring Alternative Visions*, London: Falmer Press.

Davis, D., Kimmet, T. and Auty, M. (1993) *HSC Personal Development, Health and Physical Education*, Melbourne: Macmillan.

Dreyfus, H. and Rabinow, P. (1982) *Michel Foucault: Beyond Structuralism and Hermeneutics*, Chicago: University of Chicago Press.

Edley, N. (2001) 'Analysing masculinity: interpretative repertoires, ideological dilemmas and subject positions', in M. Wetherell, S. Taylor and S. Yates (eds) *Discourse as Data: A Guide for Analysis*, London: Sage.

Evans, J., Davies, B. and Penney, D. (1996) 'Teachers, teaching and the social construction of gender relations', *Sport, Education and Society* 1(2): 165–84.

Fairclough, N. (1989) *Language and Power*, London and New York: Longman.

Fairclough, N. (1995) *Media Discourse*, London: Edward Arnold.

Fitzgibbon, L., Ruskin, R. and Cross, T. (1992) *Outcomes: Studies in Personal Development, Health and Physical Education*, Milton, QLD: Jacaranda Press.

Foucault, M. (1972) *The Archaeology of Knowledge*, New York: Pantheon.

Foucault, M. (1997) *Ethics: Subjectivity and Truth*, New York: The New Press.

Gard, M. and Wright, J. (2002) 'Managing uncertainty: obesity discourses and physical education in a risk society', *Studies in Philosophy and Education* 20(6): 535–49.

Giddens, A. (1991) *Modernity and Self-Identity: Self and Society in the Late Modern Age*, Cambridge: Polity Press.

Kirk, D. (1997) 'Schooling bodies for new times: the reform of school physical education in high modernity', in J.-M. Fernandez-Balboa (ed.) *Critical Aspects in Human Movement: Rethinking the Profession in the Post-modern Era*, Albany: SUNY Press.

Lee, A. and Poynton, C. (eds) (2000) *Culture and Text*, Sydney: Allen and Unwin.

Luke, A., O'Brien, J. and Comber, B. (1994) 'Making community texts objects of study', *Australian Journal of Language and Literacy* 17(2): 139–49.

Lupton, D. (1995) *The Imperative of Health: Public Health and the Regulated Body*, London: Sage.

Lupton, D. (1996) *Food the Body and the Self*, London: Sage.

Parker, R., Patterson, J. and Hearne, D. (2000) *Health Moves I*, second edition, Melbourne: Heinemann.

Peterson, A. and Bunton, R. (eds) (1997) *Foucault, Health and Medicine*, London and New York: Routledge.

Rhineberger, C., Davis, R. and Hewitt, P. (1994) *Lifewise: Book 2*, Melbourne: Thomas Nelson Australia.

Scheurich, J.J. (1997) *Research Method in the Post-modern*, London: Falmer Press.

Silverman, K. (1983) *The Subject of Semiotics*, Oxford: Oxford University Press

Taylor, S. (2001) 'Locating and conducting discourse analytic research', in M. Wetherell, S. Taylor and S. Yates (eds) *Discourse as Data: A Guide for Analysis*, London: Sage.

Usher, R. and Edwards, R. (1994) *Post-modernism and Education*, London: Routledge.

Wright, J. (1995) 'A feminist post-structuralist methodology for the study of gender construction in physical education: description of a case study', *Journal of Teaching in Physical Education* 15(1): 1–24.

Wright, J. (2000) 'Disciplining the body: power, knowledge and subjectivity in a physical education lesson', in A. Lee and C. Poynton (eds) *Culture and Text*, Sydney: Allen and Unwin.

Wright, J. and Burrows, L. (2003) '"Being Healthy": the discursive construction of health in New Zealand children's responses to the National Education Monitoring Project', *Discourse* 25(2) (in press).

Wright, J., MacDonald, D. and Groom, L. (2003) 'Physical activity and young people: beyond participation', *Sport, Education and Society* 8(1): 17–33.

Part II

The social context
of physical education
and health

3 Sociology, the body and health in a risk society[1]

John Evans and Brian Davies

The social context of physical education and health

This chapter offers a way of reading and interrogating some of the developments that have occurred in physical education and health curricula (PEH) in recent years, drawing heavily on the theoretical work of Michel Foucault and Basil Bernstein. We suggest that in order to understand the form, content and function of these developments in schools and classrooms, we need set them within the context of a range of global social forces and trends relating to 'health' and 'the body', at the same time dealing explicitly with issues of pedagogy, power and control (see Chapters 2 and 14).

The past twenty-five years have been a period of considerable socio-economic and cultural change, accompanied by 'monumental efforts to undertake significant educational reform' (Hargreaves 1999: 340) in schools and in initial teacher education (ITE). In England and Wales we have witnessed the arrival of a National Curriculum for physical education and similar initiatives have occurred in Australia, New Zealand, USA and elsewhere, many foregrounding 'sport' and/or 'health' agendas amongst their goals. Fundamental changes in the form and organisation of economic activity affecting both the nature of and the relationships between paid work, unpaid work and leisure, have occurred throughout the Western world. These changes in the economic base have had a profound impact on the socio-cultural infrastructure of society, dramatically altering relationships between men and women and making problematic conventional conceptions of masculinity and femininity in the work-place, home and at leisure. Conventional beliefs and value systems (including the once powerful grand narratives of socialism, feminism, religion and morality) have, if not broken down, been thoroughly stirred or shaken. Concomitantly, a resurgence of interest in notions of self-help, 'community' and religious, ethnic and national identity has occurred, perhaps reflecting a search for social, psychological and ontological certainty or security and as ways of countering these globalising trends (Castells 1997). Some of these changes have been reflected in significant educational reforms in many countries, including the re-rigging of more strongly state-controlled markets represented by movement towards more locally or self-managed schools. Such neo-liberal policies embody expectations that educational systems should operate more on the lines of the market, treating parents and pupils as 'consumers' of education. The curriculum is now considered more a package of quality-controlled consumer goods than a set of rights to educationally worthwhile experiences, its requirements 'being defined less in terms of content to be covered and time to be allocated to that content, than in terms of standards, targets or outcomes that must be achieved' (Hargreaves 1999: 340). In conditions such as these, the value of any particular school curriculum often seems to be determined less by its educational merit than by its potential use value in exchange for vocational rewards or success in sport. How these changes are reflected in formal education and schooling remains a story to be told.

On one view, these changes reflect the Macdonaldisation of society to which Ritzer (2000) refers; moving inexorably toward a totally regulated bureaucracy in which schools, like universities, become increasingly like fast food establishments offering a diet that, putatively, both defines and satisfies everyone's basic needs. In the UK, for example, the National Curriculum has ensured that, in principle, a child can attend any one of the state sector's school outlets knowing that the PE and any other curriculum on offer is, rhetorically, at least, 'the same' as in every other. Unsurprisingly, in these conditions teachers (and pupils) find it easier to describe the fine detail of *what* curriculum content they should be teaching (and learning) than to give appropriate educational, philosophical or sociological reasons *why* they are doing so in the way that they are. The many and varied responsibilities laid upon teachers presage a homogenised and standardised, predictable, curriculum made up of skills and competencies. It has been accompanied by an inexorable erosion of their ability and authority to define and control the nature of valued knowledge in respect of children's and community needs.

On another view, centralisation runs counter to current social trends which seem to require that we accept more, not less, responsibility for all aspects of our lives. In this perspective, coincident with deregulation of the economy, political instability, the threat of global terrorism and the globalisation of knowledge, information and entertainment have together engendered greater social, moral and scientific uncertainty. With it, according to some analysts, new levels of risk impact deeply on our daily lives. In Giddens' (1999a: 2) view, such risk, especially 'manufactured risk' ('human environments of uncertainty' created by the advances of science and technology) is now not just one of the most important issues in the social sciences today; it is central to what our lives are about, so that what it means to have self-identity, 'how we relate to the diversity of information about diet, food, on the one hand and the global economy on the other, the Asian crisis, ecological problems – in their own way are all risk environments' (ibid.: 5). In this view, the world is now not only full of surprises and unintended consequences, it is also a world of 'deregulated uncertainty' where advances in science and technology accompany an erosion of 'tradition' in the western world (Turner 2002: 4). And as there is no higher authority to call on for direction in our lives, a society living on the 'other side of nature and tradition', argues Giddens (1999b), is one that calls for less centralisation and a greater level of individual decision-making in everyday life. 'We' now seem to be faced with countless choices (over relationships, diet, procreation, looks, sexuality, etc.) where previously there were few, or none.

Ironically, this has made life more uncertain and less comfortable psychologically. As Giddens points out, '(w)herever you have choice you have risk because you're confronting an open future'. And in many of 'the new risk situations, calculations of probability are not possible because there is no historical experience with which to make calculations' (ibid.: 6). The upshot of this, he says, is that in the 'new moral climate of risk we tend to get an oscillation between accusations of scare-mongering on the one hand and accusations of cover-ups on the other' (ibid.). BSE ('mad cow disease') and 'obesity disease', as others will contend (see Chapters 5, 6 and 9), are good examples of this, though evidence of doubt and uncertainty is not readily apparent amongst policy-makers and others who help manufacture 'obesity scares' or teachers who trade on them in schools (see Evans 2003).

The idea that human beings should be more autonomous and responsible for their own health and safety, individually and collectively, has paralleled the rise of 'manufactured risk'. At one level, this trend is clearly reflected in the massive expansion in Western economies of 'health industries', variously purveying specialist 'expertise', cure-all drugs and vitamins, health and exercise advice, or surgical body modification techniques, to help individuals take care and control of their lives. At another, it is seen in the heightened emphasis given to health issues in government polices and in physical education and the wider school curriculum in recent years in the USA, UK, Australia, New Zealand (see Penney and Chandler 2000) and elsewhere, that increasingly privilege, alongside 'performance', body-centred 'perfection codes' celebrating individual responsibility, autonomy and self-surveillance and control. In the UK, for example, it is variously expressed in the 'new' PE curriculum as Health Related *Education*, in New Zealand and Australia as Health and Physical Education, all trading on elements of child-centredness to achieve their aims and ideals. There is a dark side to this development, as we will later see.

We share Turner's (2002) view that both these seemingly contradictory views of an increasingly regulated and deregulated social world are plausible and register trends that find expression in complementary, rather than contradictory, ways in the school curriculum, especially in PEH. Far from effecting greater autonomy amongst teachers and pupils, the decentralising, diversifying, benchmarking, standard-setting British educational state is now more rather than less powerful, constraining and in control.

Sociology and health as social control

Socio-economic change has also had some impact on developments within social theory. Since the early 1980s, a number of social theorists (for example, Lyotard, Rorty, Jameson, Foucault (see Best and Kellner 1991; Lyon 1994), variously referred to as either 'post-modernist' or 'post-structuralist' (see Chapter 2), and recently the ideas of Bourdieu (e.g. Light and Kirk 2000; Holroyd 2003) have exerted considerable influence on research, including socio-cultural research in physical education and sport in schools (see Fernandez-Balboa 1997; Kirk 1998, 1999a, b; Wright 2000; Gard and Wright 2001; Glyse *et al.* 2002; Ronholt 2002).

Together these theorists have provided a substantial challenge not just as to how we think and write about the social world but also as to how it is we claim to know it and as to the status and nature of the knowledge itself. Issues of representation have been brought to the fore. The work of Foucault, in particular, has captured the imagination. On the one hand it has prompted a rich vein of writing on 'the body', education policy and the social construction of identities in classroom life. On the other, it has influenced the study of medicine, health and illness in society and schools (see the seminal work of Turner 1984, 1997; Featherstone 1982; Shilling 1993b). This, at least in part, may itself be a reflection of the broad socio-economic changes described above. In Turner's (1984, 1997) view a variety of new influences have all underscored a sociological interest in 'the body': growth in consumer culture; the development of new lifestyles emphasising consumption and leisure; increased commercial and consumerist interests in the body; contemporary emphasis on keeping fit, the body beautiful and the putative postponement of ageing by involvement in physical activity and sport; increased life expectancy pressing the body to become the focus for medical control and intervention; and feminist criticism of conventional socio-cultural systems that have generated heightened sensitivities to gender, sexuality, and biology. In some respects there is a deep irony to this. As Berger (2001) pointed out, in contemporary Western culture images are everything and abound everywhere. 'Never has so much been depicted and watched . . . Appearances registered, and transmitted with lightening speed.' Yet with this, he says,

> something has innocently changed. They used to be called physical appearances because they belonged to solid bodies. Now appearances are volatile. Technological advances have made it easy to separate the apparent from the existent. And this is precisely what the present system's mythology continually needs to exploit. It turns appearances into refractions, like mirages: refractions not of light but of appetite, in fact a single appetite, the appetite for more. Consequently – and oddly, considering the physical implications of the notion of *appetite* – the existent, the body, disappears. We live within a spectacle of empty clothes and unworn masks.
>
> (Berger 2001: 12)

Thus, the heightened interest in 'the body', of knowing who and what we are supposed to be, within a contemporary culture of increased anxiety and risk, may itself be regarded not only as a contingent intellectual epiphenomenon, in part a quest for ontological security in an ephemeral world, but co-opted and constrained by the interests of post-modern capitalism. At times this intellectual movement has seemed so besotted with corporeal issues that important and enduring agendas of ethnicity, class, gender, ability, poverty and oppression appear to have been sidelined, though it may be fairer to claim that they have simply been reconfigured in 'new' and innovative ways (Cooper 1995).

Teachers as health experts

The idea that, as the global economy has developed into a culture of risk, so nation states have developed new, regulatory systems of social control that work on 'the body' and the self, has serious implications for the curriculum and pedagogies of schools and ITEPE (see Pronger 2002). As Turner (1997) points out, welfare and health systems in Western societies are now a complex mixture of risk culture and Macdonaldisation of services. We expect not just quick-fix solutions to all our health needs but also to receive the knowledge and expertise that will inform us as to what future actions are needed to avoid falling prey to illness and disease, the 'risks' of living in a fast-changing post-modern world. Knowledge of and about health has become an inherent and inseparable mechanism of 'body control'. This claim, no doubt, may seem oddly at variance with the thinking of professionals who believe that they are primarily concerned to alleviate suffering and improve individual health through 'health promotion' in the curriculum of schools, rather than social control. However, in this view, the notion of 'generalised risk' in the environment has, in effect, led to greater surveillance and control through the promotion of preventative medicine (Lupton 1997). 'Epidemics', such as AIDS and 'the obesity crisis', have helped create a socio-political climate within which intervention and control of populations and individuals by medical practitioners or health experts including teachers in schools 'are seen as both necessary and benign' (Turner 1997: xix). As the individual is confronted with a complex diversity of alternatives, especially in relation to lifestyle, so 'feelings of anxiety and 'crisis' become an endemic 'normal' part of the individual's experience' (Giddens 1991: 181–5, quoted in Petersen 1997: 191). And once the individual is cut loose from traditional commitments and support relationships he or she must chose between a diverse array of lifestyles, sub-cultures and identities and 'enter into the process of his or her own self-governance through processes of endless self examination, self care, and self improvement' (Petersen ibid: 194). In these social conditions it seems that only the knowledge produced by science and especially epidemiology, mediated through the actions and discourses of 'expert' medical and health professionals, including teachers in schools, can help ensure that populations and individuals achieve the expected new degrees of self-responsibility, self-discipline and control:

> The complex system for managing and regulating populations that is indicated in the goals and targets strategy is informed, and technically facilitated, by advances in the statistical calculation of risk, employing sophisticated techniques of epidemiology. Epidemiology has become so central to the public health endeavour of identifying, reducing exposure to, or eliminating 'risk' that it has become almost synonymous with the public health enterprise itself. It has a broad agenda which makes use of vast numbers of practices such as case studies, quantitative analysis and laboratory experiments, and contemporary epidemiologists work closely with public policy groups and public health departments to help track populations and to educate all populations.
>
> (Petersen 1997: 197)

This, we suggest, is the very stuff of understandings, for example, of obesity and other 'diseases' that feed the practices of teacher educators, teachers and other professionals in PEH in schools (see Chapters 5, 9 and 12). To some, this approach is substantially flawed (see Le Fanu 1999; Evans 2003). As Lupton (1995: 67) points out, the recourse to epidemiology, regarded by those involved in health promotion as invaluable, provides 'only a veneer of scientific legitimacy, objectivity and expertise'. Importantly, though, in these circumstances, the role of the 'expert' health professional or pedagogue is thrust to the fore, as is the status of the scientific disciplines (e.g. psychology, biology, exercise physiology) that inform them (see Pronger 2002). The new-found 'expertise' of the teachers in contemporary PEH in the UK, Australia, USA, New Zealand and elsewhere, is therefore central to the exercise of power for at least three reasons. First,

> by locating the authority of claims in 'scientificity' this serves to distance systems of self-regulation from formal forms of political power. Second, 'expertise' can be mobilised within political argument wherein it can play a particular role in the development of programmes of government. Third, expertise has a salience for the 'self-regulating capacities of subjects' in that it ties their subjectivity to 'truth' and in this respect it has a potent ethical dimension.
>
> (Nettleton 1997: 215–16)

'Social facts' are drawn on by politicians not only to describe what individuals and populations currently are in terms of their health conditions but also what they ideally ought to be if schools and other government agencies are allowed to intervene. The roles played by the biological, behavioural and health sciences within sport science and ITE programmes in the UK and elsewhere in the creation of 'expert' knowledge' and, concomitantly, 'expert' professionals, are instrumental in processes such as these (Pronger 2002; Tinning and Glasby 2002; Leahy and Harrison, Chapter 9).

Pupils, self surveillance and health

These changes have also had an impact on how we are meant to think about young people in schools. The idea of the 'individual-as-enterprise' (Petersen 1997: 198) has emerged as a basic premise of neo-liberal rationality:

> A manifestation of this is to be found the phenomenon of 'healthism', described by medical sociologists (Greco, 1993: 357). Healthism posits that the individual has choice in preserving his or her physical capacity from the event of disease. In the event that one is unable to regulate one's own lifestyle and modify one's risky behaviour then this is, at least in part, 'a failure of the self to care for itself'.
>
> (Greco 1993: 361, quoted in Petersen 1997: 198)

'Healthism', as a particular form of 'bodyism' in which 'a hedonistic lifestyle is paradoxically combined with a preoccupation with ascetic practices aimed at the achievement or maintenance of appearance of health, fitness and youthfulness' (Dutton 1995: 273, quoted in Petersen 1997), is of particular interest here (see also, Kirk 1993, 1999b). The discourses of health and health care, expressing new body-centred perfection codes (Chapter 14), driven by the interests of business and the economy and informed by the bio sciences and psychological theories and practices, have contributed massively to policy developments and practice in PEH settings in recent years in Europe, USA, Australia, New Zealand and elsewhere. We have witnessed a reconfiguration not only of the PE curriculum and pedagogies around health and body perfection but also of our understandings of the 'individual child'. In the 'new' child/body-centred health-related curriculum the pupil is no longer thought of as relatively 'docile', a 'passive recipient of advice and health care but as one who, at least rhetorically, possesses the capacity for self-sur-veillance and control, responsibility, rationality and enterprise' (Nettleton 1997: 214): qualities that are embodied and have routinely to be displayed. Indeed, Ogden (1995) has argued that so pervasive and powerful is the impact of psychological theory on policy and practice that we could be forgiven for reaching the conclusion that 'it is not environmental factors, or bacteria, or viruses *per se* that cause illness; the critical factor resides in individuals, their willingness to take decisions and appropriate evasive action' and, more particularly, in managing their self-control (Nettleton 1997: 214). The replacement of educational aims and principles in PEH with food and 'weight concerns' and the ideological and pedagogical desire to make children and young people active, fit and thin is one reflection of this trend (Evans 2003).

Health and body hierarchies

Nowhere are these tends more pervasive or pernicious than in the analysis of how the massive socio-economic changes alluded to above have impacted on our core relations to exercise and food. Westernised cultures seem besotted with 'the body', size, shape and form. Multi-million pound health industries have emerged putatively to help people live longer, stay healthy, and engage in body 're-design'. In these conditions, discourses of 'obesity' and 'self-starvation' (for example, anorexia nervosa and bulimia) seem to work symbiotically as topics of public concern presented quite inaccurately in the popular and academic press as 'diseases' of epidemic proportion of modern humankind. Beardsworth and Keil (1997: 174) point out the ironies in relation to the latter disorders. Although the food supply has become more secure and plentiful, at least in the Western world, a substantial proportion of the population now claims to be on a diet, trying to avoid eating the range of foods now available. They also note that as average body weight increases in the general population, the preferred body image in the media, entertainment industry and commercial and industrial organisations emphasises the slim, slender and underweight. Moreover, the second half of the twentieth century is associated with a rise in eating disorders arising from weight loss so extreme as to endanger health and even life (anorexia nervosa), or from a pattern of unrestrained eating (bulimia nervosa) threatening the health of the sufferer. Much of the available data also suggests that many of those involved in dieting and eating disorders of this kind are women, that is, 'the people who are "normally" responsible, or will as adults become responsible, for the selection, preparation, and serving of food'. This leads Beardsworth and Keil to remind us that, as Brown and Jasper (1993) argue so cogently, 'if we are to contribute anything to the analysis of such issues we should find answers to these questions: 'Why weight?' 'Why women?' and 'Why now?'' (loc. cit.). How these trends are reflected in teachers thinking about 'the body' in schools and, in their recognition and reward of 'ability' and health behaviour in PEH, should be of more than just our passing concern. There is some evidence to 'suggest' (see Doyle and Bryant-Waugh 2000, for a cautionary comment on this) that we are facing a rising level of pathological body dissatisfaction and eating disorders, especially anorexia nervosa and bulimia nervosa, amongst young women, particularly in the 13–19 age range, and, increasingly, young men, in the UK and elsewhere in Western cultures (see Grogan 1999). Yet, as is pointed out in Chapter 11, very little sociological attention has been given to how schools may be implicated in the aetiology and development of these conditions, especially when performance and perfection codes intersect (see Chapter 14).We are reminded of Giddens's (1999b: 5) observation that 'the dark side of decision making' is the rise of addictions and compulsions in relation to work, exercise, food, sex, especially amongst the middle classes. Addiction comes into play he says, 'when choice, which should be driven by autonomy, is subverted by anxiety'. This is a commonplace cocktail of emotions experienced by pupils in many schools today given the heightened expectations placed on young women and men 'to succeed' and the quite alarming levels of assessment and examinations to which they are subjected within a curriculum that offer endless option choices but few means of ownership of knowledge or pedagogical control. Bruch (1973: 82), drawing on her work with young people suffering from anorexia nervosa, wrote:

> growing girls can experience . . . liberation as a demand and feel that they have to do something outstanding. Many of my patients have expressed the feeling that they are overwhelmed by the vast number of potential opportunities available to them . . . and [that] they have been afraid of not choosing correctly.
> (Quoted in Lask 2000: 73)

Are such conditions of ill-health constructed by or exacerbated in the cultures of healthism, performance and perfection manufactured in and outside schools? Do PEH curricula leave pupils feeling valued, included, competent, comfortable and in control of their bodies health; or feeling neglected and alienated from their corporeal selves? Do they help propel some toward disordered eating and ill-health? (see Chapter 12).[2] Has 'ability' been reduced to a display of shape, weight and exercise concerns? Answering these questions requires a much more critical stance than is currently the case towards the core assumptions and beliefs of the behavioural, health and bio sciences that feed conceptions of the 'valued body' and its 'correct usage' into the curriculum of PEH in schools (Pronger 2002). We need to pay particular attention to the way in which contemporary ideals of body shape, image and the discourse of 'obesity' influence the policies and practices of teachers and pupils' embodied self, identity and health and divert attention both from the educational purposes of physical activity and the social and cultural conditions that shape and constrain individual lives (Evans 2003).

Theorising health: Foucault, warts and all

The work of Petersen and Bunton (1997), Turner (1984 and 1997) and Lupton (1995, 1997) in particular, is of great interest here in respect of these issues, particularly for those wishing to consider the potential of Foucault's analysis for the analysis of these health and body themes. Indeed, we share Turner's (1997) view that Foucault's work, combined with Ulrich Beck's (1992) notion of 'risk society', offers a paradigm for understanding health discourses and, in particular, the new epidemiology of disease, such as HIV, or obesity, in late modern or post-modern society.

Foucault's work, concerned essentially with the problematisation of the fundamental domains of experience in Western culture, such as madness, illness, deviancy and sexuality, is difficult and elusive, not least because its focus developed and changed over time. Foucault sought to illustrate how subjectivity, our sense of the body and self, is constituted in and through a wide range of discourses and practices within fields of power, knowledge and truth (see Best and Kellner 1991 and Jan Wright, Chapter 2). He was fundamentally, though far from exclusively, interested in issues of social control. However, as Turner (1997) stressed, his understanding of control has to be situated within a theory of power, where '*governmentality*' acted as the bridge between 'regimes of discipline' and 'the production of the self' (Turner 1997). In Turner's view, 'governmentality' referred to 'a system of power which articulates the triangular relationships between sovereignty, discipline and government' (ibid.: xiii) emerging, according to Foucault (1991), in the eighteenth century when governments required a whole series of specific *savoirs* ('knowledges', always referred to in the plural by Foucault) to help regulate and control populations. As Tyler (1997: 79) points out, in his later work, Foucault defined 'governmentality' as the 'contact' between 'technologies of power' which determine the conduct of individuals and submits them to certain ends or domination and 'technologies of the self'

> (W)hich permit individuals to effect by their own means or with the help of others a certain number of operations on their own bodies and souls, thoughts, conduct and way of being, so as to transform themselves in order to attain a certain state of happiness, wisdom, perfection, or immortality.
>
> (Foucault 1988: 18)

This raises problematic issues concerning the relationships between the constraining/determining features of 'governmentality' and the 'agency' implied in the notion of 'technologies of the self'. However, the rationale of modern government, according to Tyler (1997: 78), is to maximise the capacities of populations: an act of facilitating the development of certain characteristics considered 'good' or 'desirable' and of eliminating or minimising others. Power and knowledge are, thus, 'always inevitably and inextricably interconnected so that any extension of power involves an increase in knowledge' (Turner 1997: xiii), an insight that has proved enormously useful and important for medical sociologists and others concerned with health issues, in their attempt to understand the forms of power assumed by medical and other health practices inside and outside schools.

Foucault saw power not as residing in the interests of particular groups or individuals but as 'a relationship', '[i]n reality power means relations, a more or less organised, hierarchical co-ordinated cluster of relations' (Foucault 1980: 198). This view assumes that people are unequal and that power, though wide-spread and dispersed, is thus concerned with domination and subjection. Notions of relational power and social relations supplant 'resource based' analyses of power as something that particular classes or groups possess, typically found, for example, in Marxian and other earlier social theories. In the Foucauldian view, neither power nor subjectivity has meaning or existence outside a particular relationship between social forces. It is 'localised, dispersed, diffused and typically disguised through the social system, operating at micro, local and government levels' (Turner 1997: xi). In effect, it is embedded and ultimately embodied in the day-to-day practices of, for example, the medical profession, social workers and teachers in schools. In this view, which is not without its critics, power exists through 'disciplinary practices which produce particular individuals, institutions and cultural arrange-ments' (ibid.: xii). It is a view that paves the way for tracing how 'discourses of subjectivity' produce identities or roles, such as the 'good' and 'bad' patient, or 'able', 'fit' or 'unfit' pupils. As we will see, the medicalisation of 'fat/weight' issues and the global export of the 'obesity problem' are illustrations of this process. Furthermore, in a Foucauldian perspective, the practices of subjection and self-formation involve the emergence of complex pedagogies of self-transformation and education that, in turn, require a particular moral order or ethos which become the organising principle of 'practices of the self'. A code evolves by which moral identities are shaped and guided (ibid.: xiii). Through education, via the medical professions and the policy rhetoric of governments and their agencies, we each learn to know what kind of good citizen in body and health we are and ought to be.

We are each and every one of us involved routinely in power relations and the discursive production of our own and others' sense of identity and self (see Wright, Chapter 2). Turning more and more in his later work to the analysis of the self, rather than the body, in the context of medical history and the development of sexuality, Foucault centred on how 'the self' was an effect of 'discourses of the self' in Western societies (Turner 1997). He provided a description of what Turner called the 'institutions of normative coercion', such as the law, religion, medicine and, we add, schools. These institutions are coercive in the sense that they discipline individuals and exercise forms of surveillance over everyday life in such away that actions are both produced and constrained by them. Significantly, this is not achieved through violent or obviously repressive action but subtle forms of control, exercising a moral authority over individuals by explaining problems (e.g. of health) and providing solutions for them (e.g. of correct diet and exercise). In this way, their coercive character is disguised and masked by their normative involvement in the troubles and problems of individuals themselves. The production, regulation and representation of bodies within contexts of disciplinary surveillance are, thus, Foucault's main concerns. The body and populations play a continuous role in the analytic structure of his work; they are the targets of the medical *gaze*, a principal *technology of power* concerned with the gathering of information, informing and creating discussion on its subject matter, prior to intervention, regulation and control. In this way, discourses, for example, about 'health' and 'ability', 'create *effects of truth* which are of themselves neither true nor false. Because of this association of a productive power with the fabrication of "effects of truth" Foucault speaks of *power/knowledge* – a phenomenon which cannot be reduced to either component' (Fox 1997: 36). The governmentality of health is, thus, a form of policing specifically designed to ensure that individuals and populations are always attuned to the requirements of the labour process and wider economic needs (see Leahy and Harrison, Chapter 9, and Tinning and Glasby 2002).

The concept of 'discourse' and its association with power/ knowledge is central in Foucault's work (Fox 1997: 35) and is used in a particular way to develop a basis for understanding what makes knowledge possible (see Chapter 2). It offers an 'archaeology' of knowledge, a method of understanding the ways in which self and society are constructed and underpinned by rules which may operate independently of subjectivity. It is, once again, a method that compels us to peel away the layers of the taken-for-granted, the orthodox and the obvious in society and school, not in search of some essential 'core reality' where none is to be found but towards more complete understandings of the nature of authority, power and control.

Some cautionary notes

This form of social theorising is not, of course, without its limits and critics. There is, argues Fox (1997: 39) the potential for the Foucauldian body to 'become a romantic subject-substitute, continually buffeted by discourse, never able to self actualise, doomed always to be the plaything of power/knowledge'. In this respect it is worth bearing in mind, with Fox and Wright (Chapter 2), that in Foucault's later writing the individual and self supplement the more usual subject and 'body'. We see a move from a concern with external 'technologies of power', to 'technologies of the self'. Now the project is how we become 'desiring subjects', in other words, how we articulate our bodies and desires within a form of subjectivity capable of reflection. 'Practices of the self mark the engagement between discourses of the social and the individual, such that power is integral to the autonomous ordering of the individual's own lives' (Fox 1997: 42). Subjectivity is achieved through discourse and discursive practices, quintessentially human activities. These complex relationships between discursive and other forms of social constraint and human agency are illustrated in the chapters that follow, especially with reference to the relationships between contemporary public debates on body shape, obesity and health (effecting a 'knowledge of the body' fed by government reports and policies, informed by epidemiology) and their inter-pretation, adoption, rejection, ultimately their 'internalisation' as part of the subjective identities of teachers and pupils in schools. Other critics (see Hargreaves 1999; Constas 1996; Lupton 1997; Moore and Muller 1999; Evans and Davies 2002 and Chapter 14) centre attention particularly on Foucault's inherent relativism and tendency to evade, rather than dismiss altogether, structural issues relating for example, to racism, gender, ability and social class.

Whether these limitations are 'real' or imaginary artefacts of the difficulty of drawing conclusions from Foucault's slippery prose is largely immaterial. We could now point to a vast array of literature that has productively applied post-structural theory to the study of gender issues, relations and hierarchies, perhaps less so race, ethnicity, ability/disability and class. The discourses of post-modernism certainly demonstrate the kind of commitment to 'the ideal of doubt' that the 'new' sociology of education in the UK once sought to appropriate as its trademark and deny to the 'old'. In this sense, as Constas (1996: 31) points out, 'postmodernism represents the reinvigoration of a sceptical attitude and should cause us to raise questions about the veracity of the frameworks used to make sense of the world' with, in our view, much of its concomitant voyeurism and atheoretical opportunism. We should also note that, whether the theoretical inclinations of researchers are interactionist, structuralist, post-structural or post-modern, they all continue to annotate the most significant single notion produced within the sociology of education to date, that the form and content of educational practice both matter greatly in determining the life chances and identities of pupils. What children learn from the school curriculum in general and PEH in particular derives not only from its content but also from the manner and mode in which it is organised and then provided and from how learning is interpreted, assessed and displayed. There is no conceivable content without transmission, no instructional discourse that is not embedded in the regulative, no education/pedagogical process independent of social control. The work of Foucault, especially when combined with that of other social theorists and particularly when anchored to a Bernsteinian grammar of the pedagogic field (Bernstein 1996, 2000), helps us look at these processes afresh.

The strength of viewing power as multifarious and multi-located, not to be reduced to a conspiratorial group or entity, such as class interests, the state or patriarchy, is that we are compelled to study the role of education and PEH in cultural re/production and social control as an 'exercise of power'. It focuses attention on the relationships between power, knowledge and pedagogy. This prompts consideration of how certain values, attitudes and norms relating for example, to health, 'ability' and sport, come to be identified as appropriate for education, and through what mechanisms people come to accept them as legitimate.

It generates questions as to what and whose discourses are privileged in the PEH curriculum, for example health-related fitness and games-teaching rather than, say, aesthetics, dance and outdoor education. What, for example, are the class, gender and ethnic origins of performance and perfection codes that are expressed in the variants of sport education and health education now found in schools? It becomes important to seek the origins of these discursive codes in wider 'regimes of truth' and the socio-political and economic interests that they serve, to see how power, as a resource, is drawn on and used by policy-makers, pupils, teacher-educators, teachers, to determine what may be thought, taught and learned. Skelton (1997) points out that a Foucauldian perspective invites us to look at schools as disciplinary institutions, organising physical space and time with structures which are designed to change and reinforce people's behaviours along designed lines. Techniques of surveillance, such as testing, observing and documenting aspects of students' personal dispositions and feelings, are central to this endeavour. In this process, students become objectified and may accept institutional definitions of themselves which enable them, subsequently, to be politically dominated as docile beings. For Foucault, then, 'the hidden curriculum of schooling would refer to those disciplinary practices that reduce individuals to docility' (ibid.: 187). If the goals of democracy and equity through education and PE are our 'good things', the work of Foucault, and other like-minded social theorists, allows us to advance some way in the direction of answering questions of this kind. But it also brings us to points where, conceptually and empirically, we are drawn to a halt by the limits of the theoretical frame and its failure to speak to the kind of issues outlined below. For us, the work of Bernstein provides an even more enlightening conceptual scheme. These are matters to which we return in Chapter 14.

Conclusion

The enduring requirement of doing the sociology of education, whether expressed in old or new ways, is that we examine the social bases of conventional practices and decision-making process, including those which grant or withhold access to valued forms and practices in contexts of PEH. It means interrogating the criteria that underpin curriculum selection, the rationales that are used to justify them, locating them not only within subject communities but also the wider organisational, social and political contexts of which they are a part. This requires theory and methods capable of making connections between embodied consciousness, human agency, culture and social structure. In the study of schooling we must seek the relations between the complexities of teachers' and pupils' cultures, their actions and intentions and their relationships with forms of curriculum organisation and content, the organisational contexts of schools and the communities and wider societies in which they are located, and with prevailing global trends. This calls for a more sophisticated view of micro-macro relationships, 'avoiding the artificial conceptual boundaries between what is inside classrooms and what is "out there"'. As Hargreaves (1999) notes:

What is 'out there' is already 'in here' in the ethnocultural diversity of students, in the technological world of virtuality through which students live their lives and which they bring to schools, in the ways that the passions and desires of minority students are relegated from the curriculum and regulated within the classroom by a Eurocentric tradition of rationalised control and so on.

(Ibid.: 351)

Our central idea must remain that we may only arrive at an understanding of the activities of teachers and teaching and what pupils learn and embody if we view them relationally and locate them historically, organisationally, institutionally and intentionally.[3] We remain a long way from having exhausted these projects in the sociology of education, physical education and health.

Notes

1   This is a development of Evans and Davies (2002) first published in Laker (2002).
2   The relationship between body dissatisfaction and eating disorders is both complex and much debated and it cannot be assumed that the former condition is a trigger to the latter. A complex array of factors is involved in propelling some towards eating disorder (see Grogan 1999; Evans *et al.* 2003).
3   We also accept that what is required is genuine rapprochement between those who wish to work with such ideas in both sociology and psychology (not to say philosophy and curriculum studies). Among psychologists, we commend the work of Ivinson (1998, 2000), who attempts to bring Bernstein and Moscovici together, and Daniels (2001a, b), who sees the work of Bernstein and Vygotsky as deeply complementary.

References

Beardsworth, A. and Keil, T. (1997) *Sociology on the Menu*, London: Routledge.
Beck, U. (1992) *Risk Society: Towards a New Modernity*, London: Sage.
Berger, J. (2001) *The Shape of a Pocket*, London: Bloomsbury.
Bernstein, B. (1996) *Pedagogy, Symbolic Control and Identity: Theory, Research and Critique*, London: Taylor & Francis.
Bernstein, B. (2000) *Pedagogy, Symbolic Control and Identity: Theory, Research and Critique*, revised edition, London: Rowman & Littlefield.
Best, S. and Kellner, D. (1991) *Postmodern Theory – Critical Interrogations*, London: Macmillan.
Brown, C. and Jasper, K. (eds) (1993) *Consuming Passions: Feminist Approaches to Weight Preoccupation and Eating Disorders*, Toronto: Second Story Press.
Bruch, H. (1973) *The Golden Cage: The Enigma of Anorexia Nervosa*, London: Open Books.
Castells, M. (1997) *The Power of Identity. The Information Age: Economy, Society and Culture*, Volume II, Oxford: Blackwell.
Constas, M.A. (1996) 'The changing nature of educational research and a critique of postmodernism', *Educational Researcher* 27(2): 26–33.
Cooper, D. (1995) *Power in Struggle*, Buckingham: Open University Press.
Daniels, H. (2001a) 'Bernstein and Activity Theory', in A. Morais, I. Neves, B. Davies, and H. Daniels (eds), *Towards a Sociology of Pedagogy*, New York: Peter Lang, pp. 99–112.

Daniels, H. (2001b) *Vygotsky and Pedagogy*, London: Routledge/Falmer.

Doyle, J. and Bryant-Waugh, R. (2000) 'Epidemiology', in B. Lask and R. Bryant-Waugh (eds) *Anorexia Nervosa and Related Eating Disorders in Childhood and Adolescence*, second edition, Hove: Psychology Press, Taylor & Francis, pp. 41–63.

Dutton, K.R. (1995) *The Perfectible Body: The Western Ideal of Physical Development*, London: Cassell.

Evans, J. (2003) 'Physical education and health. A polemic. – Or, let them eat cake', *European Physical Education Review* 9(1): 87–103.

Evans, J. and Davies, B. (2002) 'Theoretical background', in A. Laker (ed.) *The Sociology of Sport and Physical Education*, London: Routledge/Falmer.

Evans, J., Evans, R., Evans, C. and Evans, J. (2003) 'Fat free schooling: the discursive production of ill-health', *International Studies in the Sociology of Education* 12(2): 191–215.

Featherstone, M. (1982) 'The body in consumer culture', *Theory, Culture and Society* 1(2): 18–33.

Fernandez-Balboa, J.-M. (ed.) (1997) *Critical Postmodernism in Human Movement, Physical Education and Sport*, New York: SUNY.

Foucault, M. (1980) *Power/Knowledge*, New York: Pantheon.

Foucault, M. (1988) 'Technologies of the self', in L.H. Martin, H. Gutman and P. Hutton (eds) *Technologies of the Self: A Seminar with Michel Foucault*, London: Tavistock Publications.

Foucault, M. (1991) 'Governmentality', in G. Burchell, C. Gordon and P. Muller (eds) *The Foucault Effect*, Brighton: Harvester Wheatsheaf, pp. 87–194.

Fox, N.J. (1997) 'Is there life after Foucault? Texts, frames and differends', in A. Petersen and R. Bunton (eds) *Foucault, Health and Medicine*, London: Routledge, pp. 31–53.

Gard, M. and Wright, J. (2001) 'Managing uncertainty: obesity discourses and physical education in a risk society', *Studies in the Philosophy of Education* 20: 535–49.

Giddens, A. (1991) *Modernity and Self Identity: Self and Society in the Late Modern Age*, Stanford: Stanford University Press.

Giddens, A. (1999a) 'The director's lectures. Runaway world', The Reith Lectures Revisited, Lecture 2, hhttp://www.lse.ac.uk/Giddens/reith_99/week3/week3.htm (November 1999).

Giddens, A. (1999b) 'Lecture 3 – Tradition – Delhi', The Reith Lectures 1999, http://www.lse.ac. uk/Giddens/reith_99/week3/week3.htm (November 1999).

Glyse, J., Pigeassou, A., Marcellini, E., De Leseleuc, E. and Bui-Xuan, G. (2002) 'Physical education as a subject in France (school curriculum, policies and discourse)', *Sport, Education and Society* 7(1): 5–25.

Grogan, S. (1999) *Body Image*, London: Routledge.

Hargreaves, A. (1999) 'Schooling in the new millennium: educational research for the postmodern age', *Discourse: Studies in the Cultural Politics of Education* 20(3): 333–57.

Holroyd, R.A.(2003) 'Fields of experience: young people's constructions of embodied identities', unpublished thesis, Loughborough University.

Ivinson, G. (1998) 'The child's construction of the curriculum', *Papers on Social Representations: Threads and Discussions. Special Issue: The Development of Knowledge* 6(1) 21–40.

Ivinson, G. (2000) 'The development of children's social representations of the primary school curriculum' in H. Cowie and D. Van der Aalsvort (eds) *Social Interaction in*

Learning and Instruction: The Meaning of Discourse for the Construction of Knowledge, Kidlington: Pergamon Press and EARLI.

Kirk, D. (1993) *The Body, Schooling and Culture*, Deakin: Deakin University Press.

Kirk, D. (1998) *Schooling Bodies: School Practice and Public Discourse 1880–1950*, Leicester: Leicester University Press.

Kirk, D. (1999a) 'Educational reform, physical culture and the crisis of legitimation in physical education', *Discourse* 19(1): 101–13.

Kirk, D. (1999b) 'Health, the body and the medicalisation of the school', in C. Symes and D. Meadmore (eds) *The Extra-ordinary School*, New York: Peter Lang.

Laker, A. (ed.) (2002) *The Sociology of Sport and Physical Education*, London: Falmer/Routledge.

Lask, B. (2000) 'Aetiology', in B. Lask and R. Bryant-Waugh (eds) *Anorexia Nervosa and Related Eating Disorders in Childhood and Adolescence*, second edition, East Sussex: Psychology Press, Taylor & Francis.

Le Fanu, J. (1999) *The Rise and Fall of Modern Medicine*, London: Abacus.

Light, R. and Kirk, D. (2000) 'High school rugby, the body and the reproduction of hegemonic masculinity', *Sport, Education and Society* 5(1): 163–77.

Lupton, D. (1995) *The Imperatives of Health: Public Health and the Regulated Body*, London: Sage.

Lupton, D. (1997) 'Foucault and the medicalisation critique', in A. Petersen, A. and R. Bunton (eds) *Foucault, Health and Medicine*, London: Routledge, pp. 94–113.

Lyon, D. (1994) *Postmodernity*, Buckingham: Open University Press.

Moore, R. and Muller, J. (1999) 'The discourse of the "voice" and the problem of knowledge and identity in the sociology of education', *British Journal of Sociology of Education* 20(2): 189–206.

Nettleton, S. (1997) 'Governing the risky self: how to become healthy, wealthy and wise', in A. Peterson and R. Bunton (eds) *Foucault, Health and Medicine*, London: Routledge, pp. 207–23.

Ogden, J. (1995) 'Psychological theory and the creation of the risky self', *Social Science and Medicine* 40(3): 409–15.

Penney, D. and Chandler, T. (2000) 'Physical education: what futures?', *Sport, Education and Society* 5(1): 71–89.

Petersen, A. (1997) 'Risk, governance and the new public health', in A. Petersen and R. Bunton (eds) *Foucault, Health and Medicine*, London: Routledge, pp. 189–207.

Petersen, A. and Bunton, R. (eds) (1997) *Foucault, Health and Medicine*, London: Routledge.

Pronger, B. (2002) *Body Fascism. Salvation in the Technology of Physical Fitness*, London, Ontario: University of Toronto.

Ritzer, G. (2000) *The Macdonaldisation of Society*, New Century Edition, Thousand Oaks, CA: Pine Forge Press.

Ronholt, H. (2002) '"It's only for sissies . . . " Analysis of teaching and learning processes in physical education: a contribution to the hidden curriculum", *Sport, Education and Society* 7(1): 25–37.

Sadovnik, A. (1995) 'Basil Bernstein's theory of pedagogic practice: a structuralist approach', in A.R. Sadovnik (ed.) *Knowledge and Pedagogy. The Sociology of Basil Bernstein*, Norwood, New Jersey: Ablex Publishing Co.

Shilling, C. (1993a) 'The body, class and social inequalities', in J. Evans (1993) *Equality, Education and Physical Education*, Lewes: Falmer Press.

Shilling, C. (1993b) *The Body and Social Theory*, London: Sage.

Skelton, A. (1997) 'Studying hidden curricula: developing a perspective in the light of post modern insights', *Curriculum Studies* 5(2): 177–95.

Tinning, R. (1997) 'Performance and participation discourses in human movement: towards a socially critical physical education', in J.-M. Fernandz-Balboa (ed.) *Critical Postmodernism in Human Movement, Physical Education and Sport*, New York: SUNY, pp. 99–121.

Tinning, R. and Glasby, T. (2002) 'Pedagogical work and the "cult of the body". Considering the role of HPE in the context of the "new public health"', *Sport, Education and Society* 7(7): 109–21.

Turner, B. (1984) *The Body and Society. Explorations in Social Theory*, Oxford: Blackwell.

Turner, B.S. (1997) 'Foreword: from governmentality to risk, some reflections on Foucault's contribution to medical sociology', in A. Peterson and R. Bunton (eds) *Foucault, Health and Medicine*, London: Routledge, pp. ix–xxviii.

Turner, B. (2002) 'Risk society and medical technologies: towards a critical overview of Cartesian medicine', http://central.com.au/artmed/papers/turner2.html

Tyler, D. (1997) 'Foucault and the medicalisation critique', in A. Petersen and R. Bunton (eds) *Foucault, Health and Medicine*, London: Routledge, pp. 94–113.

Wright, J. (2000) 'Bodies, meanings and movements: a comparison of the language of a physical education lesson and a Feldenkrais movement class', *Sport, Education and Society* 5(1): 35–51.

4 Towards a critical history of the body, identity and health

Corporeal power and school practice

David Kirk

Introduction

The social construction of bodies has in the past two decades emerged as a topic of increasing significance in social research. This scholarly interest in the body has covered a wide and diverse range of topics and has now generated a sufficiently large literature to warrant the publication of review articles and introductory textbooks (Cranny-Francis 1995). Along with Franks (1990) we might argue about the most adequate ways in which to discuss bringing society into the body and the body into society. At the same time, there appears to be an increasingly widespread understanding of the notion that the body is as much a social as it is a biological phenomenon, existing simultaneously in culture and nature.

This new work on the body in society has already demonstrated a potential to liberate our thinking from the tyranny of Cartesian dualism (Fitzclarence 1990; Grosz 1994) and in so doing to offer persuasive arguments that the body is integral to understanding the development and constitution of society (Shilling 1993). There has, however, been a tendency for writers to remain silent on the question of the part schools and other educational institutions play in socially constructing bodies, some exceptions being Corrigan (1988), Evans (1988), Connell (1989) and Shilling (1991). This silence is particularly notable in relation to such activities in schools as sport, physical education, dance and manual arts, where one might have imagined there would be ample opportunity to observe such processes at work in starkly explicit forms (Gard 2001; Kirk 2003). Indeed, there is a considerable and long-standing stock of knowledge on how organised forms of physical activity might contribute to the better physiological, biomechanical and neurological functioning of children. Even though educational researchers have investigated how children's participation in organised physical activities contributes to inequities within the gender order (Wright 1997) and various forms of social disadvantage (Evans 1993), the body has sometimes been overlooked in these investigations.

Shilling (1991) is one sociologist who has explored these links between the social construction of the body and educational practices. He does so by drawing substantially on Bourdieu's notion of 'the habitus', which Shilling claims is located within the body, every gesture and physical act betraying an individual's class-dependent social location and orientation to the world. Shilling has shown how the body and the bodily or physical capital invested in it play key roles in the production of social inequalities and how school physical education and sport contribute significantly to this process. Pointing out the class and gender dimensions of these inequalities, he suggests that while physical capital can be turned to economic and social gain, social class location delimits the range of opportunities available for such conversion. Thinking of activities such as rugby union, polo and lacrosse, Shilling claims that 'children from (the dominant) classes tend to engage in socially elite sporting activities which stress manners and deportment and hence facilitate the future acquisition of social and cultural capital' (Shilling 1991: 656).

Indeed, in his comprehensive overview of a range of sociological writing dealing with the body, Shilling (1993: 129) argues that the social construction of bodies needs to be located within particular social locations, within the habitus, and through the development of taste. He argues that, for growing numbers of people from particular social class, age and ethnic groups, the body has, since the early 1990s, emerged as an individual project underpinned by two propositions. The first is the widespread and commonplace acceptance of the idea that the body is malleable, a view supported by growing knowledge and technical expertise of means of intervening in and substantially altering the shape and look of bodies. The second is a growing awareness of the body as an unfinished project that can be pursued to some kind of resolution according to the lifestyle choices people make. Shilling argues that contemporary preoccupations with the body as a project are set apart from various treatments of the body in pre-modern societies by the conflation of physical appearance and self-identity, wherein the body is the flesh-and-blood manifestation of social and, more recently, individual identity.

At the same time, a problem with much of this work is that it has tended, in the main, to lack a historical perspective, with some notable exceptions (e.g. Foucault 1977; Turner 1992; Dutton 1995). One of the consequences of this becomes all too apparent when we consider Lowenthal's (1985: 4) claim in *The Past is a Foreign Country* that 'nostalgia is today the universal catchword for looking back'. According to Lowenthal, lack of detailed attention to historical evidence allows pasts to be manufactured so that they can be enjoyed nostalgically. Not only does this process construct pasts that are often used to legitimate oppressive practices in the present, it also obscures the relationships between past, present and future by asserting that the past is a foreign place that can only be comprehended dimly, a place somehow richer yet simpler and better than the present.

Gough (1986: 2), following the work of Slaughter on futures research, has advocated a form of curriculum research that develops a relational analysis of past, present and future. He argues that history and futures study are important because they help us to avoid 'the temptation of withdrawing into the narrow confines of an attenuated and bounded present . . . and looking to past and future as an escape from the present'. Musgrave (1988) argued that growing interest in curriculum history since the late 1980s has been marked by a shift in motivations from a need to simply understand the past to a desire to participate more effectively in complex practical situations in the present. This practical use of history immediately signals its intersection with political processes, with an incorporation of various forms of social theory and with the real-life hopes and aspirations of educational workers.

This chapter proposes that it is not possible to grasp the process of socially constructing the body through school and related practices without the development of a critical history of the relationships between school practices and broader public discourses concerned with, among other things, corporeal power. Drawing on three specific historical examples in Australian schools between the 1880s and the present, I argue (elaborating an argument of Foucault 1980 that is more fully developed in Kirk 1998) that school practices have been part of broader practices of corporeal power which, since the mid to late 1800s, have become increasingly diffused, individualised and internalised in Australian and other similar Western societies. In order to understand the forms physical education, school sport and health education have taken in particular places at specific times, I suggest it is important to understand the prevailing forms of public discourse in which they were embedded.

On the basis of a critical, relational history of school practices and public discourses, I will argue that the school in contemporary Australia and perhaps in other Western nations is currently struggling to maintain its original, modernist institutional form. This form had as its goal the production of compliant and productive bodies. To illustrate the potential of a critical, relational history of the role of school practices in the production of the body in society, I will argue that the emergence of forms of physical activity in Australian schools since the early 1900s is closely associated with the construction of the docile body within modernity (Giddens 1990). This development was informed by the notion that the body was disciplined and energised through mass educational, medical and other interventions to be economically productive and politically acquiescent. Moreover, it was informed by the idea that the body is the most intimate manifestation of social and self-identity. I will then suggest that since the end of the Second World War there has been a shift in forms of corporeal regulation and normalisation to a looser form of power over the body, moving towards the dissemination, individualisation and internalisation of corporeal power. I will propose that contemporary configurations of bodily knowledge in schools in an era Giddens (1990) among others has labelled 'high modernity' are increasingly at risk of being discontinuous and contradictory in relation to trends in the practice of corporeal power beyond schools. The chapter concludes with some brief considerations of these discontinuous and contradictory practices for the production of young people's embodied identities.

Schooling the docile body: heavy, ponderous, meticulous and constant power

The emergence of various systems of rational gymnastics towards the end of the eighteenth century (Munrow 1955) and their eventual widespread adoption by a number of institutions, such as schools and the military, by the end of the nineteenth century, was a constituent part of the development of a range of regulative and normative practices aimed at schooling the docile body. As Foucault (1977) observed, docility did not imply subjugation of the body, since economic productivity was partnered with the effective use of the labour of compliant and healthy citizens. On the contrary, in Foucault's terms, the 'little practices' of schooling the body were meant to achieve the twin aims of 'docility-utility', without the need for the exercise of raw power through routine violent punishment (Kirk 1998).

From their first appearance in the mid 1800s, physical activities in Australian schools can be viewed as practices of corporeal regulation and normalisation that were integral to the emergence and operation of at least two institutions of modernity, surveillance (or 'the control of information and social supervision') and capitalism (or 'capital accumulation in the context of competitive labour and product markets') (Giddens 1990: 59). As Turner (1984: 161) has argued, following Foucault, from the early 1800s 'capital could profit from the accumulation of men and the enlargement of markets only when the health and docility of the population had been made possible by a network of regulations and controls'. This entanglement of corporeal regulation and normalisation with surveillance and capitalism was part of a process of reifying and constructing the modern body which had been in train since the Renaissance, through which the body was increasingly identified with personhood (Broekhoff 1972). Physical appearance was conflated with self-worth or value (Finkelstein 1991), initially defined as the classed, raced and gendered (or socially positioned) self, and later (and additionally) as the self-as-individual. By the end of the nineteenth century, we can see these notions being worked through in a range of mass corporeal regulative and normative practices described by Foucault (1977), constituting prisons, schools, factories and barracks. It is here, within this nexus of practices, that early forms of bodily practices in Australian schools can be located, particularly drilling and exercising, school medical inspection, and competitive team games. All were sites within schools of surveillance of bodies as they were shaped to meet particular social and economic ends.

The emergence of drilling and exercising, school medical inspection and competitive teams games in Australian schools exemplify in relatively highly codified forms the notion that the body is not a 'natural' phenomenon, despite the hegemony of medical and biological science. Instead, it reveals that the body is also in culture and can be normalised and regulated to suit particular social class, economic and cultural purposes. By the end of the nineteenth century in Australia and elsewhere, the use of forms of physical activity for the purposes of shaping the docile body within the context of a particular habitus was explicitly prescribed in the official discourse of educational policy-makers, manual-writers and head teachers of elite schools. There followed a period of consolidation of these school practices during the first three decades of the twentieth century, through the institutionalisation of a drilling and exercising form of physical training in government schools, of school medical inspection and of games-playing in private and government schools.

The body-shaping which took place during this period had two key features. The first of these was that children were usually treated in the mass rather than as individuals. The second was that these practices of corporeal regulation and normalisation relied in the main on securing children's compliant participation through the enforcement by teachers and other adults of precise and meticulous prescriptions and measurements detailed in texts and manuals, in the cases of drilling and exercising and medical inspection, or in the case of games-playing, through the strict application of an unwritten but all pervasive code of gentlemanly conduct.

Drilling and exercising as a codification of corporeal power

An example of the codification of ponderous and meticulous corporeal power aimed at schooling the docile body is the system of physical training in operation in Australian schools between 1911 and 1931. Physical training at this time was under the auspices of the Commonwealth Department of Defence, in association with the Junior Cadet Training Scheme (Kirk 1998). Only 12 to 14 year-old male pupils were eligible to become junior cadets. Nonetheless, Defence Department instructors ran courses for teachers based on the Junior Cadet Manual, published in 1916 by the Australian Military Forces, and in so doing, had a more or less direct influence on the physical training of girls and younger boys. Lessons in the Junior Cadet Manual drew on the Swedish system of gymnastics and were scripted in the form of tables that dealt, in a systematic way, with the major joints and muscle groups of the body. The tables themselves were organised in an immutable sequence according to the age and experience of the pupils. This amounted to an entire physical training programme with progressions, sequencing and age standards mapped out in detail.

Lessons were set out in a format that also had to be adhered to strictly. There were eight categories of activities and each lesson was constructed on the basis of a selection of exercises from each category. The categories were, in order of appearance in the lesson: (1) introduction and breathing exercises; (2) trunk-bending back and forward; (3) arm-bending and stretching; (4) balance exercises; (5) shoulder-blade exercises (abdominal exercises); (6) trunk-turning and bending sideways; (7) marching, running, jumping, games, etc.; and (8) breathing exercises. Teachers were required to memorise the precise series of exercises for each lesson, and to deliver their instructions using such commands as 'head backwards – bend', 'left foot sideways – place', 'trunk forward and downward – stretch' and 'knees – bend'. These commands were amended to 'suit Australian conditions' in 1922 and again in 1926 but the militaristic flavour persisted (Department of Defence 1922).

This same formula was still in use in the 1930s, even after the Defence Department had retired from the scene, and on into the 1940s. Correctness of performance was the overriding principle in this approach. Rosalie Virtue, the Victorian Education Department's Organiser of Physical Training between 1915 and 1938, advised teachers that 'correct starting positions and the correct performance of exercises are essential' and that '"quickeners" should be put in to keep the children mentally alert' (Education Department of Victoria 1922: 5).

'Teach only one new exercise each day', she stressed, since 'this allows repetition to obtain correctness of performance, a gradual change of table, and more work done by children.'

The scheme embodied in the various physical training manuals was, effectively, the first and last national programme of physical activity in Australian schools, though its implementation was dogged by problems from the start. The First World War caused massive disruptions due to the posting of servicemen overseas. These disruptions encouraged criticism from commentators who, as early as 1917, were referring to drill as 'a monotonous duty' (Kirk 1998: 73). They suggested that this formula for teaching physical training lessons was more likely to cause resentment rather than foster willing compliance. This was because it relied entirely on the teachers' strict adherence to the prescriptions of the manual and left no room for initiative or expression on the part of either pupils or teachers. For two years in the early 1920s the scheme was abandoned temporarily, only to be resurrected on a reduced scale following vehement protests from the state governments. While the state education departments resented the involvement of the military in their schools, the attraction of a scheme of physical training funded by the Commonwealth that, ostensibly, benefited not only junior cadets but all children, outweighed their concerns. The Department of Defence was finally forced to withdraw its services in 1931, again under protest from the states, when the scheme was suspended in 1929 by the Scullin Labour government in a climate of deepening economic and social crises.

This rather chequered career between 1911 and 1931 meant that implementation of this drilling and exercising form of physical training was uneven across the country and can hardly have been wholly effective. Nevertheless, these pedagogical practices in schools, appearing as they did at a time when questions of national and racial identity had a potent influence on public and professional discourses, reveal highly codified and institutionalised attempts to normalise and regulate children's bodies, docile bodies that were both compliant and productive. Regardless of the actual effectiveness of drilling and exercising, its sociological significance lies in its use as a strategy of corporeal power, focusing in this case specifically on the construction of acquiescent and productive working-class bodies. Linked to school medical inspection, which was inaugurated between 1900 and 1910 in most states and which sought to map and measure an entire range of physical 'defects' among pupils (Kirk and Twigg 1994), drilling and exercising focused in a ponderous and meticulous fashion on the movements of children's bodies in space and time. This form of physical training was a codification of corporeal power through its precise definitions of physically appropriate and inappropriate activity. It shaped how and where the body might move and the range of outcomes physical activities might produce. The body constructed and constitutued by this regime of physical training linked to medical inspection was intended to be compliant but productive, a body suited to the emergence of high modernity.

The invention of physical education: the emergence of a looser form of power over the body

The 1940s marked a change in this process of corporeal regulation and normal-isation within schools, with a gradual shift from treatment of children's bodies in the mass to a greater concern for individual bodies. The new regime was also less regimented and there was little strictly prescribed movement. The reformist agenda of inspection and intervention proposed by school medical officers in the pre-First World War period, informed largely by a philosophy of positive eugenics, was watered down somewhat during the 1920s in the aftermath of the war as radical eugenicists advocated drastic solutions to the problems of feeblemindedness and other forms of 'abnormality'. Even so, the same strategies of medical inspection and the identification of 'defectives' continued to be employed well into the late 1930s (Kirk 1998).

After this point, in the early 1940s, medical inspection's link to physical activity programmes in schools was loosened by the relocation of the school medical services from state education to health departments (Kirk 1999a). This devel-opment reflected broader changes in the ways in which bodies were treated within government schools, with the emergence in the late 1930s of a new form of physical education as a comprehensive programme of physical activities that had competitive team games at its core (Kirk and Twigg 1995).

Following its successful passage through Parliament in 1941, the National Fitness Act was instrumental in establishing three-year diploma courses for specialist physical education teachers in most of Australia's universities, a devel-opment which heralded the emergence of a home-grown physical education profession. It was also during this period that a definition of 'physical education' began to be constructed out of a cluster of disparate physical activities. By 1929 in Victoria, the Minister of Education in his annual report was suggesting that physical education 'includes not merely formal physical exercises, but swimming, organised games, rhythmic exercises, folk dancing, practical hygiene, and remedial exercises based on the medical assessment of the needs of each child' (Victorian Parliamentary Papers 1929: 8).

This notion, that the term 'physical education' might embrace this com-prehensive range of activities, was new at this time and not widely accepted nor understood in the education community. There was, for instance, no timetabled subject called physical education in schools beyond drilling and exercising lessons. It was competitive team games that were to exert the greatest influence over the new notion of physical education as a comprehensive programme of physical activities for schools. Games were already well established in government schools by the late 1920s, with State Schools Amateur Athletic Associations being formed around 1906 in Victoria and New South Wales to organise inter-school and inter-State matches (Kirk and Twigg 1995). Only the major team games were played, plus athletics and competitions in swimming, and these activities were extra-curricular. There was no instruction in games-playing within curriculum time, though there was certainly some coaching by teachers of teams that competed in inter-school matches. By all accounts, competition was taken very seriously and, significantly, was continually justified by appeals to what Mangan (1986) has described as the 'games ethic'. Children in the schools serving Australia's social elites had been participating in organised sport competitions with each other since at least the 1880s, and this practice was embedded in versions of the English public schools games ethic. In the context of these elite schools in England, game-playing was integral to the construction of Christian manliness and to fostering leadership, and was in itself a form of corporeal normalisation and regulation suited to the particular habitus of the middle classes (Sherington 1983). This ethic was adopted with only minor modifications in elite schools for girls (Crawford 1984).

Crawford (1981) argued that, over time, the bourgeois English version of the games ethic was reconstructed in the antipodes to provide a distinctively Australian flavour. This reconstruction of the games ethic in Australia's elite schools may have reflected, as Crawford has claimed, some indigenous qualities of Australian middle-class manhood. At the same time, game-playing as a form of leadership education was not a key concern in the education of the working classes, though it may have been viewed as a means of moral improvement and of civilising the working-class body. Notions of manliness were prominent in early justifications of games for boys in government schools. According to Crawford, following the carnage of the First World War, there was a pronounced emphasis on physical development through games and other physical activities in an attempt to repair 'the national physique'. Later, through the 1920s, we find greater attention being paid to values such as cooperation, courage and playing for the sake of the team, as much as means of counteracting undesirable behaviour, like cheating, than as positive virtues in themselves. Later still, in the 1930s and 1940s, under the influence of the progressive movement in primary school education and, perhaps, in more conscious consideration of girls, in addition to boys, concepts such as self-confidence, enjoyment and play begin to be added to the list of positive qualities that games were claimed to foster (Kirk and Twigg 1995).

This reconstruction of the games ethic for use in government schools can be seen in an important series of articles that appeared in a 1941 issue of the Victorian *Education Gazette* (Education Department of Victoria 1941). The articles addressed the problem of the 'cult of athleticism' that had plagued sports contests between the elite schools, involving boisterous and sometimes violent behaviour among players and spectators alike. In similar fashion, excessive zeal and ferocious competition were not uncommon in sports contests between government schools. It was advocated, in contrast, that games are the means by which every child can be given an interest in physical activity. Children should be taught to gain satisfaction from seeing their own improvement in performance and not necessarily from competing.

Appeals of this sort to the higher qualities to be developed through games-playing were commonplace in official government policy statements throughout the 1920s and 1930s. However, the notion that games could benefit the majority of children, not merely the socially privileged or physically talented, added a new twist that ran counter to some of the earlier elitist connotations of the games ethic.

By the end of the Second World War, this view of games-playing was the generative force behind a definition of physical education as a comprehensive programme of educational physical activities, and sport, in the form of major team games, was firmly lodged at the heart of this notion of physical education.

In 1946, a textbook for physical education prepared for use in Victorian schools, known as 'the Grey Book', crystallised this new concept of physical education (Education Department of Victoria 1946). In the foreword to this new Victorian textbook, comprehensive physical education was contrasted with the drilling and exercising form of physical training the Grey Book sought to displace, arguing that 'formal exercises are artificial, unrelated to life situations, and generally lacking in interest; they also completely ignore the very important influence that the emotions exert on the physical well-being of the individual' (ibid.: vi). The writer of this foreword went on to map out the key dimensions of this definition of physical education that continue to have currency today. 'Enjoyment and enthusiasm' were recognised as of central importance to the beneficial effects of participation in physical activity, in contrast to the formality of the former regime of drilling and exercising.

The influence of the progressive, child-centred movement in primary education is also strongly in evidence. Adopting the notion that play is a natural activity for children, the writers of the Grey Book commented 'every child has the right to play, and this right must be restored to all children who have lost it' (ibid.: vii). In a significant conceptual leap, the writers went on to equate 'play', within this new notion of physical education, with playing competitive team games, and, in one stroke, conflated the key elements of the middle-class games ethic with an educational progressivist notion of play, through the idea that all children in government schools had the right to participate in competitive team games. This continues to be a significant conjoining of concepts underpinning contemporary physical education programmes in Australia, since it positioned sport as pivotal to the educational legitimation of physical education. Few other conceptualisations have the symbolic power of this particular discursive configuration (Kirk 1998).

One other relationship remained to be constructed at this time. This was the nexus between the specialist physical education teacher's role in timetabled lessons and competitive sport in schools. With growing numbers of specialist advisers in the primary school sector and specialist physical education teachers in the secondary schools in the 1940s–1960s, it was now possible to provide instruction for all children in the skills considered to be prerequisite to games-playing. The specialists took on this role with considerable enthusiasm. In so doing, physical education had to be conceptualised as the base of a pyramidal structure that had elite sport competition at the top. The majority of children participated in school physical education, while only a few talented individuals survived to reach the pinnacle of the pyramid (Evans 1990). Physical education lessons provided the so-called fundamental motor skills of running, throwing, jumping, kicking and so on, and these were then applied within an ascending scale of competitive contexts in inter-school, inter-district, inter-state and international sport.

Contemporary physical education: a looser form of power?

The invention of physical education as a comprehensive programme of physical activities, which brought to the fore sport-related skills and formed the foundation for competitive sport, and its implementation in schools after the Second World War, was part of a liberalising movement in primary school education. From the earliest forms of physical activities in schools in the late 1800s to the arrival of comprehensive physical education in the 1940s, we can see marked contrasts in the ways in which anticipated outcomes were expressed. For instance, the Victorian Inspectors of Drill argued in 1889 that 'with a compulsory system of drill, incipient larrikinism would receive a severe check, and the military spirit of the colony would be greatly fostered' (Victorian Parliamentary Papers 1890: 264), while some sixty years later the writer of the foreword to the Grey Book stressed the right of all children to play alongside their enjoyment and well-being. The shift in corporeal power signalled by these changes was further elaborated in school programmes over a forty-year period between the 1940s and the 1970s. The emphasis changed from treating the mass of bodies to the individual body, evidenced in new teaching methods of individualised skill and fitness development, and from external prescription and enforcement to internal motivation to participate, evidenced in the concern for children's enjoyment of physical activities and the development of positive attitudes and lifelong participation.

Notwithstanding this shift, the institutional imperatives of schooling continued to demand that children be taught the same material in age-graded classes, delimiting the implementation of individualised approaches to students' learning that the liberation from drilling and exercising seemed to herald. While there may have developed a looser form of power over bodies in physical education and sport lessons in the post-Second World War period, schooling continued to award teachers the key role of ensuring children's participation. Indeed, in many secondary schools, physical educators continued to be perceived within the wider school community as enforcers of discipline through semi-regimented, command style teaching methods (Woods 1979). Feminist scholars have been critical of the perceived links between sport-based physical education and male violence (e.g. Kenway and Fitzclarence 1997; Waite 1985). Moreover, as team games increasingly became the dominant feature of school physical education programmes, the individualism of liberal progressivism coexisted in uneasy tension with the need for sublimation of individual needs to the needs of the group or, in this case, the team.

Contemporary physical education and sport in schools has only recently been forced to come to terms with this legacy of corporeal normalisation and regulation brought about mainly by an acceleration of interest during the 1970s, 1980s and 1990s in what Featherstone (1982) called 'body management' within the population at large. Current treatment of the body in schools continues to frame the mass practices of developing sport skills and physical fitness within a liberal humanist philosophy of enjoyment, choice and lifelong participation. In the last decade we have witnessed the widespread adoption by physical educators of notions such as active lifestyle as key goals of their programmes, mirroring developments in popular physical culture more broadly.

While the pedagogy and organisation of school programmes differ little from the practices of the immediate post-war period in terms of treating children's bodies in uniform ways, the range of activities now available in schools has broadened considerably. Students in many secondary schools have greater choice of activity than ever before. These developments, as logical elaborations of the discourse of comprehensive physical education, are clearly less prescriptive and meticulous in their treatment of children's bodies in time and space than their forerunner, drilling and exercising. They seem to represent a looser form of power over the body, even though their operation is circumscribed by, and sometimes contributes to, the institutional priorities of schooling.

New times in the 1980s and 1990s brought shifts in popular physical culture that have scarcely been acknowledged by school physical education, while the broad, institutional practices of schools have remained rooted in the corporeal logic of the 1950s (Kirk 1999b). New regulative and normative practices associated with the representation and management of the body brought into question the continuing cultural relevance of these school practices. These cultural practices take the malleability of the body and the conflation of the body with self-identity well beyond the means available to physical education and sport. The acceleration of interest in body management as an unfinished project predicated on lifestyle choices has diffused, internalised and individualised corporeal power much more fully and profoundly than physical education in schools.

For example, since at least the mid to late 1980s, there has been an increasing visibility of the body in popular cultural forms such as the television advertisement, revealing the extent to which the body itself has become a commodity (Fitzclarence 1990). Media sport, as a hybrid of live sports contests and television, has greatly added to the length of time bodies confront the viewer and voyeur. It is significant that body shape is often the pivotal point of focus in contemporary corporeal discourse since it is visual media, in both its televisual and popular magazine forms, which have been the main conduits for transmission of images and representations of the body. The 'normal' body for many women in Australia and elsewhere in the West is now much more slender than it was in the 1950s. Moreover, the conjunction of representations of bodies with the consumption of products (through advertising) has created desire for corporeal normality and a consequent willingness to submit to self-imposed regulatory regimes such as dieting and exercising.

In this regard, Susan Bordo (1990: 85) has argued that slenderness is the dominant, desired body shape in contemporary Western cultures, particularly among women. Signalling the gradual internalisation of surveillance, she suggests that the slender body is a manifestation of normalising strategies which ensure 'the production of self-monitoring and self-disciplining "docile bodies", sensitive to any departure from social norms, and habituated to self-improvement and transformation in the service of these norms'. However, the looser form of power mentioned by Foucault (1980) does not necessarily mean greater freedom for individuals, according to Bordo. Since the quest for slenderness marks an internalisation of the process of social regulation, Bordo is interested in representations of the slender body as analogous to the social body and a symbol of power and power relations, especially among and between men and women. She suggests that,

> the 'correct' management of desire in (consumer) culture, requiring as it does a contradictory 'double-bind' construction of personality, inevitably produces an unstable bulimic personality-type as its norm, along with the contrasting extremes of obesity and self-starvation. These symbolize the contradictions of the 'social body' – contradictions which make self-management a continual and virtually impossible task.
>
> (Bordo 1990: 88)

In high modernity (Giddens 1990), these contradictions appear to be taking the form of a crisis as the body as a project begins to confront the limits of malleability (Shilling 1993). This project of body management is being played out to the point where biological and genetic factors, as well as the ultimate fate of the death of the body, have brought into sharp focus some of the limitations and dangers of the modernist conflation of the body with self-identity. The excesses of the cults of slenderness (Tinning 1985) and appearance (Lasch 1991) discussed by Bordo are hyper-real examples of the playing out of the project of body management, resulting in the increased incidence of eating disorders, over-exercising, and the widespread prevalence of anxiety about body shape (Kissling 1991; Koval 1986).

These corporeal dimensions of high modernity are, in certain respects, merely a working out of practices constituting and constructing the malleable, modernist body. They also conflate the conforming and productive body with social identity, though in high modernity the body and self-identity are increasingly conflated also (Giddens 1991). School physical education and sport may be in crisis, at least in part because they represent a series of modernist bodily practices concerned with normalising and regulating children's bodies through methods and strategies which are perhaps already culturally obsolete. Some researchers argue that a significant number of adolescents are preoccupied with physical activity as recreative sport and entertainment, but at the same time disapprove of their physical education and sport experiences in schools (e.g. Tinning and Fitzclarence 1992). This is hardly surprising given the hyper-real representations of sporting bodies through media sport and, in particular, the collages of sporting action that have become a regular feature of mainstream commercial television sports shows and on satellite television beamed into public places, described by Bradbury (1993) as the pornography of sport. These images present an objectified performing body that is a seductive counter-example for young people to the mundane, abstracted and routinised bodily practices of school physical education and sport lessons.

Conclusion

The apparent disjunction between corporeal practices in schools and those in other social sites, such as media sport and exercise gymnasia, points to a lack of uniformity in the development and diffusion of corporeal power. This unevenness presents particular difficulties for theorising about the body in society. The example presented here of the cultural lag between physical education and sport programmes in schools and recent developments in popular physical culture suggests the existence of countervailing trends in the operation of corporeal regulation and normalisation. Given Shilling's sensible observation that social location, the habitus, and the development of taste each play a part in the particular ways in which bodies are socially constructed and constituted, carefully contextualised historically informed studies of embodiment in a range of social settings might provide useful perspectives on practices of corporeal regulation and normalisation and the elaboration and diffusion of corporeal power.

The possibility that there are definite limits to the extent to which bodies might be shaped biologically and culturally offers some perspective on the question of the continuing cultural relevance of school physical education and sport programmes. Use of critical history as a key dimension of relational analysis suggests that perhaps only radical alteration to the institution of schooling might permit physical education practices to articulate more coherently with corporeal practices in other sites. Alternatively, school physical education and sport might continue a decline, to be replaced by individualised programmes of physical activity run by private companies that children participate in only if they can afford to pay. Given the high commercial stakes of media sport and the emergence from Australian tertiary institutions of increasing numbers of sport and exercise scientists in place of physical education teachers, this commodification of school programmes coupled with the commodification of bodies may arrest the decline of physical activity programmes in schools. It is open to question whether these new institutional practices will continue to be enmeshed in the modernist institutions of surveillance and capitalism, and whether the looser form of power they might embody will be individually and socially productive means of corporeal normalisation and regulation.

Through the use of a critical history we can understand the process of schooling bodies to be layered, complex, contradictory and contested. A necessary constituent of the process of schooling bodies is both their empowerment and their regulation. Following the work of Foucault in particular, we can mention empowerment in the sense that practices such as physical education provide opportunities for young people to develop and realise particular movement capacities of their bodies. We can speak of regulation in the sense that the development of some forms of movement expertise inevitably delimits other movement capacities young people might develop. By bringing school practices under detailed examination through critical, relational history, one might begin to address such policy dilemmas. One can seek out the connections between these school practices and other related practices within the wider public domain, take seriously the effects of these practices on young people, and rethink the means by which teachers, policy-makers and the general public are educated about the whole range of consequences of school practices, in particular those physical practices that have been by and large ignored or marginalised in sociological studies of the body and education.

References

Bordo, S. (1990) 'Reading the slender body', in M. Jacobus, E. Fox-Kellner and S. Shuttleworth (eds) *Body/Politics: Women and the Discourse of Science*, New York: Routledge.

Bradbury, M. (1993) 'The pornography of sport', *The Age*, 10 July: 6.

Broekhoff, J. (1972) 'Physical education and the reification of the human body', *Gymnasion* 9: 4–11.

Connell, R.W. (1989) 'Cool guys, swots and wimps: the interplay of masculinity and education', *The Oxford Review of Education* 15(3): 291–303.

Corrigan, R. (1988) 'The making of the boy: meditations on what Grammar School did with, to, and for my body', *Journal of Education* 170: 142–61.

Cranny-Francis, A. (1995) *The Body as Text*, Carlton: Melbourne University Press.

Crawford, R. (1981) 'A history of physical education in Victoria and NSW 1872–1939: with particular reference to English precedent', unpublished Ph.D. thesis, La Trobe University.

Crawford, R. (1984) 'Sport for young ladies: the Victorian independent schools, 1875–1925', *Sporting Traditions: Journal of the Australian Society for Sport History* 1: 61–82.

Department of Defence (1922) *The Junior Cadet Training Textbook*, Melbourne: Government Printer.

Dutton, K. (1995) *The Perfectible Body: The Western Ideal of Physical Development*, London: Cassell.

Education Department of Victoria (1922) *Education Gazette and Teachers' Aid*, January, Melbourne: Government Printer.

Education Department of Victoria (1941) *Education Gazette and Teachers' Aid*, July, Melbourne: Government Printer.

Education Department of Victoria (1946) *Physical Education for Victorian Schools* Melbourne: Government Printer.

Evans, J. (1988) 'Body matters: towards a socialist physical education', in H. Lauder and P. Brown (eds) *Education in Search of a Future*, Lewes: Falmer Press.

Evans, J. (1993) (ed.) *Equality, Education and Physical Education*, Lewes: Falmer Press.

Evans, J. (1990) *Sport in Schools*, Geelong: Deakin University Press.

Featherstone, M. (1982) 'The body in consumer culture', *Theory, Culture and Society* 1: 18–33.

Finkelstein, J. (1991) *The Fashioned Self*, Cambridge: Polity Press.

Fitzclarence, L. (1990) 'The body as commodity', in D. Rowe and G. Lawrence (eds) *Sport and Leisure: Trends in Australian Popular Culture*, Sydney: Harcourt Brace Jovanovich.

Foucault, M. (1977) *Discipline and Punish: The Birth of the Prison*, London: Allen and Unwin.

Foucault, M. (1980) *Power/Knowledge: Selected Interviews and Other Writings*, Brighton: Harvester.

Franks, A. (1990) 'Bringing bodies back in: a decade review', *Theory, Culture and Society* 7: 131–62.

Gard, M. (2001) 'Dancing around the "problem" of boys and dance', *Discourse: Studies in the Cultural Politics of Education* 22: 213–25.

Giddens, A. (1990) *The Consequences of Modernity*, Oxford: Polity Press.

Giddens, A. (1991) *Modernity and Self-Identity: Self and Society in the Late Modern Age*, Cambridge: Polity Press.

Gough, N. (1986) 'Curriculum inquiry: questions from futures study', paper presented to the Annual Conference of the Australian Association for Research in Education, University of Melbourne, November.

Grosz, E. (1994) *Volatile Bodies: Towards a Corporeal Feminism*, Sydney: Allen and Unwin

Kenway, J. and Fitzclarence, L. (1997) 'Masculinity, violence and schooling: challenging "poisonous pedagogies"', *Gender and Education* 9: 117–34.

Kirk, D. (1998) *Schooling Bodies: School Practice and Public Discourse 1880–1950*, London: Leicester University Press.

Kirk, D. (1999a) 'Health, the body and the medicalisation of the school', in C. Symes and D. Meadmore (eds) *The Extra-Ordinary School: Parergonality and Pedagogy*, New York: Peter Lang.

Kirk, D. (1999b) 'Embodying the school/ schooling bodies: physical education as disciplinary technology', in C. Symes and D. Meadmore (eds) *The Extra-Ordinary School: Parergonality and Pedagogy*, New York: Peter Lang.

Kirk, D. (2003) 'Beyond the academic curriculum: the production and operation of biopower in the less studied sites of schooling', in B. Baker and K. Heyning (eds) *Dangerous Coagulations? The Uses of Foucault in the Study of Education*, New York: Peter Lang.

Kirk, D. and Twigg, K. (1994) 'Regulating the Australian body: eugenics, anthropometrics and school medical inspection in Victoria, 1909–1915', *History of Education Review* 23: 19–37.

Kirk, D. and Twigg, K. (1995) 'Civilising Australian bodies: the games ethic and sport in Australian government schools, 1904–1945, *Sporting Traditions: Journal of the Australian Society for Sport History* 11: 3–34.

Kissling, E. (1991) 'One size does not fit all, or how I learned to stop dieting and love the body', *Quest* 43: 135–48.

Koval, R. (1986) *Eating Your Heart Out*, New York: Penguin.

Lasch, C. (1991) *The Culture of Narcissism*, New York: Norton.

Lowenthal, D. (1985) *The Past is a Foreign Country*, Cambridge: Cambridge University Press.

Mangan, J.A. (1986) *The Games Ethic and Imperialism: Aspects of the Diffusion of an Educational Ideal*, Harmondsworth: Viking.

Munrow, A.D. (1955) *Pure and Applied Gymnastics*, London: Arnold.

Musgrave, P.W. (1988) 'Curriculum history: past, present and future', *History of Education Review* 17: 1–13.

Sherington, G. (1983) 'Athleticism in the antipodes: the AAGPS of New South Wales', *History of Education Review* 12: 16–28.

Shilling, C. (1991) 'Educating the body: physical capital and the production of social inequalities', *Sociology* 25: 653–72.

Shilling, C. (1993) *The Body and Social Theory*, London: Sage.

Tinning, R. (1985) 'Physical education and the cult of slenderness: a critique', *ACHPER National Journal*, 107: 10–14.

Tinning, R. and Fitzclarence, L. (1992) 'Postmodern youth culture and the crisis in Australian secondary school physical education', *Quest* 44: 287–304.

Turner, B.S. (1984) *The Body and Society: Explorations in Social Theory*, Oxford: Blackwell.

Turner, B.S. (1992) *Regulating Bodies: Essays in Medical Sociology*, London: Routledge.

Victorian Parliamentary Papers (1890) *Reports of the Minister of Public Instruction, 1889–90*, Vol. 95, December, Melbourne: Government Printer.

Victorian Parliamentary Papers (1929) *Reports of the Minister of Public Instruction, 1928–9*, Vol. 134, December, Melbourne: Government Printer.

Waite, H. (1985) 'Playing a different game: toward a counter-sexist strategy in physical education and sport', *Education Links* 25: 23–5.

Woods, P. (1979) *The Divided School*, London: Routledge & Kegan Paul.

Wright, J. (1997) 'A feminist poststructuralist methodology for the study of gender construction in physical education: description of a study', *Journal of Teaching in Physical Education* 15: 1–24.

5 An elephant in the room and a bridge too far, or physical education and the 'obesity epidemic'

Michael Gard

Introduction

> The general goal of physical education is to help individuals achieve optimum personal development and contribute to the goals of society. The importance of physical activity in developing a healthy lifestyle must be understood by society and its children. The vitality of a country is directly related to the fitness and energy of its citizens.
>
> (Pangrazi and Dauer 1995: 1)

> It is within this conversation that we locate the whole re-articulation of lifestyle in the 1980s as part of a policing of the crisis of the Welfare State, through a policing of the body, through a 'strengthening of the superego' (Ingham 1985: 50). Through exercising smart lifestyle choices, the individual becomes personally responsible for his or her own quality of own life. The language of lifestyle is one of independence and self-sufficiency; it signifies pleasure, freedom, success and mobility. In this sense, practices in physical culture provide a personal freedom and the opportunity to share in the good life . . .
>
> (Howell and Ingham 2001: 337)

The *idea* that we are all getting fatter, regardless of age, sex, class, ethnicity or nationality, has been received, if not with glee, then at least with enthusiasm by people championing a startling diversity of causes. Some geneticists have claimed that fatness is primarily a problem for molecular biology and, not surprisingly, implore governments to direct more research funds their way (Hope 2002; Pirani 2002). Neo-Darwinists have announced it as proof that our modern lifestyles are out of step with our prehistoric and biologically determined natures (Engel 2002; McMichael 2002). 'Family values' advocates have seen it as yet another lamentable outcome of fragmented modern families which they claim no longer partake in wholesome, communal family meals nor take time to enjoy idyllic (and calorie-burning) walks and picnics (Shanahan 2002). And for those with an anti-global-corporation bent, increasing obesity is yet another ill which can be blamed on US-based multi-national fast food chains (Bunting 2002; Nestle 2002; Schlosser 2001; Tabakoff 2002). In each case, there is an obvious willingness to calmly accept the proposition that an 'obesity epidemic' is sweeping the world and now poses a serious global health problem.

And so it is with physical education. Sidestepping the tricky question of why they have not to this point been able to keep the masses waistlines under control, physical educators have responded to the recent avalanche of popular and academic interest in obesity by claiming special expertise in the area of weight control (for example, see Brown and Brown 1996; Fox 1994; Halawa 2001; Hills 1991; Kidd 1999; Sleap *et al.* 2000). And yet it is this claim to special expertise which demands of physical education a more critical approach to the issue of population overweight and obesity. While others may be excused for taking scientists at their word, the last forty years have witnessed an increasing prominence of the language and subject matter of science within physical education teacher training and classroom practice (McKay *et al.* 1990; Pronger 1995; Swan 1993), and it is this self-styling which disqualifies physical education's passive acceptance of scientific knowledge claims. If nothing else, a passive orientation towards scientific knowledge would at least seem out of step with contemporary discussion about the need for *students* in universities and schools to exercise critical judgement when evaluating the knowledge claims of others.

In the remainder of this chapter I propose to offer a critical perspective on the so-called 'obesity epidemic' and its relationship with the knowledge base and practice of physical education. In doing so, I will pursue three general lines of argument. First, I will suggest that the idea that Western societies are in the grip of a *generalised* crisis of obesity, affecting 'everyone everywhere', is at least controversial and probably mistaken. Second, I will argue that belief in the 'everyone everywhere' prognosis draws its intellectual and moral inspiration from a post-Keynesian, neo-liberal view of the individual. Third, I will explore the apparent and potential fallout of a physical education explicitly aligned with the 'war on obesity'. Bringing these three threads together, I will conclude by offering an outrageously speculative analysis which locates the politics of the 'obesity epidemic' within an internationally political context.

A contemporary crisis?

There are a number of very peculiar things about the 'obesity epidemic' literature. For example, some scientists writing in the field now seem prepared to accept that per-capita food consumption has either remained stable or gone down in Western countries over the last fifty years or so (Bouchard 2000; Hill and Melanson 1999) and that people are deriving a lower proportion of their total caloric intake from fats (Ernst *et al.* 1997; Stephen and Sieber 1994). From here, there are few alternatives other than to argue that general levels of physical activity have gone down so much that overweight and obesity have increased *despite* lower food intake. And yet of the thousands of papers published in this area, not one exists to support the claim that Western populations are less active now than in the past. Instead, it is assumed by scientific writers to be axiomatic (for a striking example, see Bouchard and Blair 1999). In my view, this is a considerable weakness in the idea that modern Western lifestyles have caused an explosion in obesity. For example, if, as we are told, technology and modern appliances are partly to blame, why are those people who own more of them, the more affluent, less obese than those who can afford fewer of them?

In other words, if the diseases said to be associated with overweight and obesity are 'diseases of affluence', why are the most affluent less likely to suffer from them? And why now? Despite there being ample evidence that Western societies have been *continuously* concerned about overweight and obesity for over 100 years (Sobal and Maurer 1999; Stearns 1997), contemporary writers tend to look back to the end of a mythical golden period, around the 1950s, in which Western people were generally 'trim, taut and terrific'. And so a familiar and recurring historical phenomenon emerges in which those concerned about the size and shape of Western bodies look nostalgically into the past and find a lost ideal, rueing what they have now become. In each moment, it has been (and remains) the lifestyles and gadgets of *present* Western living which are to blame, whether they have been pianos, telephones, radios, televisions, video recorders, computers or video games. And yet nobody has stopped to notice that Western lives, particularly those of the urban middle classes, have been changing for the best part of two centuries. So, in precisely what respect is middle-class Western life of 2003 *more sedentary* than that of the 1950s or the 1920s? What exactly is it about the past ten or twenty years that is significant? Without a satisfactory answer to this question, generalised demonising of contemporary (as opposed to earlier forms of) Western life is defenceless against the charge that it is nothing more than a rehearsal of an old moral panic.

Despite these difficulties, many of the scientists writing in this area claim that overweight and obesity, particularly amongst children, have accelerated in the last ten to twenty years (for example, see Deckelbaum and Williams 2001; Micic 2001). This is despite the proliferation of government, club and community-based sport and exercise initiatives, and what appears to have been a sharp escalation in the level of people's 'knowledge' (leaving to one side the complex question of whether this 'knowledge' is 'true' or 'untrue') about the value of exercise and dietary restraint in maintaining bio-medical health over recent decades. Indeed, a number of scientific writers concede that *recreational* physical activity has probably increased in recent decades (for example, Bouchard 2000).

Readers may have already guessed where the search for the 'obesity epidemic's' cause now turns; faced with a reduction in food intake and an increase of recreational physical activity, the 'last-man-standing' is so-called 'incidental physical activity', the energy it takes to lead 'normal' day-to-day lives. Put simply, the argument is that the reduction in incidental physical activity over the last few decades has been so great that it outstrips the improvements that have been made in diet and recreational physical activity (for examples of this argument, see Bouchard 2000; Jebb and Moore 1999). This seems an extremely ambitious claim and one which enjoys no empirical support in the literature. Unfortunately, this line of reasoning, hamstrung by its dogged determination to conceive of human body weight exclusively in terms of the difference between 'energy-in' and 'energy-out', also places its proponents in the worst of all possible empirical dilemmas. This is because, of all the variables which feed into the 'energy-in/energy-out' model of body weight, incidental physical activity is the most difficult to measure. On the one hand, very small study samples can be measured using elaborate and expensive equipment which can be carried around by research participants. But the fact that participants know that their physical activity is being measured casts doubt on the validity of these data, and small samples severely reduce their representativeness. On the other hand, large samples can be researched using inexpensive instruments, such as self-reports and diaries, but these are notoriously unreliable, particularly with children.

It is interesting to note that despite (or perhaps because of) the difficulties of measuring population averages for incidental physical activity, not to mention the complete absence of longitudinal comparative studies, the 'self-evident' fall in incidental physical activity is asserted over and over again in the scientific literature (Bouchard and Blair 1999; Hill and Melanson 1999; Koplan 2000). Some even go so far as to confidently quantify the average daily caloric expenditure of our prehistoric ancestors in order to show how current sedentary lifestyles are out of synch with our biological natures (Leonard and Robertson 1997). Given the profound difficulties of calculating these averages for people who are alive *today*, this is, to say the least, a bold claim.

While the dangers of simply assuming and asserting that modern life causes obesity are numerous, one telling example is worth exploring briefly. When searching for explanations, 'obesity epidemic' writers are prone to point the finger at 'technology', particularly television, videos and computer games (see Hill and Melanson 1999; Koplan 2000; Salbe and Ravussin 2000). Here the argument goes that the more time people spend using these machines, the less time they will spend being physically active. This argument is particularly popular amongst those interested in childhood overweight and obesity. No doubt this logic springs from a view of the body as itself a machine, and a kind of financial-accounting approach to the 24 hours of every day we have at our disposal; ergo 'time spent doing this equals less time doing that'. However, this logic is flawed, as Marshall *et al.* (2002: 5) point out:

> One hypothesis is that involvement in sedentary behaviour limits the time available for participation in health-enhancing physical activity. Most data do not support this hypothesis and cross sectional and prospective data between TV viewing and adiposity show inconsistent and weak associations. Sedentary behaviours appear to be able to coexist with physical activity, with each having a unique set of determinants.

In fact, Marshall *et al.*'s (2002) own study of approximately 2,300 North American and English children suggests that the more sedentary children (particularly boys) are, the more active they are. In other words, if there is a connection between technology and physical activity, it is in the opposite direction to that which is routinely *assumed* elsewhere in the literature. Elsewhere, in their review of the research concerned with sedentary behaviour, body composition, childhood physical activity levels, they conclude:

> A recent review of correlates of physical activity of children and adolescents concluded the relationship between TV/video games and physical activity to be indeterminate among 4–12 yr olds and zero among 13–18 year olds. The current review examined these studies more closely, located additional evidence and concluded that the relationship, across all age groups, is best described as zero (73% of effect sizes show no association).
>
> (Marshall *et al.*, in review: 10)

My purpose here is not to pit one group of scientists against another and to claim that one is closer to the 'truth'. Instead, my argument is that the 'obesity epidemic' literature is replete with untested assertions, the ideological significance of which I now want to discuss. Because if it were just that this literature was guilty of lazy assumptions, this would constitute an important but hardly decisive critique. What is most pressing about this issue is that it is an example of how reductionist science leads at best to ineffective solutions, and at worst to oppressive social policies

An epidemic?

To this point, I have suggested that, in the context of the scientific literature, the 'obesity epidemic' is a phenomenon without a cause. Because the human body is conceived of as a vessel whose weight is determined by the difference between energy intake and energy expenditure, attention is focused on what *individuals* do: their *lifestyles*. And when the existing empirical data provide no obvious clues about *how* modern lifestyles are contributing to the 'obesity epidemic' (in fact, as we saw, much of the data suggests we should be witnessing a *reduction* in obesity), the causal explanation is said to be 'self-evident'. Flegal's (1999: S512) conclusion that we know 'remarkably little' about the causes of obesity stands in stark contrast to the majority of scientific writers who exhibit so little doubt that they have already moved confidently to discussing solutions.

Some readers may be equally frustrated with the generalised claims of 'obesity epidemic' writers and the generalised ways in which *I* sought to critique them in the previous section. I did so because I wanted to show how the flaws in 'obesity epidemic' thinking are evident even *on their own terms*. But what if we were to approach the issue from a different angle, one which sought to ask *which* people are most likely to be obese and *why*?

There is now ample evidence that levels of overweight and obesity are neither uniform between (Flegal 1999; Seidell 2000; Wang *et al.* 2002) nor within individual countries (Averett and Korenman 1999; Flegal 1999; Grundy *et al.* 1999; Hill and Melanson 1999; Wardle *et al.* 2002). But while these disparities are regularly noted in passing, their significance is rarely discussed (although see Schoeller and Kushner 1996 for a brief discussion of obesity amongst African-Americans). An obvious exception to this is Flegal (1999) who notes the significant over-representation of African-Americans and Hispanics in the ranks of the overweight and obese in the US. Flegal (1999: S512) concludes:

> From a population perspective, it may be useful to focus less on the 'agents' of diet and physical activity and more on the 'environment' of social and economic organization and cultural values. The work of economic and social historians, sociologists, and anthropologists may lead to a better understanding of the social forces at work.
>
> (Ibid.: 512)

This is certainly not to suggest that overweight and obesity do not afflict members of the more affluent classes. However, my argument is that it is the scientific language of the 'energy-in/energy-out' discourse and the use of terms such 'epidemic' and 'pandemic' (Radford 2002; Seidell 2000) which seem to preclude any serious discussion of social division and, in fact, serves to conceal it. In 2002, the Premier of the Australian state of New South Wales convened an 'obesity summit' which brought together experts from a wide range of scientific fields. While the summit proposed a number of anti-obesity initiatives, the focus was squarely on individualised measures which took no account of differing rates of obesity amongst different social groups. In fact, the measures that were suggested were almost totally directed at a kind of mythical, decontextualised individual who simply needed to change his or her 'lifestyle'. Moreover, it targeted the two elements of the 'energy-in/energy-out' discourse, food intake and recreational physical activity, which, as we have seen, some scientists suggest are *least* significant in the 'obesity epidemic'.

To use an expression currently popular in American journalism, there would appear to be 'an elephant in the room'; that is, a very obvious conclusion about which nobody dares to speak. When it comes to diagnosing the problem, it is claimed that individuals' dietary and recreational habits are not the decisive factor. Yet when it comes to suggesting solutions, dietary change and increased recreational physical activity appear to be the only solutions on offer. Moreover, the idea that the 'obesity epidemic' is affecting 'everyone everywhere', regardless of social divisions, leads to a generalised demonisation of 'modern Western lifestyles'. But there is no such thing as *a* 'modern Western lifestyle', only different kinds of socially and economically shaped forms of life under varying modes of capitalism. And these different forms of life are symbolically and materially linked to particular body aesthetics, consumption patterns, diets and attitudes towards exercise and other 'health'-related practices. If the affluent middle classes are *the* embodiment of modern Western life there is no 'obesity epidemic' and, in fact, there is no case for modern Western life to answer. You need only stroll along the streets and into the cafés, health clubs, restaurants, supermarkets and shopping centres of the fashionable districts of Sydney, New York and London to see how simplistic the idea of a generalised global 'obesity epidemic' is. And as you stroll, try to remember that scientists are asking us to believe that approximately one in two Western people are so fat as to endanger their health.

The mirror of modernity

As a number of historians have documented, anxiety about what Western life does to the minds and bodies of those who live it is not particularly new. For example, Stearn's *Fat History* (1997), which compares the development of 'fat-phobia' in the United States and France during the twentieth century, argues that anxiety about overweight began not as a medical or public health concern but as a compensatory response to the erosion of other forms of moral censure. In particular, he points to increased middle-class consumption and wealth accumulation, the expanding role of women in public life and changing attitudes towards sexual conduct as developments which flew in the face of older moral norms and which called for new forms of visible restraint. More generally, it is clear that the body, its shape and its capacities have been tightly linked to Western notions of 'nationhood', 'progress' and 'civilisation', at least since the late 1800s (for example, see Kirk 1998a; Mangan 2000). While white people have often waxed lyrical about the beauty, grace, strength and utility of 'native' bodies, there has been a corresponding lament about the moral, intellectual and physical degeneration of the 'civilised' 'white man'. And just as the body has been laden with cultural significance, so too have the forms of physical activity which Western societies have devised. This is an important point because, while physical educators (including myself) will often talk about the inherent joy of physical activity, there is nothing pre-given about the forms of physical activity we do; they all have histories.

Physical education is no exception. Indeed, it is difficult not to come to the conclusion that, while, on the whole, very much a minor player in Western educational history, it owes its emergence and continued existence to moments of crisis, whether military, political or social. Is it going too far to suggest that physical education is merely an expression of a nagging concern that 'progress' is bad for you? If, as some theorists maintain (for example, Beck *et al.* 1994), modernity brings with it a reflexivity, a kind of looking in the mirror, which inevitably evokes both celebration and horror, then organised, rule-bound, (supposedly) productive forms of physical activity, such as physical education, are more a product of the latter than the former.

It is partly physical education's symbolic status as a therapeutic institution that creates the conditions in which its reinvigoration seems an appropriate response to the alleged global explosion of overweight and obesity. But what evidence is there that curriculum-based physical activity in schools is an efficacious response?

It is a measure of physical education's symbolic status as a place where children's bodies are shaped and disciplined that it is so blithely invoked when people look around for potential obesity cures. For example, sports scientists and medical researchers (such as Hill and Melanson 1999; Salbe and Ravussin 2000) have no apparent trouble in claiming either that less physical education causes more obesity or that more physical education causes less obesity, despite the existence of published research which sharply contradicts these views (for example, see Green 2002). It is particularly noticeable that when these claims are made in academic journals, they pass without supporting evidence. This is unsurprising since no evidence exists. In fact, only a small number of studies which have sought to measure the amount of vigorous activity physical activity students do in physical education have been published, all of which offer no comfort to the idea of a physical education-led 'war on obesity' (Simons-Morton *et al.* 1993; Sleap and Warburton 1996; Stratton 1997; Warburton and Woods 1996; Yelling *et al.* 2000). It is interesting to speculate about whether these papers which appear in educational journals are ignored by medical and sports science researchers because they simply (and incorrectly) *assume* that physical education involves levels of exertion likely to result in weight loss, because they are worried by what they might find, or because of sheer disciplinary insularity.

There is, of course, no shortage of studies which show that specific fitness and weight reduction programmes can have an affect on the body weight of children. However, these programmes, usually consisting of pre-planned, repetitive, continuous, moderately high-intensity exercise, pose a profound dilemma for physical education since they do not require three- or four-year trained university graduates to administer them. In fact, there is the distinct possibility that a future funding body, say a national government, might decide that a comprehensive physical education, complete with specialist teachers, syllabus documents, a varied curriculum and occupying significant space in school timetables, is an appalling extravagance when all we are trying to do is reduce body weight. And it will be of little solace that the goal of reducing body weight was one that physical education chose for itself.

In the short term there is the important question of how children experience physical education programmes which are designed to combat overweight and obesity. The research that exists suggests that an impossibly fine line separates activity which will have an effect on children's body weight and activity which is boring, stressful, humiliating and ultimately counter-productive, particularly for overweight and obese children. Some physical educators will counter this problem by saying that their goal is to 'plant the seeds' for future healthy lifestyles using 'fun' physical activity, rather than trying to whip children into shape here and now. The problem with this response is that it enjoys little empirical support while also saddling physical education with the most difficult of all possible goals. The amount of physical activity that people do is largely circumscribed by their social circumstances at any given moment and it is naïve (even insulting) to suggest that, if people are sedentary during particular periods of their life, it is because they are ignorant of the alternatives or have simply not got into the 'habit' of exercise. And then there are the obdurate problems alluded to earlier; first, that even for many 'active' people, recreational physical activity makes up a very small percentage of overall caloric expenditure, hence the consistent research finding that exercise programmes make only a minute difference to body weight; and second, that recreational physical activity may have increased in recent years at precisely the same time, we are told, as obesity has become more prevalent.

We now find ourselves in a situation where it is virtually impossible to think of physical education as not in some way relevant to the body shape and bio-medical health of Western citizens, and, at the same time, virtually impossible to make an argument to substantiate this relevance. One alternative would be for physical educators to withdraw completely from debates about body weight and health. Another, more positive, response would be to think more critically about this issue and what our role is or might be.

In earlier work (Gard and Wright 2001), my colleague Jan Wright and I sought to explore some of the unsupported assumptions that scientific researchers tend to make when writing about obesity, as well as the way in which knowledge claims which are controversial in the scientific literature can end up being presented as facts by physical education scholars. Taking up similar issues, Evans (2003) also advocates a critical orientation to bio-medical knowledge about obesity and health more generally and, in particular, asks us to think about the kinds of relationships being fostered between children, their bodies and physical activity by a physical education dominated by discourses of epidemic, risk, self-surveillance and a negation of pleasure (see also earlier contributions from McKay *et al.* 1990; Kirk 1996). In part, this work takes up the now well-established critiques of Western science articulated across a range of academic traditions, such as sociology, feminism and postcolonial studies. Indeed, there now exists a multitude of theoretical resources with which physical educators might interrogate their discipline's knowledge base and pedagogical practices. The potential prize for doing more of this kind of work is a physical education which speaks with its own voices, rather than one which is subservient to other epistemological, economic and political agendas. On the other hand, it is not a trivial matter that physical education has a stake in both liberal/humanistic educational traditions as well as what we might call the scientific 'world view' of the body; it is almost by definition interdisciplinary, a resource which we have scarcely begun to exploit. In this chapter, I have tried to make a small contribution to new and emerging cross(perhaps even anti)-disciplinary agendas and debates about the place of physical activity and the role of physical educators in the world.

A conclusion?

While there are doubts about the degree to which the so-called 'obesity epidemic' really is the 'global' phenomenon it is claimed to be, it has clearly become an important discursive resource in the legitimation of a number of academic disciplines, industries and public health policy agendas. Indeed, a complex feedback loop in which academics, entrepreneurs, funding bodies and governments are simultaneously constructing and responding to this alleged crisis is now in full swing. Almost inevitably, it seems, schools have also been drawn into the obesity vortex. It comes as no surprise that a number of obesity researchers (such as Booth and Samdal 1997; Epstein and Goldfield 1999) now see schools, particularly via physical education, as a key site for intervention. The issue that I have sought to highlight in this chapter is the tendency for physical education to be positioned, largely by those outside the discipline, in ways which take no account of the realities of classroom physical education or the socially embedded ways in which people relate to and experience their bodies and physical activity (Giles-Corti and Donovan 2002).

Over the last ten years Kirk (particularly 1994 and 1998b) has written extensively about what has come to be called the 'crisis' of physical education. In general, he has argued that, if there is a crisis, then it is discursive in nature; that is, tied up with the politics of meaning and knowledge and the increasingly ana-chronistic place traditional sports-based approaches to physical education occupy within the movement and body cultures of contemporary Western societies. While agreeing with much of Kirk's analysis, I would argue that there are other dimensions to the crisis (if crisis is the right word), both discursive and more concrete, which need to be considered.

First, many (if not all) of the basic premises which underpin 'common-sense' understandings of body weight, health and physical activity are under (in some cases extreme) empirical pressure. These include the ideas that high levels of recreational (as opposed to incidental) physical activity make you healthier, that physical activity is an effective and safe way to lose weight, that it is healthier to be thin rather than fat, or that modern Western life (as opposed to other forms of life) leads to increased sedentary behaviour, increased obesity and poor health. It is almost as if the more research we conduct on these phenomena the less we know. And while it has become fashionable to talk about the 'excesses' of 'extreme' post-modernism, it is intriguing to wonder whether those of us who are interested in body weight, health and physical activity are not smack bang in the middle of the ultimate post-modern swamp, where the 'scientific method' turns out to be ill-suited to the subject of our enquiry. Where would physical education go if its scientific aspirations turned out to be illusory? In this case its discursive crisis would be profound indeed.

Second, as I have suggested above, there remains the distinct possibility that the 'war on obesity' will turn out to be a bridge too far. If history tells us anything, it is that physical education's contribution to the health of nations is, at best, impossible to assess and, at worst, marginal or zero. This is unlikely to change, given its low status in schools and the increasingly crowded curriculum. The questions that physical educators need to ask are whether this is a job we want and what will happen when it becomes clear that others can do the job just as well for less pay and with a great deal more industrial flexibility. This is an important point despite the fact that some physical education practitioners may go on teaching in the same way as before, happy to ignore predominantly academic debates about obesity which go on around them. In this context, silence will be taken to mean consensus and, unless a credible alternative vision for physical education can be articulated, we may end up having to explain our failure in a job for which we did not apply.

The third point to consider is the extent to which physical education can or should be seen as another arm of public health policy. As a number of authors (such as Crawford 1980; Howell and Ingham 2001) have suggested, the modern construction of a 'healthy lifestyle' which leads to improved bio-medical health, and the idea that the job of health educators is to produce informed (individual) health decision-makers, both owe their emergence to the decline of welfare state politics and Keynesian economic theory. This is not to say that it is an entirely new phenomenon for people to be seen as responsible for their own well-being. What it means is that, by virtue of its apparently apolitical posture, physical education, as a discipline which seeks to simultaneously blame and empower the individual, is highly political. This political allegiance is reflected in the bodies of knowledge which have come to dominate physical education curricula in schools and teacher education programmes in universities and the practices which are thereby legitimated. But it is also reflected in the language of 'healthy lifestyles', a concept championed in the public health rhetoric of Reaganite and Thatcherite Western governments.

And there is something else. Why is that people are able to talk about a *global* 'obesity epidemic' when the problem appears to be much more acute in the United States than anywhere else? Why is it that small rises in obesity in India or South Africa are read as evidence of a global *pandemic*? Why are lower levels of obesity outside of the US read as evidence that these countries are suffering from the same disease as the US, rather than a different disease or no disease at all? In short, why are differing levels of obesity around the world virtually ignored by the experts as they try to understand what is going on? Is it because many Western people (especially in Australia) now automatically assume that we are a part of the US, and that their problems are ours, or that 'Western' means 'of the US'? It is apparent that few have stopped to ask these questions. Once again, the general notion of a 'Western lifestyle' as the problem is profoundly misleading and many extremely affluent Western countries have comparatively low levels of obesity.

And so I want to conclude by proposing some admittedly speculative but intriguing lines of analysis and research. Is it possible that rather than being a simple question of 'energy-in/energy-out', Western obesity is more accurately described as connected to the deregulation of economies, the idea that capitalism should be allowed to produce whatever products will turn a profit regardless of their effect on people, the mass production and distribution of food where keeping costs low is the primary goal, the stratification of society into the very rich and the very (sometimes working) poor, the commodification of exercise and health such that they become products to be conspicuously consumed, and the claims that citizens are best served by non-interventionist governments and that individuals working in isolation will solve all social problems? If these factors are not the primary drivers of obesity, and they may not be, the task of explaining the very different levels of obesity in different Western countries remains almost completely unaddressed. Stearns' (1997) work is the only sustained attempt that I am aware of, and yet it is severely limited by its reliance on cultural stereotypes to explain material outcomes.

I began this chapter with a quote from a standard primary physical education text book in which the American authors asserted that 'The vitality of a country is directly related to the fitness and energy of its citizens'. What are we to make of this quote given the current state and distribution of global economic and cultural power , on the one hand, and the prevalence of overweight and obesity in different parts of the world, on the other? In other words, how much longer can we live with the assertion that a nation's future is tied to the cardiovascular fitness, body shape, athleticism and 'vitality' of its citizens? Dare we wonder how this claim would sound in the villages of Kenya, Tanzania and Ethiopia? What exactly are we telling ourselves about the origins of our privileged Western place in the world if and when we repeat this claim?

At present, an uncritical acceptance of physical education's role in the 'war on obesity' is naïve, both because it ignores the possible ramifications for physical education as a discipline, and because it has the potential, at best, to conceal important social divisions and, at worst, to exacerbate them. And it may also be that we are unwittingly aligning ourselves with a particular strain of Western life and political governance for which we would otherwise have little sympathy.

References

Averett, S. and Korenman, S. (1999) 'Black-white differences in social and economic consequences of obesity', *International Journal of Obesity and Related Metabolic Disorders* 23(2): 166–73.

Beck, U., Giddens, A. and Lash, S. (1994) *Reflexive Modernization: Politics, Tradition and Aesthetics in the Modern Social Order*, Cambridge: Polity Press in association with Blackwell Publishers.

Booth, M.L. and Samdal, O. (1997) 'Health-promoting schools in Australia: models and measurement', *Australian and New Zealand Journal of Public Health* 21: 365–70.

Bouchard, C. (2000) 'Introduction', in C. Bouchard (ed.) *Physical Activity and Obesity*, Champaign, IL: Human Kinetics.

Bouchard, C. and Blair, S.N. (1999) 'Introductory comments for the consensus on physical activity and obesity', *Medicine and Science in Sports and Exercise* 31(11): 498–501.

Brown, W.J. and Brown, P.R. (1996) 'Children, physical activity and better health', *ACHPER Healthy Lifestyles Journal* 43(4): 19–24.

Bunting, C. (2002) 'Healthy diet? Eat your words', *The Times Higher*, 15 March: 16–17.

Crawford, R. (1980) 'Healthism and the medicalization of everyday life', *International Journal of Health Services* 10(2): 365–88.

Deckelbaum, R.J. and Williams, C.L. (2001) 'Childhood obesity: the health issue', *Obesity Research* 9, Supp. 14: 239S–43S.

Engel, M. (2002) 'Land of the fat', *Guardian*, 2 May: 2.

Epstein, L.H. and Goldfield, G.S. (1999) 'Physical activity in the treatment of childhood overweight and obesity: current evidence and research issues', *Medicine and Science in Sports and Exercise* 31(11): 553–9.

Ernst, N.D., Obarzanek, E., Clark, M.B., Briefel, R.R., Brown, C.D. and Donato, K. (1997) 'Cardiovascular health risks related to overweight', *Journal of the American Dietetic Association* 97: S47–S51.

Evans, J. (2003) 'Physical education and health: a polemic or let them eat cake!', *European Physical Education Review* 9(1): 87–101.

Flegal, K.M. (1999) 'The obesity epidemic in children and adults: current evidence and research issues', *Medicine and Science in Sports and Exercise* 31(11): S509–S514.

Fox, K. (1994) 'Understanding young people and their decisions about physical activity', *British Journal of Physical Education*, Spring: 15–19.

Gard, M. and Wright, J. (2001) 'Managing uncertainty: obesity discourses and physical education in a risk society', *Studies in Philosophy and Education* 20(6): 535–49.

Giles-Corti, B. and Donovan, R.J. (2002) 'The relative influence of individual, social and physical environment determinants of physical activity', *Social Science and Medicine* 54(12): 1793–812.

Green, K. (2002) 'Physical education and 'The Couch Potato Society' – Part One', *European Journal of Physical Education* 7(2): 95–108.

Grundy, S.M., Blackburn, G., Higgins, M., Lauer, R., Perri, M.G. and Ryan, D. (1999) 'Physical activity in the prevention and treatment of obesity and its comorbidities', *Medicine and Science in Sports and Exercise* 31(11): S502–S508.

Halawa, A. (2001) 'Prevalence of childhood obesity: a rampant epidemic in our schools', *Pennsylvania Journal of Health, Physical Education, Recreation and Dance* 71(2): 32–5.

Hill, J.O. and Melanson, E.L. (1999) 'Overview of the determinants of overweight and obesity: current evidence and research issues', *Medicine and Science in Sports and Exercise* 31(11): S515–S521.

Hills, A. (1991) 'Childhood obesity: strategies for control', *ACHPER National Journal* 132: 14–15.

Hope, D. (2002) 'Premier's obesity solution "rubbish"', *Australian*, 23 September: 3.

Howell J. and Ingham, A. (2001) 'From social problem to personal issue: the language of lifestyle', *Cultural Studies* 15(2): 326–51.

Jebb, S.A. and Moore, M.S. (1999) 'Contribution of a sedentary lifestyle and inactivity to the etiology of overweight and obesity: current evidence and research issues', *Medicine and Science in Sports and Exercise* 31(11): 534–41.

Kidd, B. (1999) 'The economic case for physical education', in G. Doll-Tepper (ed.) *Proceedings of the World Summit on Physical Education*, Berlin, November 3–5: 95–104.

Kirk, D. (1994) '"Making the present strange": sources of the current crisis in physical education', *Discourse: Studies in the Cultural Politics of Education* 15(1): 46–63.

Kirk, D. (1996) 'The crisis in school physical education: an argument against the tide', *ACHPER Healthy Lifestyles Journal* 43(4): 25–7.

Kirk, D. (1998a) *Schooling Bodies: School Practice and Public Discourse 1880–1950*, London: Leicester University Press.

Kirk, D. (1998b) 'Educational reform, physical culture and the crisis of legitimation in physical education', *Discourse: Studies in the Cultural Politics of Education* 19(1): 101–12.

Koplan, J.P. (2000) 'The obesity epidemic: trends and solutions', *Sports Medicine Bulletin* 35(3): 8.

Leonard, W.R. and Robertson, M.L. (1997) 'Comparative primate energetics and hominid evolution', *American Journal of Physical Anthropology* 102(2): 265–81.

Mangan, J.A. (ed.) (2000) *Superman Supreme: Fascist Body as Political Icon – Global Fascism*, London: Frank Cass.

Marshall, S.J., Biddle, S.J.H., Gorely, T., Cameron, N. and Murdey, I. (in review) 'Couch kids? Relationships between sedentary behaviour, body composition and physical activity among youth', *British Medical Journal*.

Marshall, S.J., Biddle, S.J.H., Sallis, J.F., McKenzie, T.H. and Conway, T.L. (2002) 'Clustering of sedentary behaviours and physical activity among youth: a cross national study', unpublished paper, Loughborough: Loughborough University.

McKay, J., Gore, J.M. and Kirk, D. (1990) 'Beyond the limits of technocratic physical education', *Quest* 42(1): 52–76.

McMichael, T. (2002) 'Not knowing what makes us tick has made us sick', *Australian*, 17 September: 9.

Micic, D. (2001) 'Obesity in children and adolescents – a new epidemic? Consequences in adult life', *Journal of Pediatric Endocrinology & Metabolism* 14, Suppl. 5: 1345–52.

Nestle, M. (2002) *Food Politics: How the Food Industry Influences Nutrition and Health*, Berkeley: University of California Press.

Pangrazi, R.P. and Dauer, V.P. (1995) *Dynamic Physical Education for Elementary School Children*, Boston: Allyn and Bacon.

Pirani, C. (2002) 'A great weight of hope in one pill', *Weekend Australian*, 31 August– 1 September: 21.

Pronger, B. (1995) 'Rendering the body: the implicit lessons of gross anatomy', *Quest* 47(4): 427–46.

Radford, T. (2002) 'World health "threatened" by obesity', *Guardian*, 18 February: 8.

Salbe, A.D. and Ravussin, E. (2000) 'The determinants of obesity', in C. Bouchard (ed.) *Physical Activity and Obesity*, Champaign, IL: Human Kinetics.

Schlosser, E. (2001) *Fast Food Nation: What the All-American Meal is Doing to the World*, London: Allen Lane.

Schoeller, D.A. and Kushner, R.F. (1996) 'Increased rates of obesity among African Americans confirmed, but the question of why remains unanswered', *Ethnicity and Health* 1(4): 313–15.

Seidell, J.C. (2000) 'The current epidemic of obesity', in C. Bouchard (ed.) *Physical Activity and Obesity*, Champaign, IL: Human Kinetics.

Shanahan, A. (2002) 'Why fat is a family issue', *Sunday Telegraph*, 15 September.

Simons-Morton, B.G, Taylor, W.G., Snider, S.A. and Huang, I.W. (1993) 'The physical activity of fifth-grade students during physical education', *American Journal of Public Health* 83(2): 262–4.

Sleap, M. and Warburton, P. (1996) 'Physical activity levels of 5–11-year-old children in England: cumulative evidence from three discreet observation studies', *International Journal of Sports Medicine* 17(4): 248–53.

Sleap, M., Warburton, P. and Waring, M. (2000) 'Couch potato kids and lazy layabouts: the role of primary schools in relation to physical activity among children', in A. Williams (ed.) *Primary School Physical Education: Research Into Practice*, London: Routledge/Falmer.

Sobal, J. and Maurer, D. (eds) (1999) *Weighty Issues: Fatness and Thinness as Social Problems*, Hawthorne: Aldine de Gruyter.

Stearns, P. (1997) *Fat History: Bodies and Beauty in the Modern West*, New York: New York University Press.

Stephen, A.M. and Sieber, G.M. (1994) 'Trends in individual fat consumption in the UK 1900–1985', *British Journal of Nutrition* 71(5): 775–88.

Stratton, G. (1997) 'Children's heart rates during British physical education lessons', *Journal of Teaching in Physical Education* 16(3): 357–67.

Swan, P.A. (1993) '"This is really important, you need to know this": hierarchies of subject knowledge within physical education teacher education and student intention', unpublished Ed.D. thesis, Deakin University.

Tabakoff, J. (2002) 'Slam the brakes on fast food before health problems get any worse', *Sydney Morning Herald*, 13 August: 11.

Wang, Y., Monteiro, C. and Popkin, B.M. (2002) 'Trends of obesity and underweight in older children and adolescents in the United States, Brazil, China, and Russia', *American Journal of Clinical Nutrition* 75(6): 971–7.

Warburton, P. and Woods, J. (1996) 'Observation of children's physical activity levels during primary school physical education lessons', *European Journal of Physical Education* 1(1): 55–65.

Wardle, J., Waller, J. and Jarvis, M.J. (2002) 'Sex differences in the association of socio economic status with obesity', *American Journal of Public Health* 92(8): 1299–304.

Yelling, M., Penney, D. and Swaine, I.L. (2000) 'Physical activity in physical education', *European Journal of Physical Education* 5(1): 45–66.

6 The discursive production of childhood, identity and health

Lisette Burrows and Jan Wright

Introduction

Contemporary critical psychological and post-structural theorists (Baker 2001; Dahlberg *et al*. 1999; Malaguzzi 1993; Morss 1996; Sloan Canella 1997; Weedon 1997; Wyn and White 1997) write about childhood as a relational concept, that is, our ways of thinking about concepts like childhood and identity are 'constructed and reconstructed within specific contexts – contexts which are always open for change and where the meaning of what children are, could be, and should be cannot be established once and for all' (Dahlberg *et al*. 1999: 57). From this point of view, what being a child means is repeatedly being renegotiated in relation to a range of other people (for example, parents, teachers, peers) in their lives and in relation to institutional and cultural discourses. In this chapter, we draw on this approach to examine how childhood is currently being constructed and reconstructed in relation to corporeal discourses that define the healthy child. We are particularly interested in the ways this knowledge, as produced in the popular media, medical and public health knowledge, is taken up in schools and initial teacher training in physical education (ITTPE) to fashion particular policies and practices applied in the best interests of children's health and well-being.

Discourse about young people's health has, until recently, tended to focus on concerns about drug-taking, alcohol consumption, becoming pregnant, contracting sexually transmitted diseases, being violent and committing suicide (Department of Health 1992; Education Review Office 1996), that is, issues that are linked in cultural and institutional discourse to the social, and the emotional, to young people's capacity to say no, to resist peer pressure and so forth (Bunton *et al*. 1995; Kelly 2000). Currently, new health risks have been articulated – ones that position young people, and particularly children rather than adolescents, less as social beings and more as biological, physical bodies at risk of the forms of ill-health which have been linked to overweight and obesity (Gard and Wright 2001). We argue in this chapter that media reporting of epidemiological and related research associated with a so-called obesity epidemic together with an on-going representation of young people as at risk of a range of health-inhibiting habits and products, serves to create a panic which constructs particular ways of looking at and acting upon children. Such constructions of childhood support normalising processes and processes of surveillance (Gore 1995) that are not in children's nor parents' interests and which have effects on school programmes, policies and the allocation of funds. As educators we are interested in the ways such constructions of child-hood feed in to education policy and practice, including the making of curriculum, the allocation of resources and the positioning of parents, teachers and children in relation to child health and identity.

In the first part of this chapter, we discuss ways of thinking about childhood that have prevailed at particular junctures throughout history. We do this to show that far from being a static category with universal meaning, childhood has meta-morphosed in tandem with the shifting societal, economic and political concerns of particular temporal and geographical locations. Next, we turn our attention to the particular mix of bio-medical, popular and bureaucratic 'truths' that seems to be driving health imperatives in schools. While we recognise that many of the concerns that have previously been associated with adolescence are finding purchase with children (e.g. drugs, alcohol and suicide), in this chapter we will focus on the ways in which the child becomes the centre of concerns associated with a relationship between health, weight and physical activity. Drawing on news media and a range of other-out-of school sources, we interrogate the ways in which the discursive truths associated with this relationship shape curriculum policy and practice in health and physical education. Finally, we examine the consequences of institutionalising particular constructions of a healthy child for the positioning of those at the centre of teaching – young people.

Ways of thinking and knowing children

'What is a child?' is a question central to debates, not only in professional circles, but increasingly amongst the public at large. As James and Prout (1990) argue, the mismatch between the ideal of childhood and the reality depicted in media coverage dealing with issues around child sexual abuse, the ravages of war and so on is preying on the consciousness of many who hitherto had retained images of childhood as innocent, safe, happy and protected.

Visions of childhood have always been closely articulated with images of an ideal society (Hendrick 1997; Sommerville 1982). Shamgar-Handelman (1994) maintains that the function of childhood has always been to produce 'good' children, yet at particular temporal junctures, children have been treated more like 'little adults' when economic circumstances have required that they function as cheap factory labourers, for example. When concerns about the moral degen-eration of society have been high on societal agendas children have been recast as either innocent amoral beings in need of adult supervision and guidance or alien sinners to be watched, controlled and constrained from running amok (Hendrick 1997; Marshall and Marshall 1997). When justifications for institutionalising schooling as a compulsory activity for children have been required, the child has been constructed as a special brand of being, inhabiting his/her own world and in need of specialised training (Stainton Rogers and Stainton Rogers 1992, 1995).

Throughout history, different demands have been made of children depending on the cultural and political lenses through which they have been regarded. Wyn and White (1997), for example, have clearly shown how the relatively recent Western conception of adolescents as 'risk-takers' and 'problems' is linked to the proliferation of 'agencies' and 'services' designed to minimise risk and ameliorate 'youth' problems. They argue for a notion of 'youth' as a relational and historical construct. That is, childhood is a discursively produced identity, the dimensions and constituents of which have changed and continue to change over time.

> Being a 'young person' does have real implications, but its meaning is tied to historical and specific circumstances and the ways in which relations of social divisions are played out.
>
> (Wyn and White 1997: 3)

As Burman (1994) contends, more often than not, disparate models of childhood have coexisted and competed rather than superseded each other in sequential fashion. Which particular image of childhood has been most fervently embraced at any particular time is a function of the interrelationship of a complex web of factors ranging from the compatibility of religious tenets with philosophical tracts on the child, to the intermeshing of economic and political imperatives with theories about the suitability of categories of children for schooling (Jenks 1995). It is when revolutionary changes in the long-range goals of a society have occurred that the most definitive statements about the character of childhood and relationship of family to state have emerged. In other words, the value systems of any society have been lived out in its treatment of children (James and Prout 1990). While conceptions of childhood and dominant social visions do not coexist in a one-to-one causal relation, we suggest that currently Western societies, at least, are influenced by several dominant cultural narratives that work to constitute children, their identity and their health in specific ways.

Children at risk

From the romantic vision of childhood as 'innocence' promulgated by French philosopher Rousseau, through to the nineteenth-century middle-class ideals of childhood as a period of 'helplessness' and more recent developmental psychological representations of childhood as a period of 'dependency', successive periods have shared a vision of childhood as a 'distinct period of human life with particular needs for stimulation, and education' (Burman 1994: 53). Throughout history a protective stance towards children has been justified by arguments pertaining to this relative 'innocence' and 'immaturity' of youth, their 'not-yet-developed' capacities to reason, think, behave in grown-up ways and a need to protect them from unsavoury aspects of adult civilisation (Burman 1991; Sommerville 1982; Stainton Rogers and Stainton Rogers 1992).

Contemporary child health concerns retain a discursive commitment to 'protecting children' yet now attempt to do so in a sociopolitical, economic and cultural context that is increasingly characterised by uncertainty (Giddens 1994). Drawing on Giddens' analysis, Kelly (2000) argues that the identification of risk factors and populations at risk (including children) can be understood as techniques for regulating the dangers and contingencies associated with this uncertainty. He suggests that a raft of preventative technologies have been mobilised to deal with the unpredictable, to protect against risk, the contingency of illness, unemployment and so forth.

In this context, what is likely to be identified as a health 'risk?' Given the need for certainty, as Gard points out in the previous chapter, epidemiological and bio-medical research provides the expert testimony for a validation for the establishment of new health 'risks' and the sustenance of 'old' ones. Population surveys, laboratory experiments and increasingly large-scale case studies are increasingly being used to assist researchers and public health departments to track the health risks and dispositions of child populations (Petersen 1997). The 'scientific' findings arrived at through these studies are selectively taken up by the media, simplified and disseminated to the wider public.

Media constructions of the child

Over a period of six months in 2001, media articles concerned with the relationship between children, physical activity and weight were collected from a range of broadsheet and tabloid newspapers and magazines in Australia, Canada and New Zealand. The media articles were analysed for the ways in which particular notions of the child were constructed in relation to institutional and cultural discourses.

In most cases the validity of claims was established through reference to epidemiological reports and/or the testimony of prominent health researchers. Typically, once the extent of the epidemic was established, developmental discourses were drawn on to explain both the reasons for the 'problem' *and* the solution to the epidemic. That is, according to most of this reporting, it is in the bodies of children that the decline evidenced in adulthood can be identified and arrested.

'Early intervention' was invariably emphasised as the key way to address the obesity epidemic. Statements and headlines such as 'Children who get a good start remain good' (Goff 1995: 6), 'Overweight children often become overweight adults . . .' (Powell 2000: 6) and 'War on obesity begins in infancy: Even Teletubbies try to reduce teletummies' (Young 2001: 3) urge adults to monitor the habits, behaviours and bodies of children and infants, to watch out for aberrant eating patterns, excessive weight gain and disinclinations to exercise. In much of this reporting children are simultaneously positioned as innocent victims (for example, of the fatty food industry, technology, neglectful parents) and as contributors to escalating national health bills (through increasing rates of obesity-related illness).

> One in four Australian children is overweight. Slower, stiffer, heavier – they are the cotton wool generation . . . Overweight children often become

overweight adults, and a child who is overweight faces all sorts of potential long-term health problems

(Powell 2000: 6)

The notion that health issues established from research conducted in largely Anglo-American contexts may be applied to *all* children is central to the construction of the kind of panic mobilised in the articles. That is, in reporting on the rising incidence of childhood obesity, children are typically represented as universally 'at risk'. In addition, headlines of the article typically suggest a competition whereby nations and states aspire to stand out as having the greatest incidence of children at risk of being overweight, thereby competing for the title of the 'fattest nation'. For instance, the headline for an article in the *Sydney Morning Herald*'s FIT supplement states, 'A big country: Australians are getting bigger and soon we may be the world's fattest nation'. The text that follows reads:

> Australia is now a close contender for the title of the fattest nation on earth and is well on course to take the title in the near future. According to the Australian Institute of Health and Welfare's latest physical activity report, obesity rates of 64 per cent for men, 50 per cent for women and 10 per cent for children put Australia only 1 per cent behind the US as having, on average, the world's fattest people.

(Powell 2000: 10)

In a *Marie Claire* extract, 'Weight of a nation', Alix Johnson (2001) draws on the expert testimony of National Heart Foundation Nutrition Research Fellow, to emphasise the magnitude of the problem:

> Dr David Crawford, National Heart Foundation Nutrition Research Fellow at Deakin University, has been researching the epidemic of obesity for the last 10 years. 'Epidemic is not too strong a word', he insists. 'Being overweight is affecting all people, all strata of society. By 2025, nearly every Australian adult will be overweight. As it is, one in five is obese – think of that in millions'.

(Johnson 2001: 234)

In Canada, the *Globe and Mail* newspaper reports, 'We are among the biggest eaters in the world and nowhere is the problem more apparent than St Catharines, Ont., the fattest city in the country' (Picard 2001: F1).

The emotionally charged discourses constituted in such reporting are often further amplified by an appeal to collective reponsibility for, and ownership of, children. Phrases like, 'How did *we* let this problem [obesity] get so big?' (Johnson 2001: 234); and 'Fat for life? Six million kids are seriously overweight. What can *families* do?' (Cowley and Begley 2000: 1) position the state and community as culpable for children's health and well-being.

Mediating and managing risk

Within the context of health promotion and public health campaigns the aggregate of risk factors appears to be expanding by the day and children are centrally positioned as targets for intervention by multiple agencies, each with an investment in alleviating one or other category of risk, albeit often for different reasons. The targeting of children as a site for intervention is nothing new (Sloan-Canella 1997) yet the proliferation of publicly funded and private agencies participating in the production of healthy children *is* a relatively recent occurrence (Kelly 2000; Seedhouse 1997; Valentine 2001).

One of the key private deliverers of health education in Australia and New Zealand is Life Education. Life Education educators facilitate sessions with children on topics ranging from alcohol, drugs and pregnancy, nutrition and the nervous system, to self-esteem and friendships. Included among Life Education resources is an exercise that links longevity to eating habits, weight and exercise, an activity that links character to somotatype and resources that encourage children to distinguish between health and unhealthy food (Life Education Trust 1996, 1997).

In the Otago region of New Zealand alone, almost all primary school classes, from new entrants to form 2, are visited once a year by Life Education's mobile classroom[1] and both children and teachers are supplied with Life Education materials and resources for on-going study. The Life Education Trust programme has tailored its teaching resources to link directly to the aims and objectives of the Health and Physical Education in the New Zealand Curriculum syllabus. Thus, many primary school teachers find the materials both accessible and applicable to their school-based programmes. Indeed, it would appear that for some schools, Life Education visits are the extent of the health education programme offered.

National Heart Foundation resources are also being increasingly taken up in primary and secondary schools to assist young people to learn about the con-stituents of a 'healthy' diet and the 'risks' associated with specific types of food (Wright and Burrows in press). Medical discourses that fuel these resources invoke 'good' food and 'bad' food binaries and provide clear directions regarding both quantity and quality of food to be ingested by the young (Lupton 1996). Links between 'healthy eating' and 'disease prevention' have always been a focus of school-based nutrition programmes. However, while once a well-fed plump child signified a 'well child', contemporary popular and medical discourses around food, at least in Western developed countries, are prevalently linked to child obesity concerns. The family is an obvious site of acculutration into norms and expectations around eating practices (Lupton 1996; Valentine 2001), yet in the context of an avowed 'obesity epidemic' schools are increasingly being regarded as 'the' key sites for nutrition education and intervention.

What each of these outside agencies share is a commitment to a notion that there is an unproblematic relationship between particular behaviours and health risks, both now and in the future, and that providing children with information about those risks *will* help them to make decisions to promote their own and others' health. These commitments are reiterated in many New Zealand government health reports (e.g. Ministry of Health 1998, 2000).

The role of the health and physical educator

The proliferation of bio-medical knowledge about obesity, its recontextualisation in popular media, and the concerns about 'declining physical activity rates' of children and their 'lack of fitness' (Public Health Commission 1994) provide further justification for many physical educators' already strong commitments to the role of deliberate physical activity in mediating multiple health risks. Obesity in childhood is linked in both popular media and public health accounts to poor performance at school, truancy, bullying, social ostracism, poor self-esteem, and mental health problems (Flegal 1999; Knight 2002; Powell 2000).

The location of the 'source' of the obesity epidemic in childhood has meant that teachers, and schools in general, have been positioned and have positioned themselves as pivotal agents in the production of the non-obese child – a role that requires persistent monitoring of children's bodily weight and size, the establishment of normative categories to enable 'at risk' pupils to be identified *and* a range of practices designed to prevent or remediate the onset of obesity (e.g. fitness plans, nutritional advice). In addition, these kinds of understandings about the role of the school in physical activity feed into particular ways of thinking about physical education as conflated with physical activity.

In Britain, for example, Tony Blair and several ministers are supporting proposals to extend the school day to enable pupils to perform two hours of daily physical exercise and sport. These proposals are touted as part of a radical plan to tackle childhood obesity or as one reporter put it, to 'curtail the rise of "couch-potato culture"' (Campell 2002). Barry Gardiner, the Labour MP for Brent North in London who is championing the British plan, explains the benefits for children in the following way:

> Isn't it better to have children still in school at four o-clock either playing or learning than at home watching television, eating crisps and doing nothing more strenuous than reaching for the remote control, or hanging around in the streets causing trouble?
>
> (Quoted in Campbell 2002)

Reminiscent of the widespread concern in the 1950s and 1960s about uncontrollable youth (Marshall and Marshall 1997), the above passage clearly indicates that the ends envisaged by mandating daily physical activity are not simply tied to making pupils healthier, but also link to agendas around reducing youth crime, cutting truancy and managing the misbehaviour of 'latch-key' pupils and other errant youth. As Kelly (2000) points out, this kind of discourse rehearses 'historical truths which construct youth in terms of deviancy, delinquency and deficit' (p. 469) while simultaneously providing further justification for the surveillance of populations of young people.

The pedagogic family

Contemporary health discourses position children themselves as the key target for intervention, yet as many critical analysts have discerned (Burman 1994; Morss 1996; Urwin 1985; Walkerdine 1984) the proliferation of health risks associated with childhood has contributed to a burgeoning attachment of discourses of blame and responsibility to families. As Kelly (2000: 468) puts it, 'the family, as the setting of nurturance, care and child/adolescent development, is increasingly responsibilized [*sic*] for the care of the youthful self.'

This responsibilisation of family is not new. In the practices of social work, psychiatry and educational psychology, families have long been regarded as crucial sites for the inculcation of developmentally appropriate practices. The 'good parenting' produces 'good children' discourse is embedded in child development literature, hospitals, childcare centres, schools, in each of the manifold institutions and professions that service families (Burman 1994; Morss 1996; Stainton Rogers and Stainton Rogers 1995). What *is* relatively new is the expansion of the boundaries and responsibilities of the family so that almost every disposition and behaviour of children is potentially amenable to family regulation (Kelly 2000).

The 'catch 'em early' discourses around childhood obesity provide a powerful exemplar of the particular surveillant positions and culpabilities for parents and families that can be invoked. While obesity in adults is ordinarily linked to moral laxity, i.e. an individual failure to take responsibility for the shape and substance of one's own body, with children, and particularly with very young children (e.g. the infants who watch Teletubbies), much of that responsbility shifts to parents, and as Burman (1991) would argue, mothers in particular. The relations constituted between parents and children in the following reportage clearly locate children as dependent and vulnerable 'victims' and parents as failing to exercise their duty to direct and control the habits of their young:

> Professor Norton said the message for parents was to restrict the number of hours their children sat in front of the television or computer screen: 'It's the easy option for parents. It's such a good baby-sitter,' he said. 'You have to have parents understand the message and turn the TV off.'
>
> (O'Neill 2001: 3)

> Sadly, TV is an effective babysitter for, say, single parents or parents who don't have money to spare for childcare.
>
> (Powell 2000: 6)

As extract 2 illustrates, it is often those parents who are already 'othered' in the normalising discourses of parenting (i.e. single parents, parents on low incomes) who are further marginalised by these moral imperatives to regulate children. And the surveillance, judgement and correction of children's practices extends beyond that of monitoring television watching. In obesity discourse families are constructed as an apparatus for control and surveillance of the type and quantity of physical activity children engage in, their opportunities for participation in sport and leisure pursuits and their access to appropriate health-enhancing resources.

Food intake is posited as something to be closely monitored by parents in relation to child obesity prevention. Parenting manuals like the British guide *Eat it Up* (Haslam 1987, cited in Lupton 1996) provide advice on how to make mealtimes fun, how to subtly influence the food preferences of children and be 'tough in the supermarket'. Mobilising the developmental discourses referred to above, many of these dictates draw causal links between eating habits formed in childhood and those responsible for rising rates of obesity in adulthood. As the main provider of food, at least in childhood, parents are positioned as 'responsible' for the inculcation of children's 'healthy' eating habits.

Parents are increasingly required to reinvent themselves as 'experts' involved in the surveillance, judgement, correction and regulation of children, activities that facilitate little space for what many would agree are the pleasures of parenting – playing with your child, sharing a meal of fish and chips, watching a movie on the couch. The anxiety and guilt associated with the role of 'professional parent' has been well documented (see Mayall 2001; Urwin 1985; Walkerdine 1993), yet as the following extracts from newsweeklies and papers suggest, the certainty with which relationships between children's health and family responsibility are established leaves parents in little doubt about who and what is the 'threat' to preferred futures:

'Child health begins at home' (Stott 1997: 5)

'What your children should eat' (Patty 2001: 3)

'Raising young couch potatoes' (Dekker 1995: 23)

Conclusion

As we have seen, the discursive constructions of childhood re-produced in corporeal discourses that currently define the 'healthy child' and the correlative positions elaborated for parents, teachers and politicians are in fact very concrete. The construction of childhood as a human condition currently under threat from a range of lifestyle, medical, interpersonal, economic and environmental 'risks' (Lupton 1999) creates power positions for adults and especially for health and physical educators. Experts in the fitness and nutrition industries are all constituted as legitimate regulators of children's bodies and souls. Further, parents themselves are increasingly being constructed as 'experts' crucially involved in the production and maintenance of their children's health.

We suggest that the identities constructed *for* children within contemporary panics around childhood obesity, especially, are 'dangerous' ones. First, the deleterious consequences of insitutionalising particular body images as 'normal' and therefore 'desirable' have been well documented in feminist literature (Bordo 1990; Markula 1997; Vertinsky 1994). Links between physical attractiveness and body shape regularly drawn in mass consumer culture are reinforced in the discourse of an obesity epidemic. A 'health' imperative is added to the 'beauty' imperative so that the requirement for young people to assess their bodies, to change their shape to fit the norms of contemporary society seems even greater. A persistent self-monitoring of bodily inputs (e.g. food, sleep, tobacco, alcohol, exercise) and outputs (e.g. body shape, size and weight) is called for not only to protect the physical self from risk but also to achieve the kind of body that signals status, moral worth, emotional stability, wealth and a 'normal' identity (Crawford 1980). As Atrens (2001) suggests, this self-surveillance and the guilt/anxiety it produces is not necessarily useful in the production of a 'healthy' self. Nor does it allow much space for enjoying the pleasures associated with consuming foods, drinking wine and other activities which in current discourse are positioned as dangerous 'indulgences'.

Second, norms are not merely useful devices for distinguishing preferred patterns of growth and development from abhorrent ones, but rather their very presence *does* something. They structure parents' and teachers' observations of their children/students. They invite comparison between children and they set up relations of competition amongst parents/teachers. As we have endeavoured to show in this chapter, they inspire all manner of professional interventions in the name of the child and at a wider level they invoke particular models of political organisation, such as welfare provisions, family policy and health policy (Burman 1994).

What is missing when childhood is positioned as 'the' site of prevention in public health discourse is any discussion of the positions available to children in constituting their identities as 'healthy' and 'unhealthy'. Research on the health beliefs of young people (Bendelow *et al.* 1998; Mayall 1994; Morrow 2001; Williams and Bendelow 1998) suggests the possibility that from children's perspective, health looks and feels very different from the visions upheld by teachers, parents and other health promoters, yet rarely are health promoters either cognisant of this or prepared to engage young people themselves in the identification of health issues that they feel are important to them. The work of Oliver (2001), Oliver and Lalik, Chapter 8 and Leahy and Harrison, Chapter 9 points to some of the manifold problems associated with deriving health programmes for children premised on adult understandings of what being a healthy child entails.

Ethnographic work with children may well assist us to begin to conceive of a healthy identity as more than a measure of a child's capacity to negotiate an aggregate of risk factors. Genealogical studies that track the variant ways that child health has been conceptualised over time and place may contribute to a recognition of the ethnocentrism and cultural specificity of many contemporary understandings about 'at-risk-children'. In the context of Western countries, a more reflexive attitude to the ways our own practices as health and physical educators buy into established panics over issues like childhood obesity and a commitment to recognising the consequences of continuing to privilege particular constructions of children and youth at risk for those at the centre of health educative work – children – will be important to our on-going attempts to educate in socially just ways.

Note

1 In 1999, 97.5 per cent of primary schools had been visited at least once by the Life Education truck (Nicholson 2000, personal communication).

References

Atrens, D. (2001) *The Power of Pleasure*, Sydney: Duffy and Snellgrove.

Baker, B. (2001) 'Moving on (Part 2): power and the child in curriculum history', *Journal of Curriculum Studies* 33: 277–302.

Bendelow, G., Williams, S.J. and Oakley, A. (1998) 'Knowledge and beliefs about health and cancer prevention: the views of young people', *Health Education* 96(6): 23–33.

Bordo, S.R. (1990) 'The body and reproduction of femininity: a feminist appropriation of Foucault', in A. Jaggar and S. Bordo (eds) *Gender/Body/Knowledge*, New Brunswick: Rutgers University Press.

Bunton, R., Nettleton, S. and Burrows, R. (eds) (1995) *The Sociology of Health Promotion: Critical Analyses of Consumption, Lifestyle and Risk*, London: Routledge.

Burman, E. (1991) 'Power, gender and developmental psychology', *Feminism & Psychology* 1(1): 141–153.

Burman, E. (1994) *Deconstructing Developmental Psychology*, London: Routledge.

Campbell, P. (2002) 'British school day could rise to 10 hours', *Observer*. Available: http://www.observer.co.uk/ (5 April 2003).

Cowley, G. and Begley, S. (2000) 'Fat for life? Six million kids are seriously overweight. What families can do', *Newsweek*, July 3: 1.

Crawford, R. (1980) 'Healthism and the medicalisation of everyday life', *International Journal of Health Services* 10: 365–88.

Dahlberg, G., Moss, P. and Pence, A. (1999) *Beyond Quality in Early Childhood Education and Care: Postmodern Perspectives*, London: Routledge.

Dekker, D. (1995) 'Raising young couch potatoes', *Evening Post*, November 8: 23.

Department of Health (1992) *Adolescent Health: Potential for Action*, Wellington: Department of Health.

Education Review Office (1996) *Sexual and Reproductive Health Education in New Zealand Schools*, Wellington: Education Review Office.

Flegal, K.M. (1999) 'The obesity epidemic in children and adults: current evidence and research issues', *Medicine and Science in Sports and Exercise* 31: S509–S514.

Gard, M. and Wright, J. (2001) 'Managing uncertainty: obesity discourses and physical education in a risk society', *Studies in the Philosophy of Education* 20: 535–49.

Giddens, A. (1994) *Beyond Left and Right*, Cambridge: Polity.

Goff, P. (1995) 'Children with a good start remain good', *New Zealand Herald*, November 6: 9.

Gore, J. (1995) 'On the continuity of power relations in pedagogy', *International Studies in Sociology of Education* 5(2): 165–88.

Hendrick, H. (1997) *Children, Childhood and English Society 1880–1990*, Cambridge: Cambridge University Press.

James, A. and Prout, A. (eds) (1990) *Constructing and Reconstructing Childhood: Contemporary Issues in the Sociological Study of Childhood*, London: Falmer Press.

Jenks, C. (1995) 'Decoding childhood', in P. Atkinson, B. Davies and S. Delamont (eds) *Discourse and Reproduction: Essays in Honor of Basil Bernstein*, New Jersey: Hampton Press.

Johnson, A. (2001) 'Weight of a nation', *Marie Claire*, October: 233–5.

Kelly, P. (2000) 'The dangerousness of youth-at-risk: the possibilities of surveillance and intervention in uncertain times', *Journal of Adolescence* 23: 463–476.

Knight, K. (2002) 'Small fries', *Sunday Star Times*, July 14: D2.

Life Education Trust (1996) *Take Home Work Book 4*, Wellington: Life Education Trust (NZ).

Life Education Trust (1997) *Take Home Work Book 7*, Wellington: Life Education Trust (NZ).

Lupton, D. (1996) *Food, the Body and Self*, London: Sage.

Lupton, D. (1999) *Risk*, New York: Routledge.

Malaguzzi, L. (1993) 'For an education based on relationships', *Young Children* 11: 9–13.

Markula, P. (1997) 'Are fit people healthy? Health, exercise, active living and the body in fitness discourse', *Waikato Journal of Education* 3: 21–39.

Marshall, J. and Marshall, D. (1997) *Discipline and Punishment in New Zealand Education*, Palmerston North: Dunmore Press.

Mayall, B. (ed.) (1994) *Children's Childhoods: Observed and Experienced*, London: Falmer Press.

Mayall, B. (2001) 'The sociology of childhood: children's autonomy and participation rights', in A.B. Smith, M. Gollop., K. Marshall., and K. Nairn (eds) *Advocating for Children: International Perspectives on Children's Rights*, Dunedin: University of Otago Press.

Ministry of Health (1998) *Towards a National Child Health Strategy: A Consultation Document*, Wellington: Ministry of Health.

Ministry of Health (2000) *The New Zealand Health Strategy*, Wellington: Ministry of Health.

Morrow, V. (2001) 'Using qualitative methods to elicit young people's perspectives on their environments: some ideas for community health initiatives', *Health Education Research: Theory and Practice* 16(3): 255–68.

Morss, J.R. (1996) *Growing Critical: Alternatives to Developmental Psychology*, London: Routledge.

Oliver, K. (2001) 'Images of the body from popular culture: engaging adolescent girls in critical enquiry', *Sport, Education and Society* 6(2): 143–64.

O'Neill, S. (2001) 'Good sports: Suzie O'Neill on keeping your children active – and happy', *Sydney Morning Herald*, November 8: 3.

Patty, A. (2001) 'Poor diet, exercise put young at risk', *Sydney Morning Herald*, November 8: 3.

Petersen, A. (1997) 'Risk, governance and the new public health', in A. Petersen and R. Bunton (eds), *Foucault, Health and Medicine*, London: Routledge.

Picard, A. (2001) 'Fat city', *Globe and Mail*, October 6: F1.

Powell, S. (2000) 'One in four Australian children is overweight – Slower, stiffer, heavier – they are the cotton-wool generation', *Weekend Australian*, May 27–8.

Public Health Commission (1994) *Our Health, Our Future. The State of the Public Health in New Zealand*, Wellington: Public Health Commission.

Seedhouse, D. (1997) *Health Promotion: Philosophy, Prejudice and Practice*, Chichester: John Wiley and Sons.

Shamgar-Handelman, L. (1994) 'To whom does childhood belong?', in J. Qvortrup, M. Bardy, G. Sgritta and H. Wintersberger (eds) *Childhood Matters: Social Theory, Practice and Politics*, Aldershot: Avebury.

Sloan-Canella, G. (1997) *Deconstructing Early Childhood Education: Social Justice and Revolution*, New York: Peter Lang.

Sommerville, J. (1982) *The Rise and Fall of Childhood*, London: Sage.

Stainton Rogers, R. and Stainton Rogers, W. (1992) *Stories of Childhood: Shifting Agendas of Child Concern*, Hempel Hempstead: Harvester Wheatsheaf.

Stainton Rogers, R. and Stainton Rogers, W. (1995) *Social Psychology: A Critical Agenda*, Cambridge: Polity Press.

Stott, C. (1997) 'Sick bodies, sick minds: child health begins at home', *New Zealand Herald*, November: 19.

Urwin, C. (1985) 'Constructing motherhood: the persuasion of normal development', in C. Steedman, C. Urwin and V. Walkerdine (eds), *Language, Gender and Childhood*, London: Routledge.

Valentine, G. (2001) *Social Geographies: Space and Society*, London: Pearson Education.

Vertinsky, P.A. (1994) 'Gender relations, women's history and sport history: a decade of changing enquiry: 1983–1993', *Journal of Sport History* 21(1): 1–58.

Walkerdine, V. (1984) 'Developmental psychology and the child-centred pedagogy: the insertion of Piaget into early education', in W. Henriques, C. Hollway, C. Urwin, C. Venn and V. Walkerdine (eds), *Changing the Subject: Psychology, Social Regulation and Subjectivity*, London: Methuen.

Weedon, C. (1997) *Feminist Practice and Poststructuralist Theory*, second edition, Oxford: Basil Blackwell.

Williams, S.J., and Bendelow, G. (1998) '"Monsters in the body": Children's beliefs about cancer', in S. Nettleton and J. Watson (eds) *The Body in Everyday Life*, London: Routledge.

Wright, J. and Burrows, L. (in press) '"Being healthy": The discursive construction of health in New Zealand children's responses to the National Education Monitoring Project', *Discourse*.

Wyn, J. and White, R. (1997) *Rethinking Youth*, St Leonards: Allen and Unwin.

Young, K. (2001) 'War on obesity begins in infancy', [Internet]. *Ottawa Citizen*. Available: http://www.ottawacitizen.com/national/010307/5054309.html 2001.

7   The body and health in policy

Representations and recontextualisation

Dawn Penney and Jo Harris

Introduction

In this chapter we seek to highlight the importance of policy as either a powerful source of stability and inequity in schools and societies, or alternatively, of active resistance and change. We argue that embedded in policies and played out in current practices[1] of physical education ('health and physical education') are incentives to pursue *particular* lives that are repeatedly being constructed as both healthy and desirable (for all) and that these lives presume the greater value and desirability of some bodies over others. They are, therefore, inherently inequitable and excluding. In hoping to counter these trends, we present policy as a force for prompting and supporting steps towards more socially critical practices in physical education that challenge and extend established thinking and actions.

At the heart of our discussion is the idea that policy features first, many and interrelated texts, each of which needs to be viewed as consciously produced and as having the inherent potential to direct (and thus narrow or broaden) views and understandings, and second, a constant interplay between texts and the contexts in which they are made, read and remade (Ball 1990, 1993). We focus particularly on physical education in England to relate some of the subtleties of the policy process and to debate the opportunities and barriers to any broadening of the 'body' and 'health' images and understandings that can legitimately be expressed and promoted in physical education and sport in schools. We also make reference to policy developments in New Zealand. This comparative perspective is designed to highlight a narrowness in thinking about the body and health that, despite accompanying rhetoric suggesting a commitment to the development of lifelong learning and inclusion in education, remains largely unquestioned and uncritically accepted amongst policy-makers and practitioners in England. However, we also acknowledge that official texts arising in New Zealand have their own discursive boundaries and tensions and far from guarantee uniformly more inclusive practices in schools.

Unfinished policy, ongoing potential

Before turning our attention to specific policy developments in physical education, we will expand upon the conceptual underpinnings of our analysis. We are attempting to integrate concepts presented by Bernstein (1990, 1996, 2000) with those central to the presentation of policy as a dynamic, relational and on-going struggle over meaning, developed particularly by Stephen Ball and colleagues (Ball 1990, 1993; Bowe *et al.* 1992). The key commonality here is a concern to focus upon and better understand 'relay' – the transfer or transmission of policy texts, the transformation of them in that process and thus, the on-going and contested production and reproduction of knowledge and understandings, values and interests. Bernstein (1990) explains 'Education is a relay for power relations to it . . . We know what it relays, but what is the relay? We know what it carries but what is the structure that allows, enables it to be carried?' (pp. 168–9). In Ball's (1993) view 'The challenge is to relate together analytically the *ad hocery* of the macro with the *ad hocery* of the micro without losing sight of the systematic bases and effects of *ad hoc* social actions' (p. 10). What exactly is the extent and nature of the connections between the formal documentary texts so often seen as 'policy' with the curriculum practices of teachers and experiences of pupils within and beyond schools?

A critical starting point is 'to recognise that the policies themselves, the texts, are . . . not necessarily clear or closed or complete. The texts are the product of compromises' (Ball 1993: 11). Furthermore, they are the subject of on-going struggles and compromises as they pass between various agencies and individuals involved in policy and curriculum development. Their very nature and their constant de- and re-contextualisation, presentation and re-presentation, means that 'gaps and spaces for action are opened up' (ibid.: 11). Yet there is a constant need to reflect critically upon the extent and nature of the gaps and spaces and how particular individuals are variously positioned to explore and exploit them. There are always limits to the opportunities for creativity in interpretations and responses to policy texts. Thinking and actions are not and never can be completely deter- mined. Rather, circumstances are created 'in which the range of options available in deciding what to do are narrowed or changed' (ibid.: 12). A reading is made and a response is actively constructed, but none of this is in circumstances of our own making. As Ball (1993) emphasises, any text 'has an interpretational and representational history' and furthermore, 'its readers and the context of response all have histories. Policies enter [and interact with] existing patterns of inequality' (p. 11). Policy analysis thus demands 'not an understanding that is based on constraint or agency but on changing relationships between constraint and agency' (ibid.: 13–14).

In this chapter we engage with these complexities in exploring policy texts produced by central government but also their 'enactment' or re-presentation in what Bernstein (1990) terms the 'official pedagogic recontextualising field' (ORF) and 'pedagogic recontextualising field' (PRF) and then, the 'secondary context' in which the focus is upon schools and teachers within them. Both the ORF and PRF are associated with the movement of texts / practices from the 'primary context' (concerned with the production of discourse), to the 'secondary context' (concerned with reproduction).[2] The ORF includes 'specialized departments and sub-agencies of the State and local education authorities together with their research and system of inspectors' (Bernstein 1990: 192), while the PRF includes university departments and research, education media and publication houses and other fields 'not specialized in educational discourse and its practices, but which are able to exert influence both on the State and its various arrangements and/or upon special sites, agents and practices within education' (ibid.: 192). In relation to physical education this prompts us to pursue the dynamics between the policy arenas of education, health and sport, and matters of 'intertextual compatibility' (Ball 1993) between parallel policy developments. Within the ORF and subsequently the 'secondary context' we examine notions of 'slippage' (Bowe *et al.* 1992) in the form and content of texts and in the meanings, understandings and interests that they promote or subordinate. In so doing we draw attention to the centrality of power relations in the relay of policy. We consider who is positioned, how, where and by whom to explore compromises and contradictions within central government policy texts, in what ways; who is able to renew struggles over meanings and understandings or equally suppress them, and with what potential impact in arenas of practice as a text is again 'delocated' and then 'relocated' (Bernstein 1990). None of these processes is neutral. Power relations are integral to the dynamics within and between Bernstein's contexts and are captured by a conceptualisation of discourse that embraces not merely the present and absent content of texts, but also the differential position and authority of individuals in relation to production and representation (Ball 1990). The policy process is fundamentally shaped by and continues to shape legitimate relations between agents and agencies, between discourses, and the forms of communication that are deemed legitimate between particular agents / agencies (Bernstein 1996, 2000; Evans and Davies, Chapters 3 and 14). In Gale's (1999) words:

> Policy discourse is like a double-hinged door; it is both productive of 'text' (understood broadly)*[3] and interpretive of it, and within this process discourse informs textual 'writings' *and* 'readings' including the latter's writerly and readerly possibilities. With respect to such possibility, discourses encode and decode policy texts in ways that constrain (and enable) their meanings . . .
>
> (Gale 1999: 395)

From this perspective we now take a critical look at the representations of the body and health in contemporary physical education policy. As indicated, our particular interest is in the discourses that are variously included, privileged, marginalised or excluded from central government texts and then, whether and in what ways the discursive boundaries or 'limitations' (Henry 1993) thus created are being extended, and may in the future be extended, in the recontextualising context. Following Henry (1993) we are open in acknowledging that

> Policy analysis is not only about the workings of policies and their deeper agenda. It is also a value-laden activity which explicitly or implicitly makes judgements as to whether and in what ways policies help to 'make things better' – acknowledging of course the contested nature of these judgements.
>
> (Henry 1993: 104)

The National Curriculum for Physical Education in England: closing the gate yet leaving doors ajar

The foreword to the latest National Curriculum for Physical Education (NCPE) requirements captures something of the tension at play in relation to our interests in prospective and potential slippage in the policy process. It stated:

> Getting the National Curriculum right presents difficult choices and balances. It must be robust enough to *define and defend the core of knowledge and cultural experience* which is the entitlement of every pupil, and at the same time flexible enough to give teachers the *scope to build their teaching around it in ways which will enhance its delivery to their pupils.*
>
> (DfEE/QCA 1999: 3, our emphasis)

Revealed here are key underlying conceptualisations that have informed the development of the National Curriculum in England and that have direct relevance to how we then see the body and health addressed within this development. Critically, a *pre-defined* body of knowledge is accorded the status of 'core', to which all pupils in state schools are entitled. The flexibility presented to teachers is in *how* they are to 'deliver' this core.

In contrast to developments in some other countries, an issue that we immediately confront in considering physical education in England is the extent to which the subject area and the professional identities of teachers associated with it, are and remain constrained by the label 'Physical Education', and not *'Health and* Physical Education' (as in New Zealand and several states within Australia) or *'Personal Development, Health and* Physical Education' (as in New South Wales in Australia). This has a direct bearing upon the ways in which 'the body' and 'health' are conceptualised by teachers and pupils. A number of extracts from recent statutory requirements for the NCPE (to be fulfilled by all state schools in England) reveal the conceptualisation of the body and health that are embedded in, legitimated and reinforced by the central government text. The images inherent in this text are:

- of the Body: as something to be appropriately prepared for physical activity; to be tuned through structured and progressively more demanding physical activity; and as the responsibility of the individual;
- of Health: as an established and agreed (rather than socially, culturally or historically specific) entity; to be gained and positively maintained through participation in physical activity; to be understood and evidenced by changes in/to the body; to be particularly considered at the beginning and end of activity.

In both instances the overwhelming focus is the disembodied, socially and culturally neutral, 'physical body'. Despite the accompanying emphasis on issues of inclusion,[4] diversity in the form of different bodies and different values in relation to health and lifestyles seems invariably denied and even actively challenged in the pursuit of the specific health, body and lifestyles that are accorded status in the text.

'The importance of physical education' is described in the following terms in the NCPE:

> Physical education develops pupils' physical competence and confidence, and their ability to use these to perform in a range of activities. It promotes physical skillfulness, physical development and a knowledge of the body in action. Physical education provides opportunities for pupils to be creative, competitive and to face up to different challenges as individuals and in groups and teams. *It promotes positive attitudes towards active and healthy lifestyles.*
>
> Pupils learn how to think in different ways to suit a wide variety of creative, competitive and challenging activities. They learn how to plan, perform and evaluate actions, ideas and performances to improve their quality and effectiveness. Through this process pupils discover their aptitudes, abilities and preferences, and *make choices about how to get involved in lifelong physical activity.*
>
> (DfEE/QCA 1999: 15, our emphasis)

The need for and desirability of positive attitudes towards 'active and healthy lifestyles' is not in question here. 'Active' and 'healthy' are uncritically linked. The choice to be made is *how* not *whether* to become involved in physical activity.

'Knowledge and understanding of fitness and health' is then identified as one of four aspects of knowledge, skills and understanding to be addressed in teaching, the other three being 'acquiring and developing skills'; 'selecting and applying skills, tactics and compositional ideas'; and 'evaluating and improving performance'. For each of four 'key stages' of education covering the primary (key stages 1 and 2) and secondary (key stages 3 and 4) phases of schooling, requirements are set out relating to each aspect and to be addressed through a stipulated range of activities applicable to the key stage (the statutory 'breadth of study'). The statutory requirements relating to the aspect 'Knowledge and understanding of fitness and health' are as follows:

Key Stage 1: Pupils should be taught:
    a) how important it is to be active
    b) to recognise and describe how their bodies feel during different activities.

Key Stage 2: Pupils should be taught:
    a) how exercise affects the body in the short term
    b) to warm up and prepare appropriately for different activities
    c) why physical activity is good for their health and well-being
    d) why wearing appropriate clothing and being hygienic is good for their health and safety.

Key Stage 3: Pupils should be taught:
   a) how to prepare for and recover from specific activities
   b) how different types of activity affect specific aspects of their fitness
   c) the benefits of regular exercise and good hygiene
   d) how to go about getting involved in activities that are good for their personal and social health and well-being.

Key Stage 4: Pupils should be taught:
   a) how preparation, training and fitness relate to and affect performance
   b) how to design and carry out activity and training programmes that have specific purposes
   c) the importance of exercise and activity to personal, social and mental health and well-being
   d) how to monitor and develop their own training, exercise and activity programmes in and out of school.

(DfEE/QCA 1999)

Finally, through stated levels of attainment, the NCPE provides descriptions of the 'types and range of performance' which pupils working at a given level 'should characteristically demonstrate' (p. 42). Essentially the levels provide an image of the types of learner and scope and nature of learning towards which the NCPE is directed. At the end of key stage 2, the expectation is that the majority of pupils will have reached level 4, and therefore, in relation to our particular interests, be able to:

- explain and apply basic safety principles in preparing for exercise; and
- describe what effects exercise has on their bodies, and how it is valuable to their fitness and health.

By aged 14, at the end of key stage 3, they are expected to have advanced to:

- explain how the body reacts during different types of exercise, and warm-up and cool-down in ways that suit the activity; and
- explain why regular, safe exercise is good for their fitness and health.

The progression is then towards increased depth of knowledge of fitness and the contribution of exercise to specific elements of fitness. The anticipation is that this knowledge will be used to enhance performance in physical activity, but more specifically and by implication, in those activities that feature in the statutory breadth of study, and that are privileged in and by those requirements. Our point here is that the programmes of study setting out the requirements for teaching at each of the four key stages detail requirements in direct relation to long-established six areas of activity,[5] not all of which have equal status or standing in the statutory order. The requirements relating to the teaching of 'knowledge and understanding of fitness and heath' are set alongside and are to be addressed within fulfilment of 'activity specific' requirements. In this relationship, the inherent strength of classification (Bernstein 1990, 1996) and the extent to which 'performance codes' (see Chapter 14) are dominant in the requirements relating to specific areas, play a key role in directing and limiting the health discourses that will feature in readings of the text. *Defining* the curriculum structure in terms of 'areas of activity' focuses thinking about the body, health, physical activity and their inter-relationships in particular ways, towards individual *performance* in sport.

A second and accompanying progression articulated in the NCPE levels is that pupils will take an increasing personal responsibility for developing and maintaining a structured programme of exercise and activity within their lives (DfEE/QCA 1999: 43–4). The surrounding curriculum structure and content (which privileges elite performance within a curriculum conceived as a collection of 'traditional' sports) is important here, influencing images and understandings of the types of exercise/activity that will feature in personal programmes and in addition, what those programmes will be primarily seen as directed towards. Green (2002: 180) has observed that 'policies that emphasise sport *per se* would mitigate [*sic*: militate] against recent trends towards the broadening and deepening of participation amongst adults'. In the development of the NCPE there has consistently been a lack of recognition that 'emphasis upon competitive sport (and particularly, traditional team games) within curricular and extra-curricular PE runs counter to developments in young people's situations and leisure patterns' (ibid.: 180). Furthermore, the images and understandings of activity, fitness and health embedded in and promoted by the focus and structure of the NCPE are strongly gendered, privileging stereotypically masculine conceptulisations of fitness, active and healthy lifestyles (Harris and Penney 2002; Hargreaves 2000).

Health and physical education in New Zealand: different boundaries, different tensions

It is only with knowledge of alternative texts that the cultural specificity of the NCPE, with its significant silences and particular orientation, becomes apparent. Comparable extracts from the Health and Physical Education curriculum in New Zealand (Ministry of Education 1999) do the talking for us in this regard. Social, cultural, environmental and, most notably, critical discourses are visible rather than excluded or subordinated. The four strands to the HPE curriculum include 'Personal Health and Physical Development' and 'Healthy Communities and Environments' alongside 'Movement Concepts and Motor Skills' and 'Relationships with Other People'. Notably the 'Personal Health and Physical Development' strand focuses attention on 'regular physical activity' but in addition, 'personal identity and self-worth'. The 'Healthy Communities and Environments' strand also engages with 'social attitudes and beliefs' and how these impact upon 'well-being'. Changing one's patterns of 'life, work, relaxation and recrea-tion' is promoted as a personal responsibility to be encouraged, but so too is the identification of inequities in relation to notions of 'healthy communities' and taking positive action to address these:

Students identify physical and social influences in the classroom, the school, the family, and society that promote individual, group, and community well-being. . . . Students are encouraged to identify inequities, make changes, and contribute positively, through individual and collective action, to the development of healthy communities and environments.

(Ibid.: 11)

The 'achievement objectives' outlined in the HPE text feature a breadth of engagement in terms of both issues and activities, which clearly go beyond the knowledge, skills and understanding set out in the NCPE. A broader view of health, as multidimensional but also socially constructed and culturally specific, is maintained in the detail of the objectives. The expectations of learning and learners display some similarities to those articulated in the NCPE but also some very obvious contrasts. At level 4 for the strand 'Personal Health and Physical Development', 'Students will':

- demonstrate an increased sense of responsibility for participating in regular, enjoyable physical activity to maintain well-being; and
- describe how social messages and stereotypes, including those in the media, can affect feelings of self-worth.

(Ibid.: 65)

At level 5 we see a subtle yet significant difference in the way in which participation in regular physical activity is portrayed and promoted in comparison to that within the NCPE. The commitment to be addressed is 'to a balanced lifestyle'. Elements of the 'Healthy Communities and Environments' reinforce an exploration rather than uncritical acceptance of what it is to be healthy, of what a healthy lifestyle will feature and of who has access to various lifestyles. For example, at level 4, it is stated that students will:

- investigate and describe lifestyle factors and media influences that contribute to common health problems across the lifespan of people in New Zealand; and
- access a range of health care agencies, recreational resources, and sporting resources and evaluate the contribution made by each to the well-being of community members.

(Ibid.: 65)

Like the NCPE, the New Zealand text has a number of silences, but of a different nature. Absent are detailed requirements relating to 'areas of activity' (and the development of skills, knowledge and understanding specific to them) which so characterise the NCPE. Yet while our reading of the New Zealand text is highly supportive of its form and content, it also needs to be acknowledged as a culturally specific reading. Salter's (2000) contention is 'that the new HPE curriculum, though intended to be (and acclaimed to be) culturally responsive, nevertheless still fails to adequately cater for Maori needs and aspirations' (p. 8). More specifically he points to what he describes as the 'progressive sanitisation' of the meaning and importance of '*hauora*' (that foregrounds the spiritual in an holistic conceptual-isation of health and well-being). In Salter's view the four-year writing period for the new HPE curriculum has seen 'a watering down and moving to the margins of a Maori dimension' (ibid.: 10) and ultimately a trivialisation and misrepresentation of *hauora*. He explains that,

> For Maori, health embodies a holistic philosophy that encompasses spiritual, mental, family, and physical dimensions along with connectiveness with the land and rootedness with one's tribal areas(s). These dimensions cannot be regarded separately, but are inter-related to form a whole on which good health depends.
>
> (Ibid.: 13)

Salter's anticipation is that the view of knowledge presented in the finalised HPE curriculum document is likely to be interpreted differently by Maori and non-Maori readers. He thus highlights that tensions and compromises embedded in this central government text can be expected to re-emerge as it is variously and repeatedly de- and relocated, and changed in those processes (Bernstein 1990). As in the case of the NCPE, policy is unfinished, nothing is guaranteed in terms of the under-standings, interests and values that will be expressed in practice.

Recontextualisation: shifting boundaries to meanings and potential actions

To view policy as a process is to acknowledge that official texts such as those above will never be the only, nor necessarily the most significant texts informing and shaping readings, responses and thus the expression of policy in practice. Many statements of policy or statutory requirements for curricula are notably minimalist. Requirements are stated but not expanded upon. Texts produced by various agencies or individuals in the 'official' and 'pedagogic' recontextualising fields (Bernstein 1990) provide crucial accompanying commentary. They provide guidance and suggestions as to the ways in which requirements might be interpreted and approached in individual school contexts, in schools' own curriculum design and in individual acts of teaching. It is here that 'slippage' takes on a real not merely abstract form. In guidance or support materials produced in conjunction with a policy initiative or new syllabus development, there is either a conscious extension of the range of discourses that might find expression in implementation, or an uncritical acceptance of the range presented in the policy text received, or some narrowing of that range. Thus in any reading and in turn re-presentation of policy, there is the scope to add or remove: to bring new or marginalised discourses to the fore, or to 'drop' discourses privileged or present in policy texts.

But as emphasised above, it is naïve to assume that all readings and emergent 'hybrid' texts (Bowe *et al.* 1992) have equal credibility in the eyes of teachers and comparable potential to shape responses to policy within schools. Power relations are maintained in and through the communications within the policy process and define its structural form. The credibility and influence of texts produced *will* depend at least in part upon who has written and/or endorsed them and where the individuals concerned are positioned in the process. Relations between agents (and their texts) within the ORF and PRF and between them and individuals (including primary and secondary teachers) in the 'field of reproduction' (Bernstein 1990) are therefore of critical importance.

Official guidance, official boundaries

Here we are concerned with what 'official' guidance materials have to say in relation to the body, health and physical activity in the context of the NCPE. A document produced by the government agency formed to undertake the revision of the National Curriculum and advise on new statutory requirements to take effect in 2000, the Qualifications and Curriculum Authority (QCA), sought to explicitly clarify a number of issues for teachers and others involved in the 'delivery' of the NCPE. 'Terminology in physical education' was an apt title for a highly authoritative text that set out the knowledge and understanding associated with 'fitness and health'. It stated:

Knowledge and understanding of fitness and health

This requires pupils to recognise and understand how their body reacts and works in different situations and activities, and increasingly to be able to use that information to help themselves. Pupils need to know and understand:

- that physical activity affects growth, development, health and personal well-being;
- how to prepare their body for activity safely and effectively;
- that different types of activity require different types of preparation;
- how different types of fitness impact upon activities and affect performance;
- how different types of activity impact upon physical fitness, health and well-being;
- that the body needs help to recover from activity;
- that the relationship between energy input and energy output is close and that an imbalance affects body size, shape, weight and health.

(QCA 1999: 7)

Subsequently the QCA produced sample 'schemes of work' as guidance materials for schools to refer to when developing their own responses to the revised NCPE requirements. Far from encouraging the exploration of 'health issues' and/or a focus upon these in implementation, the schemes effectively position health as both marginal to dominant discourses of motor skill acquisition and performance in sport, but also as entirely compatible with those discourses. The narrow conceptualisations inherent in the official NCPE text are reaffirmed and reinforced;

the potential for wider or alternative views is denied by a sustained silence. The schemes of work comprise units ('link', 'development', 'intermediate' or 'advanced') centring not on issues or particular aspects of learning, but instead, on one of the six areas of activity that make up the 'breadth of study' within the NCPE. The following learning objectives taken from units relating to dance activities illustrate the particular way in which health is defined, portrayed and positioned, and how bodies are being viewed:

Pupils should learn:

- the basic principles of preparing for dance (link unit)
- how performance is improved when preparation is carried out properly (link unit)
- what they need to do to improve their own standard of fitness in dance (development unit)
- to take responsibility for warming up and cooling down safely (development unit)
- to understand the principles used to prepare for, and recover from, dancing (development unit)
- to recognise that different types of activity require different types of fitness (development unit)
- how to continue to improve their personal fitness for dance and through dance (intermediate unit)
- to recognise and describe how regular involvement in dance activity affects their fitness, health and wellbeing (intermediate unit)
- to identify how and where they can get involved in dance activity (intermediate unit)
- to monitor exercise and fitness levels for themselves and/or others related to their dances (advanced unit)
- to devise, implement and monitor their own and/or others' exercise, conditioning and fitness programmes using principles of safe and effective exercising (advanced unit)
- to recognise and evaluate the impact fitness has on performance in dance, and dancing on personal fitness (advanced unit).

(QCA 2000)

Established boundaries to thinking and action and the key reference points for thinking and action (around discourses of performance and perfection, see Evans and Davies, Chapter 14) are reinforced rather than challenged. Attention is on the recognition and the development of a suitable response, rather than questioning, critique and exploration of potential responses. 'How' and 'where', not 'whether' are the legitimate issues to address.

Other official recontextualisation: the authoritative voice of inspectors

In England government inspectors of schools hold a position of commanding authority. Their reports on practice have direct implications for the future of schools and teachers within them. In this context, they can be regarded as key commentators on the National Curriculum's statutory requirements or more specifically, on what may or may not be deemed legitimate readings or interpretations of the requirements. Inspectors have the potential to either actively encourage or obstruct extensions to the boundaries of knowledge, skills and understanding of physical education in implementation of the NCPE. In reflecting on this scope it is appropriate to also note that the 1990s witnessed frameworks for inspection work being tightened and definite lines drawn between the inspection of schools and the provision of advisory services to schools (Evans and Penney 1994). So what are their expressed views in relation to the ways in which requirements relating to 'knowledge and understanding of fitness and health' are being addressed? Harris and Cale (2002) present a picture of inspectors as not merely legitimating but effectively accentuating the narrow conceptualisations of health inherent in the NCPE:

> Pupils know the value of a warm-up activity, such as stretching, to prevent muscles tearing. Some pupils know and locate the muscles in their legs to be stretched, for example, the hamstrings and calf muscles.
>
> All pupils have a secure grasp of the need for appropriate warm-up before physical exercise. All pupils have a good knowledge and understanding of the principles and procedures of warm-up before physical activity and are able to suggest appropriate stretches for different muscle groups. In circuit training some have developed an understanding of how to evaluate their own fitness levels. Teachers pay due regard to safety and ensure that pupils are warmed up before taking part in physical activity but pupils are rarely given the opportunity to lead this themselves.
>
> (Quotations from inspection reports,
> cited in Harris and Cale 2002)

Other comments within OFSTED's annual 'subject report' on physical education (OFSTED 2002) suggest support for some broadening of the curriculum activities included within curricula and recognition of the potential benefits of experiences of activities that are currently marginalised in the statutory NCPE text and many school curricula. Specifically, there is recognition that 'the provision of more indoor activities such as aerobics, fitness, badminton, volleyball' have been successful in countering disaffection, particularly amongst girls (ibid.: 2). Yet even here health is perceived as essentially a desirable inevitable outcome of involvement in organised sport. There is little to suggest any major shift in the discursive boundaries at play in the policy process.

Texts and recontextualisation continued

The QCA and inspectors' texts are not the only guidance materials that have been produced, not the only 'hybrid texts' that may be utilised by teachers developing the NCPE in their schools. Confines of space and the limitations of our own research prevent us from presenting an analysis of the array of commercial and other materials that have been produced by various agencies and organisations within the PRF (Bernstein 1990). Instead we turn attention to the de- and relocation of any of these texts within schools and by teachers. Our emphasis here is that readings of the statutory requirements of the NCPE or of the hybrid texts that we have discussed neither arise in nor enter vacuums. Boundaries between one policy development and others are unavoidably blurred as texts are considered and read 'in context'. Local readings always enter into a dynamic relation with wider policy, social, political and cultural contexts. In England teachers' readings of the various texts arise in and from an educational arena dominated by performance league tables and an array of measures directed towards enhanced accountability and efficiency in education. It is an arena in which views of knowledge as fixed and of pedagogical relations as uni-directional and a means of effectively and efficiently 'transmitting' this knowledge are to the fore. Furthermore the context is one in which elite performance in established 'traditional' sports retains a dominance that has been both embedded in and legitimated by the National Curriculum, and then reaffirmed and reinforced by parallel initiatives for sport development in England (see Penney and Evans 1997; Gilroy and Clarke 1997). Finally, it is a context in which initial teacher training has also and simultaneously been progressively narrowed and focused, openly restricting the scope for creative explorations of physical education curriculum content and pedagogy (see Evans 1995). Amidst a complex array of policy developments the structures and inherent power relations of initial teacher training and continuing professional development in physical education have been fundamentally changed. Most notably, the situation is now one in which sporting agencies are playing a, if not 'the', key role in shaping the future of the subject and profession.[6] It is only with this view of the complexities of policy contexts that we can understand the limits to and possibilities for 'slippage'. How then are teachers interpreting the NCPE requirements? What is the nature of their hybrid texts? Is scope for what we might term 'creative slippage' being explored, or is it overlooked, obscured from view, absent from teachers' understanding of what is both possible and acceptable in their implementation of policy?

Policies in practice: slippage (self-)contained

The NCPE is 'unfinished policy' in terms of the ways in which health will be understood and expressed in schools. In the light of the texts and contexts that we have described, it is perhaps unsurprising that narrow, gendered understandings and images of fitness, health and participation in physical activity are being actively reproduced in physical education in schools in England (Harris and Penney 2002).

We can only wonder at the on-going conservatism of 'the profession' amidst a policy process portrayed as one that is intended to influence but not determine actions. We might question the capacity of any policy texts, whether those we have described or policy developments now emerging, to influence teachers in schools.[7] The physical education curriculum and pedagogical texts that we see in many schools seem to relate more strongly to historical practices, interests and understandings that predate the development of the NCPE (Penney and Evans 1999; Curtner-Smith 1999) than to either specific policy initiatives or contemporary health needs. There is an important element of teacher-led as well as externally imposed containment of practices at play. The on-going dominance of discourses of skilled performance in physical education and sport is not confined to central government texts. It permeates the pedagogies and self-identities of many physical education teachers in England (Armour and Jones 1998; Keyworth 2001; Brown and Rich 2002). It is with these issues in mind that likely future expressions of health-centred curriculum in physical education need to be considered. Whether the implementation of the new HPE curriculum text in New Zealand or further development in the NCPE in England will prompt more critical thinking about bodies, health, physical activity amongst teachers and pupils thus remains to be seen.

Acknowledgement

This chapter has been developed from a paper entitled 'Policy, pedagogy and the politics of the body and health' presented within the Body Knowledge and Control Symposium, Australian Association for Research in Education Conference, December 2002, University of Queensland, Brisbane. Thanks go to John Evans for invaluable feedback on that paper and support for our efforts to further develop the arguments presented.

Notes

1 To some extent any discussion of policy is always hindered by language. The complexities and dynamics of 'the policy process' that we stress as always relational are in danger of being subsumed amidst portrayals of policy and practice as distinct albeit linked (Penney and Evans 1999).

2 Bernstein explains that: 'When a text is appropriated by recontextualizing agents . . . the text usually undergoes a transformation prior to its relocation. The form of transformation is regulated by a principle of decontextualizing. This process refers to a change in the text as it is first delocated and relocated. This process ensures that the text is no longer the same text:

    1. The text has changed position in relation to other texts, practices and position.
    2. The text itself has been modified by selection, simplification, condensation, and elaboration.
    3. The text has been repositioned and refocused' (Bernstein1990: 192).

3 Gale's emphasis here is to conceptualise 'action as text', (re)conceiving 'action as a form of text rather than separate from it' (p. 395).

4   The latest revision of the National Curriculum set out three principles of inclusion to be addressed in planning and teaching the National Curriculum: Setting suitable learning challenges; Responding to pupils' diverse learning needs; and Overcoming barriers to learning and assessment for individuals and groups of pupils (DfEE/QCA 1999).

5   The 'six areas' refers to the six areas of activity established within the National Curriculum for Physical Education in England: games activities, gymnastic activities, athletic activities, dance activities, outdoor and adventurous activities, and swimming activities and water safety.

6   Since 1994 the Youth Sport Trust has become an organisation very actively involved in the development of new resources and associated training for physical education and sport in schools. It is also the organisation appointed by the government to support the development of secondary schools designated as Specialist Sports Colleges that are now positioned as hubs of both curriculum and sport development in England (Penney and Houlihan 2001). In addition, there has been an increase in the involvement of National Governing Bodies of Sport (via coaching and sport development staff and the provision of resources and training) in the provision of physical education and sport for school aged children, with the aim of ensuring more coherent pathways from junior to adult participation and performance.

7   In particular we note (1) increased attention being directed towards the development of leadership skills and recognition that physical education has a role to play in introducing children to a range of roles within sporting contexts. 'Step into Sport' is a major new project focusing upon leadership and volunteering, being developed collaboratively by the British Sports Trust, Sport England and the Youth Sport Trust; and (2) moves to promote 'innovation' and provide enhanced 'flexibility' in the 14–19 curriculum across all subject areas. The government Green Paper '14–19: Extending Opportunities, Raising Standards' (DfES 2002) set out plans for major curriculum reform 14–19.

References

Armour, K. and Jones, R.L. (1998) *Physical Education Teachers' Lives and Careers. PE., Sport and Educational Status*, London: Falmer Press.

Ball, S.J. (1990) *Politics and Policy Making in Education. Explorations in Policy Sociology*, London: Routledge.

Ball, S.J. (1993) 'What is policy? Texts, trajectories and toolboxes', *Discourse: Studies in the Cultural Politics of Education* 13(2): 10–17.

Bernstein, B. (1990) *The Structuring of Pedagogic Discourse. Volume IV: Class, Codes and Control*, London: Routledge.

Bernstein, B. (1996) *Pedagogy, Symbolic Control and Identity. Theory, Research, Critique*, London: Taylor & Francis.

Bernstein, B. (2000) *Pedagogy, Symbolic Control and Identity. Theory, Research, Critique*, revised edition, Oxford: Rowman & Littlefield.

Bowe, R. and Ball, S.J. with Gold, A. (1992) *Reforming Education and Changing Schools. Case Studies in Policy Sociology*, London: Routledge.

Brown, D. and Rich, E. (2002) 'Gender positioning as pedagogical practice in teaching Physical Education', in D. Penney (ed.) *Gender and Physical Education. Contemporary Issues and Future Directions*, London: Routledge.

Curtner-Smith, M.D. (1999) 'The more things change the more they stay the same : Factors influencing teachers' interpretations and delivery of National Curriculum', *Physical Education, Sport, Education and Society* 4(1): 75–97.

Department for Education and Employment (DfEE) Qualifications and Curriculum

Authority (QCA) (1999) *Physical Education. The National Curriculum for England*, London, QCA.

Evans, J. (1995) 'Reconstructing teacher education'. *European Physical Education Review* 2: 111–21.

Evans, J. and Penney, D. (1994) 'Whatever happened to good advice? Service and inspection after the Education Reform Act'. *British Educational Research Journal* 20(5): 519–33.

Gale, T. (1999) 'Policy trajectories: treading the discursive path of policy analysis'. *Discourse: Studies in the Cultural Politics of Education* 20(3): 393–407.

Gilroy, S. and Clarke, G. (1997) 'Raising the game': Deconstructing the sporting text – from Major to Blair', *Pedagogy in Practice* 3(2): 19–37.

Green, K. (2002) 'Lifelong participation, physical education and the work of Ken Roberts', *Sport, Education and Society* 7(2): 167–83.

Hargreaves, J. (2000) 'Gender, morality and the National Physical Education Curriculum', in J. Hansen and N.K. Nielsen (eds) *Sports, Body and Health*, Odense, Denmark: Odense University Press.

Harris, J. and Cale, L. (2002) 'What do OFSTED Inspection Reports of Secondary Schools inform us about health and fitness within physical education?' paper presented at the AISEP International Conference, Spain, 2002.

Harris, J. and Penney, D. (2002) 'Gender, health and physical education', in D. Penney (ed.) *Gender and Physical Education. Contemporary Issues and Future Directions*, London: Routledge.

Henry, M. (1993) 'What is policy ? A response to Stephen Ball'. *Discourse: Studies in the Cultural Politics of Education* 14(1): 102–5.

Keyworth, S.A. (2001) 'Critical autobiography: "straightening" out dance education', *Research in Dance Education* 2(2): 117–37.

Ministry of Education (1999) *Health and Physical Education in the New Zealand Curriculum*, Wellington, New Zealand: Ministry of Education.

Office for Standards in Education (OFSTED) (2002) *Secondary Subject Reports 2000: 01: Physical Education. HMI 381*, London: OFSTED (www.ofsted.gov.uk).

Penney, D. and Evans, J. (1997) 'Naming the game. Discourse and domination in physical education and sport in England and Wales', *European Physical Education Review* 3(1): 21–32.

Penney, D. and Evans, J. (1999) *Politics, Policy and Practice in Physical Education*, London: E&FN Spon.

Penney, D. and Houlihan, B. (2001) 'Specialist Sports Colleges: A special case for policy research', paper presented at the British Educational Research Association Conference, University of Leeds, September, 2001.

Qualifications and Curriculum Authority (1999) *Terminology in Physical Education*, London: QCA Publications.

Qualifications and Curriculum Authority (2000) *Schemes of Work for Physical Education, Key Stages 3 and 4*, London: QCA publications.

Salter, G. (2000) 'Marginalising indigenous knowledge in teaching physical education: the sanitising of hauora (well-being) in the new HPE curriculum', *Journal of Physical Education New Zealand* 33(1): 6–16.

Part III

Schooling the body
Pedagogies of identity

8 'The Beauty Walk'

Interrogating whiteness as the norm for beauty within one school's hidden curriculum

Kimberly L. Oliver and Rosary Lalik

Introduction

> If the judges are White, a White girl *will* win. If the judges are Black, a Black girl *might* win.
>
> (Kisha, age 13)

These words were spoken by one of the adolescent girls who collaborated with us to study a taken-for-granted school practice known locally in the Southern US as the 'Beauty Walk'. The practice occurred as a school-sponsored fundraiser. Its format was that of a beauty pageant. Adolescent girls who were contestants in the Beauty Walk appeared on stage and stood before an audience of peers, parents, teachers and community members. Twice the group was culled publicly as some girls were selected and others excluded, based on judges' criteria for physical beauty. Ultimately a single winner was identified.

As described by Destiny and Jaylnn, two of our adolescent collaborators who studied the Beauty Walk, 'The Beauty Walk is an event that sells tickets to students, parents and friends to see 8th grade young women parade around on the stage in pretty, expensive, and fancy gowns.' As a school practice, the Beauty Walk had a long history in the community where we worked. Beginning with 5-year-old girls in kindergarten and continuing through the 12th grade, schools throughout the community held annual Beauty Walk competitions. Because the Beauty Walk was held as an annual middle-school practice, the messages circulated through the event constitute part of the schools' hidden curriculum – the unofficial knowledge that is circulated by school practices and events that lie outside the bounds of the official curriculum (Bigelow 1999).

Schools' hidden curricula have been found to be pedagogically influential insofar as they have implications for students' learning and well-being (Kenway and Modra 1992; Kirk 1998). Giroux (1981) has argued that curriculum, along with pedagogy and evaluation, is a primary message system by which schools influence learners and society. He explained that according to some theorists, 'schools function through the hidden curriculum to manipulate the student's "psychic space", those aspects of character structure that contain the possibility for emancipatory behavior and action' (p. 74). Thus analysis of the hidden curriculum is considered an essential task for radical theorists who wish to nurture 'a new conception of radical educational theory and action' (p. 72).

We learned of the Beauty Walk as Kimberly Oliver worked in the school as an educator and researcher helping girls to critique cultural messages about the female body. Together we were exploring whether the critical practices Kim encouraged enabled girls both to interrogate cultural messages about the body and to resist those messages that held negative implications for girls' health and well-being. Because there appeared to be a general acceptance of the Beauty Walk – a practice we found to be both anachronistic and abhorrent – we experienced dismay and disbelief when learning about it. Rather than ignore the practice, we decided that the Beauty Walk was an appropriate focus for the critical analysis Kim had begun with the girls. Thus Kim invited one group of girls with whom she'd been working to conduct an inquiry into the practice.

In this chapter, we describe and discuss the attention the girls paid to the role that race and racism played in the practice of the Beauty Walk. In particular, we note the girls' descriptions of cultural messages of beauty that centred on characteristics of the white body as the standard for physical beauty to be emulated and rewarded. We show how our collaborators, Brandi, Destiny, Alexandria and Jaylnn, began to question the fairness of the school's practices as they surveyed and interviewed their female peers about their views on the Beauty Walk. Additionally, we show how students at the school we studied simultaneously resisted and accepted the cultural messages about female beauty that circulated through the practice of the Beauty Walk. We highlight girls' voices throughout our descriptions.

Theoretical perspective

We came to this research inspired by our personal and professional experiences as women, university teachers and researchers attempting to develop socially just practices in the various arenas of our lives. For example, as white women aware that white hierarchical values and practices continue to percolate through US society, we work to notice and resist such values and practices in our own lives and to invent and adopt more just alternatives (Lalik and Hinchman 2001). Though we experience ourselves as agents in these matters, we recognise agency as a partial phenomenon, one limited by many factors, including the discourses and cultural practices available to us. We make no claims to innocence or absolution (Lather 1991). Rather we recognise our work as incomplete and flawed performance that requires recurring close examination and critique (St. Pierre 2000). Thus in this chapter, in addition to reporting our findings, we include a discussion of our work, pointing to several of the issues that it suggests.

Our research has been informed especially by the many adolescents who have assisted us in developing strategies for interrogating cultural messages of the body. For example, girls with whom we have worked have explained how fashion operates to complicate their young lives (Oliver 1999). They have informed us of the role that 'being noticed' plays in their relationships with boys and other girls

(Oliver and Lalik 2000). They have helped us to understand ways that they monitor their bodies to conform to standards of beauty they accept for themselves (Oliver and Lalik 2001).

Besides listening intently to girls, we have learned from writers who speak from many different theoretical perspectives. From black feminists, we have learned about the ways that black women have been overlooked and often demeaned in many conversations about feminism in the US (Collins 1990, 1998; hooks 1989, 1990; Lorde 1995). Post-structural feminists have informed us about the limitations of progressive conceptions of freedom and agency and progressivism's ignorance of the role that power and surveillance play in the development of the modern citizen (Kelly 1997; Lather 1991; McRobbie 1994; St. Pierre 2000; Walkerdine 1990). Anti-racist scholars have pointed out our responsibilities as Whites to interrogate ways that our taken-for-granted practices as Whites may interfere with our rhetorical stance as anti-racist teachers and researchers (Dyer 1997; Kincheloe *et al.* 1991; Scheurich 2000). Critical race theorists have encouraged us to question current mainstream contentions that racial equity has been achieved within US society (Delgado and Stefancic 2000; Ladson-Billings and Tate 1995; West 1994). Given these many sources of insight and theory, our research should not be understood as an attempt at unity in the service of theory. That is, we are not trying to create an impression that a single theory has informed our work or that we have been attempting primarily to develop theory or even test a single theoretical framework. Rather, we have used theory much as a *bricoleur* might use materials at hand to address a problem (Denzin and Lincoln 1994). 'The bricoleur produces a bricolage, that is, a pieced-together, close-knit set of practices that provide solutions to a problem in a concrete situation' (p. 2). The solution changes in response to a dynamic environment that includes changing resources and the evolving understanding of the *bricoleur*. Thus our work is well described as practical action in an effort to help the girls with whom we work learn how to critique cultural messages about the body, develop healthy practices in their own lives, and begin to imagine and create a more just world. To achieve these ends we have used multiple theoretical perspectives in planning, conducting and researching our work with girls. Throughout this work we have also paid particularly close attention to the views of the adolescents with whom we have worked.

Cultural messages of the female body are a focal point for the practical action of critique we seek to develop for our collaborators and ourselves. As has been explained by Walkerdine (1990), cultural messages about female bodies have long been persistent and ubiquitous. Through those messages female bodies have been pathologised. They have been found insufficiently developed for sophisticated reasoning; they have been 'hystericized and medicalized' (p. 33) and even found to be 'dangerous'. Thus historically women have been found unfit for membership in prestigious scientific societies, for participation in competitive physical events such as the Olympics, and for the rigours of life as chief executive officers of major corporations. Their bodies have been described as deficient and their dress and sexual practices have been closely regulated – a tendency that in mainstream culture is often referred to as 'the double standard.'

Exploring these patterns, Fine and Macpherson (1992) reported girls' awareness of many of these messages about the female body. During a series of conversations at dinner, four teenagers told these researchers, 'They are often reminded of their bodies as a public site (gone right or wrong), commented on and monitored by others – male and female' (p. 185). Further they reported painful descriptions of 'the violence of racism on the female body' (p. 190) that girls of colour had experienced. Reminding readers of how girls experience their bodies at the intersection of gender and culture, Fine and Macpherson elaborated:

> Gender determines that the young women are subject to external surveillance and responsible for internal body management, and it is their gender that makes them feel vulnerable to male sexual threat and assault. Culture and class determine how – that is, the norms of body and the codes of surveillance, management, threat, assault, and resistance available to them.
>
> (Fine and Macpherson 1992: 185–6)

Because of our attention to cultural messages about the female body, we have developed a sustained interest in critical literacy, though as feminists, this interest remains somewhat sceptical (Luke and Gore 1992). Scholars who describe literacy as a transformational process for developing the knowledge, skill and moral courage to change one's self and one's society in the interests of justice and equity have encouraged our interest. Prominent among these scholars is Paulo Freire (1974), an educator who rejected mainstream characterisations of literacy as a sound/letter association process primarily involving printed texts. Instead he favoured a more robust conception of literacy in which being literate means being able to critically assess and materially transform the world.

Scholars in the US and elsewhere have interpreted and applied ideas and practices developed by Freire. For example, Shor (1992) demonstrated and described ways of supporting college students in critiquing the knowledge created by mainstream journalists and in developing strategies for producing knowledge less compromised by dominant group interests. Others have described similar efforts with middle- and elementary-school students (Alvermann *et al.* 1999; Edelsky 1999; Fecho 1998). Practical application of theory – making something happen in the actual setting that is being theorised – often falls short of expectation (Ellsworth 1992) and intention (Lather 1992). Nevertheless we agree with Gore (1993) that the efforts of those scholars who have applied these theoretical notions in real world settings remain particularly impressive. This is so because such work allows for discovery and insight, even if such learning comes at the price of realising the limits and insufficiencies of one's efforts. As Morgan (1997: 25) has warned, 'No practices are "apostolic".' That is, 'no practices are absolutely correct'. In sum, we recognise that doing applied work means leaving the safe haven of pure theorising in favour of the more complex and morally dangerous terrain of practical action.

In our efforts to help girls become critically literate, we have learned that race is a salient signifier for the adolescents with whom we have worked. Thus, increasingly it has become so for us (Oliver and Lalik 2000). In this regard, the views of hooks (1992) about the persistence of white supremacist values in US society ring true. According to hooks:

> Racial integration in a social context where white supremacist systems are intact undermines marginal spaces of resistance by promoting the assumption that social equality can be attained without changes in the culture's attitudes about blackness and black people.
>
> (hooks 1992: 10)

To counter this problem, hooks encouraged her readers to employ an 'oppositional gaze' (p. 117). She explained its relation to agency. 'Spaces of agency exist for black people, wherein we can both interrogate the gaze of the Other, but also look back, at one another, naming what we see' (p. 116). Though hooks' words are addressed to Black people, we believe that she is also challenging non-Blacks to engage in anti-racist efforts.

Speaking more directly to Whites, Scheurich (2002) argued for active attention to the problems associated with race and racism.

> In many ways, white racism is like a monster standing amid us, affecting so much of what we do – or do not do – while we, particularly white people, appear to hope that if we avoid it, ignore it, or don't look at it, it will quietly go away. It won't.
>
> (Scheurick 2002: 87)

Agreeing with Scheurick (2002) and others who argue that it is better for us whites to face the problems caused by white racism than to ignore them, Kim engaged four African-American adolescent girls, Destiny, Jaylnn, Alexandria and Brandi in a year-long study that focused on critiquing cultural messages of the female body.

The data we analysed for this chapter are part of a larger research project. Our purpose for the project was to learn ways that concerned adults can help girls critically examine the connections between the ways girls' bodies are represented in culture and the ways girls' experience their bodies. As researchers we believe that such research has potential for helping girls learn critical perspectives and skills that they can use for pursuing healthy lives in a variety of contexts within and beyond school.

Working with the girls

Our four collaborators, Destiny, Brandi, Alexandria, and Jaylnn attended Landview Middle School, an 8th grade school located in the southern region of the US. Rather than being a traditional middle or junior high school, this particular school was a result of efforts to integrate the historically racially segregated city schools. Thus, rather than having two middle schools within the city limits, the school district decided that all 6th graders would be at one school, all 7th graders at another school, and all 8th graders would attend Landview. Despite efforts at racial integration, 70 per cent of the Landview students identified as African-Americans.

As primary researcher on this project, Kim worked directly with the girls. She met with each group one day per week for 60 minutes. Kim and the girls completed 26 sessions together between September 1998 and May 1999. She began the sessions by inviting the girls to develop personal biographies, and she attempted to scaffold their completion of these biographies using a series of questions about matters such as their home lives, their personal interests, and their school involvement. She also asked the girls to create personal maps of where and with whom they spent their time. Next, Kim asked the girls to complete a series of magazine explorations and critiques. Specifically, she asked them to cut out pictures that caught their attention, pictures that made them feel good and bad about their bodies, and pictures that sent messages to girls about their bodies (Oliver 2001).

While the girls were exploring magazines, Kim gave them journals and asked them to document the times they noticed their bodies. She encouraged the girls to write about what they were doing when they noticed their bodies, as well as what they were thinking and what they were feeling. Further she asked them to write about things that made them feel good and bad about their bodies and to document places where they received messages about their bodies. Finally she asked them to photograph messages they received about their bodies. In addition to journal writing and photographic documentation, Kim involved the girls in an inquiry project. The inquiry project was designed to help the girls critically examine some aspect of their culture that implicated girls' bodies. This chapter draws exclusively on the data from the girls' inquiry project.

Inquiry project description

For the first part of the inquiry, Kim and the girls designed a survey to learn about how other adolescent girls perceived the Beauty Walk. With Kim's help, the girls created twelve survey questions designed to evoke comment and critique of the Beauty Walk. The questions were: (1) Were you in the Beauty Walk? (2) Did you want to be in the Beauty Walk? (3) Do you think the Beauty Walk is a popularity contest? (4) Why does Landview Middle School have a Beauty Walk? (5) What do girls who are in the Beauty Walk have to do to prepare for the 'Walk'? 6) How do you think the Beauty Walk makes girls feel about themselves? (7) How do you think people act towards girls who participate in the Beauty Walk? (8) Describe how the Beauty Walk might be unfair to girls; (9) Imagine you won the Beauty Walk, describe how it would make you feel about yourself; (10) Imagine you were in the Beauty Walk and you did not win. Describe how it would make you feel about yourself (11) Describe what race might have to do with the Beauty Walk; and (12) Why do they have a Beauty Walk for girls and not boys?

To learn more about the Beauty Walk, two of our four collaborators, Alexandria and Brandi, attended the event with Kim. They took field notes recording their observations about contestant and audience behaviour. Throughout the event the girls talked with Kim about their observations and reactions.

During the weeks immediately following the Beauty Walk, Kim helped the girls to distribute their survey in two girls' physical education classes. To learn more about the survey responses, each of our collaborators interviewed two respondents, asking for clarification and elaboration of their written comments. While our collaborators were conducting interviews with their peers, Kim interviewed Kemya, a non-White Beauty Walk participant. With Kim's help, Destiny, Jaylnn, Alexandria and Brandi analysed the survey data, focusing their analysis on how the Beauty Walk affected girls. During analysis, the girls focused much of their discussion on how respondents described the unfairness and discrimination involved in the Beauty Walk. This response came as something of a surprise to us in so far as our collaborators had previously not strongly objected to the Beauty Walk; nor did they seem swayed when Kim raised concerns about it. We were also surprised that so many of the respondents expressed concerns about the Beauty Walk. Given the responses of our collaborators, we had expected respondents to express more acceptance of the practice.

During the final phase of the inquiry, Kim helped the girls synthesise their learning about girls' perceptions of the Beauty Walk. To support the synthesis, Kim asked the girls to express their learning in the form of a letter to the editor of a local newspaper. Kim gave the girls a list of directions she wanted them to follow as they created their letters. These were to: (1) use the surveys and interview data to help with the letters; (2) use as much detail as possible; (3) use examples and quotes from the surveys/interviews; (4) look for how the Beauty Walk is unfair to girls and why; and (6) focus on the possible advantages and disadvantages of the Beauty Walk and why. The girls worked in pairs to compose two letters. Jaylnn worked with Destiny, while Brandi worked with Alexandria.

Interpretations

In this section, we focus on the girls' voices to develop three major themes that emerged from our data analysis.[1] We describe how the White body is the school-enforced ideal for beauty, even in this predominantly non-White school. We show how our collaborators developed a critical stance toward the Beauty Walk through their inquiry work. Finally, we show how students at the school simultaneously supported and resisted the Beauty Walk. We begin this section with a vignette describing Brandi and Alexandria's comments and records while they attended the Beauty Walk with Kim.

'A Night Among the Stars': the White body as the enforced ideal of beauty

Brandi, Alexandria and Kim walked through the gymnasium door; Kim paid the admission price of 12 dollars for herself and this group of three who had come to observe the Beauty Walk and take field notes. Two students, serving as ushers, greeted them and handed each of them a programme. Depicted on the programme cover was an image of a young White woman with long hair, wearing a fancy dress, pearl earrings, necklace and bracelet. The title on the programme read, 'A Night Among the Stars'. The three found seats amongst several Black students attending the event. As the three looked around the audience, they noted that the majority of those attending were Black. Most of these audience members were students, though a few were adults who had come to support contestants. There was a small group of White students in the audience, as well as White parents and family members of Beauty Walk participants. The White parents, teachers and administrators outnumbered the White students attending the event. There were three females who served as the judges; two were Black and one was White.

As Brandi, Alexandria and Kim sat and waited for the show to begin, they looked through the programme. Alexandria and Brandi identified the race of each of the participants. In a school with a student population that was 70 per cent African-American, one might have expected that if all things were equal, about 70 per cent of the participants would be African-American. Of the thirty-seven Beauty Walk participants, 46 per cent (seventeen girls) were non-White, while 54 per cent (twenty girls) were White.

The programme began with the 'parade of the beautiful students' during which all thirty-seven girls paraded out on to the stage together. They formed a semi-circle at the back of the stage, and faced the audience. As they filed out, Alexandria documented in her field notes, 'there was a lot of snickering from the students [in the audience]'. Each contestant took a turn walking to the front of the stage, turning around so that her back was facing the audience, waiting three seconds in that position, and then walking from one side of the stage to the other and back to her original position. As each girl took her turn, she was introduced by name and by homeroom. For example, the announcer called out, 'Kemya Reeves from Ms. Smith's homeroom', as Kemya took her turn walking across the stage. Besides naming each participant, the announcer reported each girl's age, her parent's name(s), her preferred activities, and her favourite television show. Brandi documented in her field notes that: 'The Black girls received more applause from the audience than the White girls.'

After each girl was introduced and took her turn walking across the stage, the three judges, women involved somehow in the community, selected the top eleven contestants. Typically only ten girls were selected, but on this evening two girls tied for the number ten position, resulting in a 'top eleven'. The only apparent criteria for the judges' selections were how the girls looked and how they walked across the stage. As the names of the top eleven contestants were called, each stepped forward to form a line at the front of the stage. Thus, two lines of girls were created, the back line consisting of girls who had not been selected to move to the next level of competition and the front line with the girls who would move to the next phase.

While observing the formation of the two lines of girls, Brandi, Alexandria and Kim each commented on the composition of each line with respect to race. The 'majority of the girls' in the back line – those who had been eliminated from further consideration – were 'Black'. In contrast, the 'majority of girls' in the front line – those who would continue to 'walk in beauty' in this competition – were 'White'.

Brandi documented in her notes the racial identification of the girls selected as the top eleven contestants. According to her notes, eight were White girls, two were Black girls, and one girl was interracial.

The next phase of the competition involved each of the girls responding to the judges' question, 'Who do you admire most and why?' As each of the top eleven contestants took a turn answering the question, those who had not been selected remained standing at the back of the stage. When the questioning was finished, the judges announced the top three contestants, as well as the girl who would be 'Ms Congeniality'. The second runner-up was a light-skinned interracial girl, Rachel. The first runner-up was a White girl, Carol. Ms Congeniality was a White girl, Amie. The Beauty Walk winner was Mary Anne, a White girl and the daughter of the school's Parent Teacher Association (PTA) President. Brandi described the winner. 'Mary Anne looks like a Barbie Doll.'

Based on the patterns of participation and selection, it appeared that the White body was the school-enforced ideal for beauty at this Beauty Walk competition. In a school that was predominantly African-American, it was the White girls who participated and who were selected at each level of competition. Only one non-White participant was selected among the top three contestants, and, according to Brandi and Alexandria, she appeared to be a White girl. This pattern of White girls winning and being selected in the top ten, according to Jaylnn, Destiny, Brandi and Alexandria, was no different from previous years. That is, all the years that these girls could remember, the winner was a White girl.

Resisting messages from the Beauty Walk: an interview with Kemya

Kemya described herself as a 13-year-old 'mixed' [half White, half Black] girl. She had participated in the Beauty Walk, completed a survey and talked about her experience of the Beauty Walk during an interview with Kim. To foreground Kemya's views, we present an excerpt from the interview.

Kim: I want you to explain your [survey] responses to me . . . you know how at the beginning you were really excited about the Beauty Walk and then I saw you Friday and I asked you if you had a good time and you said, 'No.' Well, tell me about it from the moment you left school to get ready.

Kemya: Okay. When I first left school I was really happy and my dress had just got back from the cleaner's 'cause it had to be pressed. And I was so excited and I went to get my hair done. And I was gonna get my nails done, but I didn't think that was, you know, they wouldn't see my hands that much. And I got my hair done, and I thought it was just so cute and then I got home and it started to fall and I was like, 'Oh my God, oh my God.' I was going crazy. And then I went to McRae's [department store] and this lady did a beautiful job on my make-up. I loved it. I thought it was so cute. And I practiced my walk like it was nothin'. Like this is my stage, it's my walk. . . . And I feel that I should have made at least the top 11. . . . I didn't think it was fair . . . because most of the girls that won, it's not necessarily a racial part, but you know, every girl that was up there [in the top 11] was blonde hair and green eyes, blonde hair and blue eyes. And Rachel, I don't even think they [the judges] knew that she was a mixed, or had Black in her because her skin was so light.

Participating without winning: exploring dynamics of equity, race and power

When we first began the inquiry into the Beauty Walk, our collaborators were not sure whether race played any part in the competition. They believed that because 'both White and Black girls were allowed to participate' the event could be considered to be fair. Nonetheless, after observing the event and surveying other girls' perceptions of the Beauty Walk, they became more sceptical about the fairness of the event with respect to race and influence.

When our collaborators analysed the survey responses and interview data, they were somewhat surprised at what they found. In particular, they noticed the concerns about racial inequity expressed by the survey respondents. One survey response regarding race captured the girls' attention and prompted much discussion: 'If the judges are White, a White girl *will* win. If the judges are Black a Black girl *might* win.'

After Brandi and Alexandria finished interviewing girls about their survey responses, they joined Kim and Kemya who were talking about the role of race in the Beauty Walk. The girls began to theorise with each other about how race operated within the school event.

Kemya: [There were] eight White girls, two Black girls, and one interracial
           girl. That's eleven.
Brandi: I think if the Black judges picked mostly White [girls] so they could
           probably could get in with the [pause] so they could fit in.
Kim: And of the Black girls [selected for the top eleven] that were up there,
           only one had dark skin.
Kemya: You couldn't tell Rachel was Black. . . . Ashley's not that dark either,
           she's a little bit darker than me, but she's not really dark.
Brandi: They could have at least had one Black [dark-skinned] girl, but they
           didn't have any. Maybe they thought since Rachel was kinda mixed,
           maybe they thought they were doin' us a favor since she was mixed.
Alexandria: My mama says that since a Black girl won homecoming queen, you
           can just forget about the Beauty Walk.
Brandi: But see, we voted [for homecoming queen], it was our [student]
           choice.
Alexandria: In most Beauty Walks or pageants it is said that the White girls
           always win.

Through this inquiry on girls' perceptions of the Beauty Walk, Jaylnn, Destiny, Brandi and Alexandria developed and articulated a discourse of the Beauty Walk that featured several forms of critique. They synthesised their critique during the final phase of the inquiry by creating a letter to the editor highlighting some of their findings and views about the Beauty Walk.

In the girls' critique, both letters explain how a school function that places girls' bodies on display discriminates based on gender, race and social class and lessens 'girls' self esteem'. As Alexandria and Brandi wrote:

To Whom It May Concern:

We're writing this letter to express our concern about the Beauty Walk. We're concerned about the following: the discrimination against girls, because of racism, and how it makes girls feel about themselves. Most girls that we surveyed think the Beauty Walk is unfair to females. Some girls don't have the money to buy needed supplies . . .'Girls show off their bodies to paying people'. People are paying to see these girls. They seem like prostitutes and the girls didn't get anything. Racism is a big issue in the Beauty Walk. One student thinks, 'If the judges are white, a white girl will win. If the judges are black, a black girl might win.' Another student says, 'Race shouldn't have anything to do with the Beauty Walk'. . . . In conclusion, we think that the BW is unfair. It raises one girl's self esteem by cutting down other girl's self-esteem. We don't think that should be taught in schools. Basically, the BW should be abolished.

Destiny and Jaylnn wrote:

Concerned students say Beauty Walk (B.W.) discriminates, is unfair, and is almost equal to prostitution. The B.W. is an event that sells tickets to students, parents, and friends to see 8th grade young women parade around on the stage in pretty, expensive, and fancy gowns. According to 8th grade girls, B.W. is 'unfair' because girls are judged by their looks not by character, talent, or any other quality. Also B.W. costs too much money. Therefore girls that do not have enough money can't afford to participate. Girls have to get their nails & hair done, buy a dress & shoes . . . Most girls don't have enough money for those kinds of things. They don't have to do these things, but they are afraid if they come as themselves, the everyday person that they are, that they really won't win. That lowers most girls' self-esteem . . . Also because only one girl wins and that makes every other girl feel 'not so beautiful.' . . . Some of the girls say that the B.W. discriminates by race because most of the time it's a white girl that wins . . . The 8th grade girls say that's 'racist.' . . . What I'm trying to say is that there's no need for a school to have such a 'bad' fundraiser for school. It makes girls feel bad about themselves or makes them have a low self-esteem about themselves if they don't win. So from now on, take this in consideration, and don't have that kind of fundraiser.

Simultaneously resisting and supporting institutionalised racism

The girls who were interviewed and surveyed frequently noted the role that race played in disadvantaging Black girls who participated in the Beauty Walk. They expressed their resistance to the racism they perceived by communicating their dissatisfaction in their written comments and in their oral discussions during interviews. Yet they simultaneously supported the institutionalised racism they perceived. This was true in as much as Black girls continued to participate in the event, though at a level less than would be expected given the demographics of the school. Further, many Black students attended the event even though each student had to pay the price of 3 dollars for admission. Thus, they provided financial support for the event. The financial success of the event was an argument for its continuation by adult champions of the Beauty Walk. It continued to be a 'money-maker' for the PTA.

Even while supporting the event in the form of participation and attendance, Black students attending the event found a way to express their resistance publicly. They enthusiastically applauded the introduction of Black participants. Further, as Kemya described, they used silence, departure and rumour to show their dissatisfaction with the outcome of the event.

Kemya: And then [when the winner was announced] the thing that was so funny, it wasn't necessarily funny. . . . It was total silence in there [in the room where the event was being held]. Total silence. After Mary Anne [the winner] started walking, everybody got up and left. I couldn't believe, I was like, 'Oh my god!' It was funny, but you know I think it kinda hurt her feelings. She was like 'Why is everybody leaving?' I think she kinda felt bad about it. And there were like all of these rumors going around . . . Her mother knew the judges all that type of stuff . . . her mom is the PTA president.

So while many of the Black students and parents were willing to fund the school event, they walked out without clapping, thus, diminishing the winner, Mary Anne, and the event itself.

Discussion

The findings of this study show that the Beauty Walk was a part of the schools' hidden curriculum that celebrated the White female body as the norm for beauty even in a predominantly Black school. Through the inquiry processes that Kim supported, our collaborators were able to critique the Beauty Walk as a cultural practice and to theorise about some of the factors that supported it. Students at the school both supported and resisted the Beauty Walk. The success of our collaborators with inquiry and the resistance we observed among students was encouraging to us. Nevertheless, we are left with several concerns about our work.

Though the girls were able to conduct an inquiry project designed to critique this school event, the research fell short of helping them learn to change the taken-for-granted school practice. We believe that girls need to have opportunities to develop alternative discourses about taken-for-granted practices that form the hidden (as well as the official) curriculum. Nevertheless, we wonder if it is helpful for them to develop these discourses without concomitantly developing strategies for political action and structural transformation (Luke 1992). We wonder whether learning critique alone might not leave adolescents with feelings of frustration and helplessness. Luke explained that the language of critique might be politically counter-productive for adolescent girls and others who must live in a school and society dominated by androcentric power structures. Thus far our work with girls has not informed us about how one moves from classroom critique to 'political action and social transformation' (p. 38).

We hoped that the letters to the editor would be a small step in the trans-formational direction – one that would inspire the girls to further action. However, the girls did not express interest in continuing on with this focus, preferring instead to refocus their inquiry on other topics. Kim followed their lead, believing that keeping girls' interests at the centre of the work was a better alternative than clinging to our interests in political action and structural transformation. We believed that persisting with our agenda was tantamount to adding yet another form of oppression to those already circulating in the girls' environment.

Another issue grew from our awareness of the racial differences between our four adolescent collaborators and us. Though we are struggling to express our anti-racist stance in our work, our history and perspectives as Whites limit us. As hooks (1992) has explained, 'observing the world from the standpoint of 'whiteness' may indeed distort perception, impede understanding of the way racism works both in the larger world as well as in the world of our intimate interactions' (p. 177). Even so, we are hopeful that by listening to our adolescent collaborators and studying the writings of anti-racist scholars we may learn to understand our limitations and develop alternative practices. hooks (1992) tells us that such a shift of location is possible. 'Understanding how racism works, he [sic] [a white person] can see the way in which whiteness acts to terrorize without seeing himself as bad, or all white people as bad, and all black people as good' (p. 177).

Note

1   Please see Oliver, K.L. and Lalik, R. (in press) for a detailed description of the data analysis.

References

Alvermann, D.E., Moon, J. and Haygood, M. (1999) *Popular Culture in the Classroom: Teaching and Researching Critical Media Literacy*, Newark, DE: IRA.

Bigelow, B. (1999) 'Probing the invisible life of schools', in C. Edelsky (ed.) *Making Justice our Project: Teachers Working Toward Critical Whole Language Practice*, Urbana, IL: National Council of Teachers of English.

Collins, P.H. (1990) *Black Feminist Thought: Knowledge, Consciousness, and the Politics of Empowerment*, New York: Routledge, Chapman & Hall.

Collins, P.H. (1998) *Fighting Words: Black Women and the Search for Justice*, Minneapolis: University of Minnesota Press.

Delgado, R. and Stefancic, J. (2000) *Critical Race Theory: The Cutting Edge*, second edition, Philadelphia: Temple University Press.

Denzin, N.K. and Lincoln, Y.S. (1994) 'Introduction: Entering the field of qualitative research', in N.K. Denzin and Y.S. Lincoln (eds) *Handbook of Qualitative Research*, Thousand Oaks, CA: Sage, pp. 1–18.

Dyer, R. (1997) *White*, New York: Routledge.

Edelsky, C. (1999) *Making Justice our Project: Teachers Working Toward Critical Whole Language Practice*. Urbana, IL: National Council of Teachers of English.

Ellsworth, E. (1992) 'Why doesn't this feel empowering? Working through the repressive myths of critical pedagogy', in C. Luke and J. Gore (eds) *Feminisms and Critical Pedagogy*, New York: Routledge.

Fecho, B. (1998) 'Crossing boundaries of race in a critical literacy classroom', in D. Alvermann, K.L. Hinchman, D.W. Moore, S.F. Phelps and D.R. Waff (eds) *Reconceptualizing the Literacies in Adolescents' Lives*, New Jersey: Lawrence Erlbaum Associates Publishers.

Fine, M. and Macpherson, P. (1992) 'Over dinner: feminism and adolescent female bodies', in M. Fine (ed.) *Disruptive Voices: The Possibilities of Feminist Research*, Ann Arbor, MI: University of Michigan Press.

Freire, P. (1974) *Pedagogy of the Oppressed*, New York: Seabury Press.

Giroux, H.A. (1981) *Ideology, Culture, and the Process of Schooling*, Philadelphia, PA: Temple University Press.

Gore, J. (1993) *The Struggle for Pedagogies: Critical and Feminist Discourses as Regimes of Truth*, New York: Routledge.

hooks, b. (1989) *Talking Back: Thinking Feminist, Thinking Black*, Boston, MA: South End Press.

hooks, b. (1990) *Yearning: Race, Gender and Cultural Politics*, Boston, MA: South End Press.

hooks, b. (1992) *Black Looks: Race and Representation*, Boston, MA: South End Press.

Kelly, U. (1997). *Schooling Desire: Literacy, Cultural Politics, and Pedagogy*, New York: Routledge.

Kenway, J. and Modra, H. (1992) 'Feminist Pedagogy and Emancipatory Possibilities', in C. Luke and J. Gore (eds) *Feminisms and Critical Pedagogy*, New York: Routledge.

Kincheloe, J., Steinberg, S., Rodriguez, N. and Chennault, R. (1991) *White: Deploying Whiteness in America*, New York: St Martin's Griffin.

Kirk, D. (1998) *Schooling Bodies: School Practices and Public Discourse 1880–1950*, London: Leicester University Press.

Ladson-Billings, G. and Tate, W. (1995) 'Toward a critical race theory of education', *Teachers College Record* 97(1): 47–68.

Lalik, R. and Hinchman, K. (2001) 'Critical issues: examining constructions of race in literacy research: beyond silence and other oppressions of white liberalism', *Journal of Literacy Research* 33(4): 529–61.

Lather, P. (1991) *Getting Smart: Feminist Research and Pedagogy with/in the Postmodern*, New York: Routledge.

Lather, P. (1992) 'Post-critical pedagogies: a feminist reading', in C. Luke and J. Gore (eds) *Feminisms and Critical Pedagogy*, New York: Routledge.

Lorde, A. (1995) 'Man child: a black lesbian feminist's response', in M.L. Andersen and

P.H. Collins (eds) *Race, Class, and Gender: An Anthology*, Boston, MA: Wadsworth Publishing Co.

Luke, C. (1992) 'Feminist politics in radical pedagogy', in C. Luke and J. Gore (eds) *Feminisms and Critical Pedagogy*, New York: Routledge.

Luke, C. and Gore, J. (eds) (1992). *Feminisms and Critical Pedagogy*, New York: Routledge.

McRobbie, A. (1994) *Postmodernism and Popular Culture*, New York: Routledge.

Morgan, W. (1997) *Critical Literacy in the Classroom: The Art of the Possible*, New York: Routledge.

Oliver, K.L. (1999) 'Adolescent girls' body-narratives: learning to desire and create a "fashionable" image', *Teachers College Record* 101(2): 220–46.

Oliver, K.L. (2001) 'Images of the body from popular culture: engaging adolescent girls in critical inquiry', *Sport, Education and Society* 6(2): 143–64.

Oliver, K.L. and Lalik, R. (2000) *Bodily Knowledge: Learning about Equity and Justice with Adolescent Girls*, New York: Peter Lang.

Oliver, K.L. and Lalik, R. (2001) 'The body as curriculum: learning with adolescent girls', *Journal of Curriculum Studies* 33(3): 303–33.

Oliver, K.L. and Lalik, R. (in press) '"The Beauty Walk. This ain't my topic": learning about critical inquiry with adolescent girls', *Journal of Curriculum Studies*.

Scheurich, J.J. (2002) *Anti-racist Scholarship: An Advocacy*, Albany, NY: State University of New York Press.

Shor, I. (1992) *Empowering Education: Critical Teaching for Social Change*, Chicago: University of Chicago Press.

St. Pierre, E.A. (2000) 'Poststructural feminism in education: an overview', *Qualitative Studies in Education* 13(5): 477–515.

Walkerdine, V. (1990) *Schoolgirl Fictions*, New York: Verso.

West, C. (1994) 'Race and social justice in America', *Liberal Education*, Summer: 32–9.

9 Health and physical education and the production of the 'at risk self'

Deana Leahy and Lyn Harrison

Introduction

Notions of risk have become increasingly central to contemporary constructions of curriculum and pedagogy in school-based health and physical education (HPE). While there is a long history of attention to 'risk' in the field of HPE, there is a marked difference in how risk is currently formulated and deployed. This chapter explores how these new 'risk discourses' operate in the HPE classroom. Theorists such as Beck and Giddens point to the globalisation of risk, arguing that risk is a central characteristic of late-modern neo-liberal countries (Lupton 1999a). Our chapter, however, specifically draws on governmental theorists to explore the broad cultural and social 'turn to risk', and the significance this has for the ways in which health and physical education curriculum and pedagogy attempts to shape and produce particular kinds of people. We explore some of the effects of 'risk discourse' for curriculum, teachers, classroom practices, and for the young people who are the target of the risk curriculum. The discussion draws from data collected as part of a larger study that sought to explore the dominant and contesting discourses that operate within school-based health education.

We will centre our discussion on an analysis of classroom data from a year 10 Health and Physical Education course that was taught at an inner city Melbourne secondary school in Victoria, Australia. A range of methods were utilised to collect data for this project. These included: teacher interviews; key informant interviews; classroom observations and an examination of curriculum documents and support materials. Texts were analysed via a form of critical discourse analysis that provides 'a way of conceptualizing and deconstructing the relations both within and between education, the body, identity and health as constructed domains' (for a more detailed overview of this methodology, see Wright, Chapter 2).

Risk, governance and health and physical education

The following excerpt, taken from the rationale of the Victorian Health and Physical Education (HPE) curriculum document, is explicit in its desire to produce a particular type of citizen:

> The Health and Physical Education KLA [Key Learning Area] provides a
> foundation for developing active and informed members of society capable of

managing the interactions between themselves and their social, cultural, organizational, physical and natural environments in the pursuit of lifelong involvement in physical activity, health and well being.

(Board of Studies 2000: 5)

In statements such as this we can see that HPE is concerned with producing a certain kind of subject: one who is 'autonomous, directed at self improvement, self regulated, desirous of self knowledge, a subject who is seeking happiness and healthiness' (Lupton 1995: 11). The concept of 'governmentality' offers a generative theoretical frame with which to explore the project of HPE in relation to producing certain kinds of subjects/citizens. Government, as understood by Foucault, is a 'contact point' where technologies of power, or domination, and technologies of the self interact (Burchell 1996: 20). Foucault describes 'technologies of the self' as those practices of the self whereby subjects constitute themselves in interaction with technologies of power. Technologies of the self

permit individuals to effect by their own means or with the help of others a certain number of operations on their own bodies and souls, thoughts, conduct and way of being, so as to transform themselves in order to attain a certain state of happiness, wisdom, perfection, or immortality.

(Foucault 1988: 18)

Mitchell Dean refers to practices of the self as the process of 'governmental self formation'. He defines this as

the ways in which various authorities and agencies [in this case HPE and its associations] seek to shape the conduct, aspirations, needs, desires and capacities of specified political and social categories, to enlist them in particular strategies and to seek definite goals.

(Dean 1995: 563)

For those who are interested in governmentality studies and practices of self-formation, the 'turn to risk' is significant (Turner 1997). As Lupton notes, a 'new prudentialism' has been identified 'in governmental discourses and strategies, which moves away from older notions of social insurance as a means of distributing risks to a focus on individuals protecting themselves against risk' (Lupton 1999b: 5). This new prudentialism produces a different way of acting on the self. It incites subjects to shape themselves in particular ways. We would suggest that school-based health and physical education is one such point of 'contact', in that it provides a key site in which the governmental imperative to produce healthy citizens is enacted via a range of pedagogical strategies and processes. The aim here is to ensure that students of HPE engage in certain technologies of the self that are both health-directed and related. The imperative to produce healthy citizens is not a new phenomenon, and we would argue that school-based health and physical education has always been about shaping a particular type of subject (Kirk 2001; Lupton

1995). In this sense, HPE as a site of governance has enduring qualities. However, we argue that in late modernity, and amid the proliferation of health and risk discourses, that this production and government of the self has taken on new forms (Peterson 1997).

Several researchers have begun to explore the significance of risk, and how it operates within the field of HPE (for example, Gard and Wright 2001; Tinning and Glasby 2002). Explorations to date, however, have largely relied on policy/ document analysis to suggest potential consequences in the classroom. Given the lack of classroom data, our research specifically sought to explore the different discourses that circulate within both the HPE curriculum and HPE classroom. Like Gard and Wright (2001) and Tinning and Glasby (2002) our data demonstrates that risk is of central importance within the HPE curriculum, and that expert know-ledges were significant in the production of risk. Thus, it is not surprising that risk and risk knowledges were also a dominant feature of the HPE classrooms we observed. What was interesting, however, is the way in which risk and risk knowledges were deployed within the classroom context. We found that risk was critical to the way in which contemporary governance was enacted, in that it worked to interpellate the students as self-governing neo-liberal subjects who understood themselves as being 'at risk'. In other words, if contemporary governance is primarily concerned with seeking 'to foster and shape such capacities so that they are enacted in ways that are broadly consistent with particular objectives such as order, civility, health or enterprise' (Rose 2000: 323) then, in the current climate, a first step in enlisting people into this process is to ensure that they understand themselves as being at risk (Tait 2000). Thus the pedagogical strategies we observed worked in complex ways to constitute the students as such.

The governmentality literature *per se* has tended to focus on 'formal systems of governance' that, not surprisingly, 'neglect the non-rational (including moral) dimensions of governance' (Moore and Valverde 2000: 515). Our focus in this chapter is on the micro-practices of risk technologies in actual classrooms. This leads us to question the primacy afforded to 'expert knowledges' in the govern-mentality literature. Like Moore and Valverde we have found that information about risks appears in a 'highly mixed format that includes scientific data presented . . . alongside moralizing melodramatic narratives' (ibid.: 515). The following discussion explores how HPE operates as a site of governance, by working to constitute the 'at risk self', and the role that both expert and hybrid risk knowledges play in such a project.

Constituting the at risk self

> . . . you think about everything that they have to face and you know, the risks out
> there to them. So we do things like nutrition and physical fitness and we also look
> at issues to do with drugs. So we are teaching them ways of looking after
> themselves, how to eat good food, be physically fit and minimise risks related to
> drugs. We give them knowledge, and then some skills and they can make informed

choices. It is the last chance we have to get at them, to show them the things they can do for themselves, so they can be healthier.

(Interview: Ms Hill HPE – Key Learning Area Manager)

The year 10 course on which this chapter draws was entitled 'Mind Your Own Body' (MYOB). Interestingly, within the title of the course, the governmental imperative of HPE is explicit. One of the fundamental assumptions that underpins the course, which Ms Hill alludes to, is that all students are at risk and that HPE has a role to play in helping students manage the risks, so they can 'look after themselves'. In the case of MYOB the course focus is on providing knowledge and skills in the topic areas of nutrition, physical fitness and drugs, with the objective being to ensure that students can make 'informed choices'. The overall aim is for students to be able to mind *their* own body (an exemplary technology of the self) in a way that is congruous with the broader health/economic concerns of neo-liberal governance of the health of populations. The underlying assumption here is that it is only a lack of knowledge and skills that prevents students from acting rationally to minimise risks. The focus is on individual responsibility for changing health behaviours and this is what characterises contemporary forms of government of the self in HPE: these are the new practices of the self. These exhortations make sense within the risk discourses operating at the micro level of the classroom because they link up with broader public health imperatives to prevent certain harms and diseases associated with nutrition, drug use and physical fitness.

Given the focus of the course, the following analysis and discussion explores the role of risk in enlisting HPE students to engage in practices of governmental self-formation. Ms Hill states in her overview of MYOB that one of their explicit aims is to provide students with 'knowledge'. We suggest that this knowledge is of a particular type and its deployment in the HPE classroom is ostensibly largely about constituting an 'at risk' subject. Within MYOB, the classroom becomes a key site where students are constituted as 'at risk', and learn to understand themselves as either already being at risk, or potentially becoming at risk (essentially at risk of being at risk!). This takes place via a number of pedagogical practices that employ a range of risk knowledges.

Once the students are identified as subjects who understand themselves as being at risk, the rationale of HPE then becomes one of working pedagogically to make sure that students engage in practices that limit risk so as to guard against becoming the unhealthy 'at risk' other. The production of risk was recursive as every opportunity to reiterate risk was taken up by the teachers, in an attempt to ensure that students would not forget they were 'at risk'.

Risk knowledges

The following analysis of classroom data explores how risk knowledges are deployed within the HPE classroom to lead students into understanding themselves as being at risk.

Expert risk knowledges

Expertise is central to the project of governance (Rose 1989), in that it renders a myriad of social fields and spaces governable through a range of practices that seek to document, calculate, classify and evaluate individuals and populations (Peterson and Lupton 1996). Hence, we currently have a proliferation of epidemiological data regarding increasing levels of obesity and the prevalence of so-called lifestyle diseases (cardiovascular disease, diabetes) which are seen as amenable to intervention. These expert knowledges are disseminated in various ways, the HPE classroom being one. In reference to our data, the deployment of expert risk knowledges via the pedagogical space of MYOB occurred in a number of ways, with the effect being to ensure HPE students attained knowledge about their 'at risk' status. The following excerpt from a nutrition classroom highlights how expert risk knowledges are deployed by the teacher, and how such knowledges are utilised in the space to engage the students in the practice of comparing the self, in this case their diet, to expert knowledges about nutrition and dietary risk.

Ms Murry: Okay today we are going to be looking at nutrition, and I want you to write everything down that you ate yesterday and today already.

Class: [General groan.]

Ms Murry: Now once you've done that I want you to go through and make a note of the following things. I'll put them on the board and go over them in a minute. Start writing down what you ate, and be honest with yourself. Be sure to note quantity.

Class: [Another groan.]

[Ms Murry turns to the board and writes down the following list: Fibre, Calcium, Cholesterol, Salt, Sugar.]

Ms Murry: Can I have your attention for a moment please? Now this is for when you have finished noting down what you have eaten. I want you to go to your text and look up each of these on the board [points to board] and find out what they do for you or to you and make some notes. Um, I want you to focus on the following [writes on board as she is talking] What is the RDI? Are you eating the RDI? and What will happen to you if you don't eat the RDI? [stops writing] So girls, basically the consequences of not eating properly, eating the things you should be eating. So, what are the risks to your health? So whether it be related to cancer, CVD [asks a question] Who knows what CVD is? [no one answers] Mmm well, it's in the book. So you might want to organise it under some goals for yourselves like this in your books, like this [compiles the following list on the board].

Goals
Reduce Fat intake
Problems which may occur if this goal is ignored:
My personal goal:
I will lower my fat intake by. . . .

[turning back to the class] So if you can do that for the others here
[pointing to the list]. You can see why you might need to change your
eating habits, if you can see what the risks are to you, yeah?

(Field notes, year 10 HPE class)

This style of activity is commonly utilised within HPE, and there are a number
of pedagogical practices used to deliver this content. Versions we have observed
include: setting of a homework task where the students monitor their food intake
in a food diary; the use of computer software for the analysis; an assessment task
where students report on their eating habits and have to explain why they weren't
inside the dietary guidelines, what the associated risks are, how they could then
improve their diet and monitoring of their health behaviour change. Although there
is much to be made out of the above classroom excerpt and the additional examples,
in this chapter we are interested in how expert risk knowledges are deployed
in this setting. Expert knowledges are used to legitimate the focus on 'healthy'
eating and the teacher uses expert nutrition and risk knowledges as a way of
engaging students in a process of self-knowing in relation to whether they are eating
'properly or not' and what the consequences are to their health if they do not. Her
specific directions require that students 'confess' their diet, to 'be honest' with
themselves and then analyse their diet in light of what expert knowledges recom-
mend. Ms Murry's final comments suggest that if students properly understand the
health risks then they will rationally change their eating behaviours. This mode of
reasoning encapsulates the pedagogical effects and governmental function of HPE,
highlighting the role risk plays within both.

Other risk knowledges

Moore and Valverde (2000) have suggested that there are many domains of
risk governance and that most of the analysis in the field of governmentality studies
to date has focused on rational and expert systems of governance. While we
acknowledge that expert scientific risk knowledges are ever present within the HPE
classroom, they are not the only risk knowledges operating. In our observations
we found that other risk knowledges operated powerfully in the classroom, and
that often the teacher and students worked in combination to produce and reproduce
these. Moore and Valverde (2000) refer to these other risk knowledges as 'hybrid
risk knowledges' where melodramatic and often mythical risk narratives (supported
by popular cultural images) are mixed with scientific information. We suggest that
these hybrid risk knowledges, which are actively produced within the classroom
contexts, are incredibly effective in constituting young people as being at risk. The
veracity of these knowledges is rarely challenged as they work persuasively to
convince the HPE students that they should regulate their health behaviours in
ways that are consistent with broader governmental objectives. The following
excerpt is an example of this:

Ms Hill: Okay what is wrong with being unfit?

Class: [All at once] You get fat, look like Homer Simpson, yuk, you could die.
Ms Hill: So well if you don't want to look like Homer it's important to exercise
             to keep fit.

(Field notes, year 10 HPE class)

The above classroom discussion draws from expert knowledges about being unfit, as well as contemporary cultural icons, in this case Homer Simpson, to try and seduce the students into the project of getting, or keeping, fit. Ms Hill overlooked the students' responses related to death and obesity, what might be deemed to be derived from 'rational' public health discourses. Instead she elected to pick up on the potential risk of looking like Homer to instil the need to exercise. It is possible to discern a 'clash' of discourses in the above excerpt. The promotion of self-esteem (allowing students to voice their opinions without fear or favour, accepting themselves as they are) has a long and not unproblematic history in the HPE classroom. The imperative to 'give voice' or 'express yourself' can be insensitive to the different identifications, self-images and body shapes young people have. It is a testament to the power and the proliferation of risk discourses that concerns about body acceptance are virtually made to disappear. In another example, this time in the topic area of drugs, we found that risk knowledges worked in complex and potentially contradictory ways. In a general discussion about harms associated with drug use, a student commented:

Student: I know a friend who bought some cocaine that had glass in it and it
               was in there so it tore up the stomach so the drug got into the blood
               stream more quickly.
Ms Woods: Well yes that is one of the dangers of buying illegal drugs.

(Field notes, year 10 HPE class)

The student attempts to draw from expert knowledges, in this case pharmacological knowledges, to tell the story about harms associated with cocaine use. What is interesting is that rather than deploy expert drug knowledges that would have questioned the account that cocaine ended up in the stomach, the teacher chose to use the student story to highlight the risks associated with illegal drug use. Here expert knowledge of drug use could have potentially undone the work of 'risk'. Instead, primacy is given to the hybrid knowledge, which conveys the 'Say no to drug use' message very effectively. A similar scenario arises in the following excerpt:

Student: Two girlfriends were in bed and they were on LSD and one of them
               bit her girlfriend's nose off she was so out of it and scared. And then
               she went to the bathroom because she thought that dragons and things
               were coming out of her back. And she picked up a slinky, you know
               those wiry springy things and she started scratching her back with it
               trying to get rid of the dragons and she sawed her head nearly off. It
               was hanging on by a thread.

Ms Murry: It is one of the risks you take isn't it with illegal drugs? You might consider that to be an extreme story and does that make you think that when you use drugs, well that won't happen to me?

(Field notes, year 10 HPE class)

Once again the student's account incorporates expert knowledges and classifications commonly used in the drug field. However, these knowledges are combined to incorporate melodramatic and exaggerated tales of the effects of drug use. Together these knowledges in the classroom produced the risk associated with LSD use. The teacher used the story to reinforce the risk of drug use. In both of the examples it is clear that if the teachers had relied on isolated expert risk discourses about drug use, their responses to the stories could have been very different. For example, if Ms Murry had challenged the slinky story with expert facts about LSD use (or even the impossibility of sawing your head nearly completely off), she would have missed an opportunity to reinforce risk discourses and the individualisation of responsibility. As well, the narrative genre works well in establishing and maintaining interest, something that expert knowledges often struggle to do, and in this way often have more purchase in classroom dialogue. The call on students' voices and experiences is also a persuasive pedagogical device.

Concluding comments

Governing in the neo-liberal context requires that people understand themselves as being 'at risk', and as we have argued, the contemporary field of HPE is inextricably tied to this project. HPE has the explicit intent of working pedagogically to ensure that young people come to learn that they are at risk and are therefore responsible for managing their risks. We have shown that the 'at risk self' is constituted and managed via the deployment, and production, of a range of risk knowledges. Some of the risk knowledges were derived from expert sources and officially enshrined within contemporary policy and curriculum; however, many were what Gore (2002: 4) refers to as 'constructed out of pedagogy itself'. So whilst we acknowledge that policy is an important site for the articulation of dominant discourses in HPE, in this case risk, we also argue that not all of the discourses deployed in HPE are enshrined in the official policy and curriculum texts. Penney and Harris (Chapter 7) refer to this as slippage between policy texts and other texts. In the classrooms, we observed how expert risk knowledges were mobilised in isolation, and as hybrid versions, to guide the students into understanding themselves as being at risk. At times the teacher's deployment of expert knowledges could have, we suggested, operated to challenge the work and effectiveness of risk discourses. This is an important point because it indicates what can and cannot be said in the HPE classroom, and attests to the extent to which the classrooms in our research were constrained by risk imperatives. Even when there were opportunities to contradict risk discourse through the use of expert knowledges, the teachers turned to melodramatic hybrid discourses to sustain the risk identity imperative. Expert knowledges, whatever form they may take, worked in concert with moralising narratives (generated by teachers, students and popular cultural images/messages) to produce the at-risk young person.

What are the chances of disrupting or troubling these practices in our HPE classrooms? A full response to this question is beyond the scope of our discussion, however, as Nick Fox (1999: 29) has argued, 'What is hazardous is often likely to be highly contested'. He maintains that risk is now a part of how we think about ourselves and our social worlds and that:

> These concepts are tied up with the values of a culture and the moral rights and responsibilities of members of that culture, and as such are implicated in how people understand themselves as reflexive, ethical subjects. Because these conceptions are contingent, the subjectivities which are created around risk, health and work are also relative: if this means that we are constrained by cultural constructions of subjectivity, it also means we can resist.
>
> (Fox 1999: 30)

While this indicates the extent to which risk discourse saturates contemporary culture, it also raises a number of important questions which are beyond the scope of this chapter. For example, we might ask, to what extent do the students of HPE take up or resist the risk messages to which they are subjected?

Finally, following Nikolas Rose (2000) we argue that HPE as a governmental space is 'assembled from a complex and hybrid range of technologies' (Rose 2000: 323), and our observations of the HPE classrooms illustrate this discursive complexity. Becoming more cognisant of the discursive complexities that make up the spaces of contemporary HPE will allow us to understand the ways in which HPE acts as a site of governance and the multiple and non-unitary effects of risk and other intersecting discourses. This chapter has mapped some of the discursive practices that might shape young people's understandings of themselves and of others, and the practices of self that HPE pedagogies foster. In order to extend our knowledge of this process, we need more research that explores classroom interactions as well as young people's experience of HPE and their lived engagement with certain practices of the self.

References

Board of Studies (2000) *Health and Physical Education: Curriculum and Standards Framework II*, Carlton: Board of Studies.

Burchell, G. (1996) 'Liberal government and techniques of the self', in A. Barry, T. Osborne and N. Rose (eds) *Foucault and Political Reason*, Chicago: University of Chicago Press.

Dean, M. (1995) 'Governing the unemployed self in an active society', *Economy and Society* 24: 559–83.

Foucault, M. (1988) 'Technologies of the self', in L. Martin, H. Gutman and P. Hutton (eds) *Technologies of the Self*, London: Tavistock.

Fox, N. (1999) 'Postmodern reflections on "risk", "hazards" and "life choices"', in D. Lupton (ed.) *Risk and Sociocultural Theory: New Directions and Perspectives*, London: Cambridge University Press.

Gard, M. and Wright, J. (2001) 'Managing uncertainty: obesity discourses and physical education in a risk society', *Studies in the Philosophy of Education* 20: 535–49.

Gore, J. (2002) 'Some certainties in the uncertain world of classroom practice: an outline of a theory of power relations in pedagogy', paper presented at Australian Association of Research in Education, Brisbane, December 2002.

Kirk, D. (2001) 'Schooling bodies through physical education: insights from social epistemology and curriculum history', *Studies in Philosophy and Education* 20: 475–87.

Lupton, D. (1995) *The Imperative of Health: Public Health and the Regulated Body*, London: Sage.

Lupton, D. (1999a) *Risk*, London: Routledge.

Lupton, D. (1999b) 'Introduction: risk and socio cultural theory', in D. Lupton (ed.) *Risk and Sociocultural Theory: New Directions and Perspectives*, London: Cambridge University Press.

Moore, D. and Valverde, M. (2000) 'Maidens at risk: date rape drugs and the formation of hybrid risk knowledges', *Economy and Society* 29: 514–31.

Peterson, A. (1997) 'Risk, governance and the new public health', in A. Peterson and R. Bunton (eds) *Foucault, Health and Medicine*, London: Routledge.

Peterson, A. and Lupton, D. (1996) *The New Public Health: Health and Self in the Age of Risk*, St Leonards: Allen and Unwin.

Rose, N. (1989) *Governing the Soul: The Shaping of the Private Self*, London: Free Association Books.

Rose, N. (2000) 'Government and control', *British Journal of Criminology* 40: 321–39.

Tait, G. (2000) *Youth, Sex and Government*, New York: Peter Lang.

Tinning, R. and Glasby, T. (2002) 'Pedagogical work and the "cult of the body": considering the role of HPE in the context of the "New Public Health"', *Sport, Education and Society* 7: 109–19.

Turner, B. (1997) 'From governmentality to risk: some reflections on Foucault's contribution to medical sociology', in A. Peterson and R. Bunton (eds) *Foucault, Health and Medicine*, London: Routledge.

10 Gendered bodies and physical identities

Robyne Garrett

Introduction

Recent writing and research on the body (Amour 1999; Bordo 1989, 1992; Frost 2001; Grosz 1995; Kirk 1993) suggests that bodies are both inscribed with and vehicles of culture. This implies that what we eat, how we dress and the way we move are not only inscribed and 'learned' but also serve as mechanisms of social control. As Arthurs and Grimshaw (1999) point out:

> . . . the body is itself the subject of constant social inscription; it is discursively constructed and 'written' on by innumerable forms of social discipline: there is no possibility of a sharp distinction between 'nature' and 'culture'.
>
> (1999: 7)

For young women in particular, the body is both socially constructed by language, visual images and binary oppositions as well as materially acculturated as it conforms to the norms and habitual practices of femininity (Bordo 1992). While young bodies provide sites for the symbolic representation of the ideal female (Wright 1998), deep-rooted ideas about what is desirable in terms of feminine beauty create powerful normalising processes that impact continuously on the way young women see themselves as well as judge those around them.

This chapter focuses on how young women experience their body in contemporary culture and specifically in relation to physical activity. It investigates the lived, embodied experiences of young Australian women in and around physical activity as well as the positioning of their body in the creation of a physical identity. The main theoretical underpinning comes from an understanding that the body is both a socially constructed 'project' as well as a biological phenomenon (Shilling 1993). A further theoretical position takes into account how self-identity is increasingly tied to bodies in contemporary society. The chapter additionally draws on the notion of 'embodiment' to explore how a physical identity is constructed and embodied into the material fabric of the young women in the study.

A feminist post-structuralist approach

Post-structuralist discussions around the body have provided alternative ways of thinking about the body and demonstrate how certain constructions are normalised over others. Foucault (1979, 1984) uses the term 'discourse' to refer to ways of thinking and speaking about aspects of reality. By being more than the communication of knowledge, discourse includes social practices, forms of subjectivity and relations of power. Depending on their availability and currency, it is through these discourses or 'vocabularies of meaning' that individuals are constituted. As Davies (1993) points out: 'In poststructural theory the focus in on the way each person actively takes up the discourse through which they and others speak/write the world into existence *as if it were their own*' (1993: 13, her italics).

Foucault views the notion of power as the constitutive forces that shape and create rather than those that destroy or oppress. He draws attention to the ways that discursive practices create powerful meanings that prescribe human activity and argues that this is a means by which culture attempts to normalise people and bodies. Hence, his notion of the body is that of a surface, acted upon by culture, inscribed with power and mediated in discourse. Foucault (1988) also identifies a form of power that he defines as 'disciplinary power', which is exercised by surveillance rather than force. Through the operation of disciplinary power people behave as if they are constantly watched. This sense is eventually internalised and contributes to an on-going state of self-surveillance or self-policing.

As the body is central to sport and physical activity, feminist writers (Hall 1996; Theberge 1987) in the area have found Foucault particularly relevant. His notions of discourse, surveillance and technologies of the self help us to gain an understanding of the ways in which modern Western society organises itself and regulates people's thoughts and behaviour through disciplinary power. His theories have been useful and relevant to this research in helping to reveal the ways in which young Australian women's bodies are constructed and inscribed with knowledge that impact on self-understanding and involvement in physical activity.

In these contexts there are dominant understandings as well as contradictions and discourses of resistance. For example, on one hand, as McDermott (2000) points out the experience of sport and physical activity can be liberating for women in terms of providing opportunities to develop a positive sense of 'physicality', which, in turn, can lead to the development of a positive physical identity. On the other however, the contradictory positioning of girls and women within sporting and physically active institutions as well as the hegemonic discourses that maintain the status of women in these institutions can have quite the opposite effect.

For Shilling (1993) and Turner (1991) however, the social constructionist perspective provides a less than complete view of the body. They suggest that the body should also be regarded as a material, physical and biological phenomenon, which cannot be reduced to social creation alone. While social relations may profoundly affect the development of bodies, bodies still remain material and biological entities. In developing a notion of 'embodiment' they allow for an analysis of the ways in which social and biological processes are inextricably linked to constitute the 'lived body'.

In keeping with this approach, this chapter attempts to go beyond an analysis of the discourses around the body for young women toward a broader understanding of how young women's lived bodies are constructed, altered and controlled through these discourses. The challenge however, has been to capture the ways in which young women experience their bodies in material and sensual terms, given that the only mechanism of description is that of language which in itself draws on discourse and socially constructed meanings.

The body and self-identity

In the affluent societies of consumer capitalism a visual identity has become almost compulsory. The work of Giddens (1991) in particular, highlights the tendency for people in high modernity to be increasingly tied to their bodies. In exploring the relationship between the body and self-identity he foregrounds bodily appearance and argues that the body actively participates in the construction of the self. Giddens also claims that responsibility for the body is placed on the individual: 'We become responsible for the design of our own bodies, and . . . are forced to do so the more post-traditional the social contexts in which we move' (1991: 102).

While cultural rules have controlled women's bodies throughout history, under an enduring 'cult of thinness' in the Western world (and increasingly with global-isation, developing countries) women are not permitted to be large nor take up space. Their subordinate status in the gender order is only exaggerated when the female identity is increasingly linked to a visual projection, which in itself is grounded in self-control and management of the body. Shilling (1993) points out that the enduring expectation of thinness removes women from active participation in society and restricts their social, physical and emotional potential. The concept has become so self-sustaining, so internalised, that no external reinforcement is necessary. As suggested by Kirk and Wright (1995) identity is then constructed through evaluations of the body as if judged by others. These are mechanisms by which identity becomes 'embodied'.

During the adolescent years young female bodies are developing physically and sexually. The ideology of 'woman as object' begins to dominate, as they increasingly become the focus of both male and female comment, gaze or criticism. The female participants in this study have learned particular interpretations of their bodies since birth through their experiences in a white, middle-class culture. They have embodied social ideas presented by this culture and these ideas have become the means by which they judge themselves and others. Thus it has been important to this research to identify how discourses around thinness have been picked up, internalised and interpreted, as well as how they have come to impact on their physical and embodied identities.

The embodiment of a physical identity

In schools we are taught how to think about and experience our bodies. They are institutions in and through which bodies are raced, classed, gendered, disciplined and shaped (Kirk 1993). For many, schooling is a site characterised by a pre-occupation with conformity, management and control over the body (Oliver and Lalik 2001; Shapiro 1994). Routine practices and procedures promote compliance and obedience and often deny the needs and potential of the body to act as an instrument of learning. With much of the educative process being confined to cognitive tasks and 'desks', a lack of space and opportunity only creates further distance between learning and the body. Instead, young people can learn powerful messages about control and the need for their body to be invisible. As Brian Fay (1987) argues there are consequences for young bodies and identities as learning is not simply a cognitive process but also a somatic one in which 'oppression leaves its traces not just in people's minds but in their muscles and skeletons as well' (1987: 146).

Bodies are gendered through social, institutional and material experiences that shape behaviour, appearance, bodily habits and desires. Through continuous bodily practice, gender is 'performed' and it is through the on-going process of gender performance that the nature and meaning of people's bodies are physically altered. Knowledge of gender becomes deeply inscribed in muscle and skeletal systems, postures, gaits and styles of movement. Connell's work (1995) on the construction of the gendered body picks up on the concept of the body as both a social and biological entity. He argues that gendered social practices do not simply negate the body but transcend and transform it. Different opportunities and thus material experiences afforded to girls and boys to engage in physical activity contribute to these transformations. It is not only that male and females think differently about their bodies, rather their bodies are physically altered through gendered practices.

For example, as Whitson (1994) points out, childhood activities teach young males to use their bodies in coordinated and forceful ways. Boys learn to develop force and transmit force through their bodies thus providing them with an accurate knowledge of their physical capacities as well as changing and strengthening their bodies. In contrast, girls are often characterised as failing to take advantage of the torque that can be generated when the entire body is engaged in forceful action. On the basis of her earlier phenomenological study of young women's movement Iris Marion Young (1980) suggests that

> for the most part, girls and women are not given the opportunity to use their full body capacities in free and open engagement with the world, nor are they encouraged as much as boys to develop specific bodily skills.
>
> (Young 1980: 153)

It is suggested that these partial and half-hearted actions are derived from social practices that have encouraged girls and women to experience their bodies as objects for others, rather than forceful, active and strong.

In taking a feminist perspective, McDermott (2000) calls for new notions of 'physicality' that correspond with how women experience themselves physically, and particularly in relation to the complex interplay of body and self perception. Kevin Young's (1997) work, incorporating a notion of physicality, gives evidence of the substantial variation and contradiction in female experiences of physical activity. His work documents the empowering and emancipatory potential of the physical use of the body by women. However, he also notes that the acceptance of dominant and gendered sporting discourses provide ambiguous meanings on 'matters of aggression, injury, femininity, and the feminist label' (1997: 303). Clearly, whilst some women are active in creating new physical identities, others continue to provide evidence of the contradictory project that is an active female body.

Bodytalk

In keeping with these concepts, this research has attempted to identify how a number of young, white, middle-class Australian women in their final year of schooling (17–18 years) came to know their bodies, their gender and their physical selves. This chapter specifically focuses on the relationship between experiences of the body and the development of a physical or self-identity. Data were collected through a series of interviews or conversations with participants, which were designed to draw out personal experiences and feelings on a range of topics. These included understanding of femininity; personal experiences of physical activity; perceptions of the body; gendered understandings; experiences of physical education; and the forms of physical activity made available (and not available) to young women.

As an outcome of these conversations 'physical stories' were mutually constructed and co-authored with participants using their language, texts and expression. Co-authoring is a method that feminists have employed in order to give up some of the control the researcher has over the research agenda and knowledge produced from it. The intent of the story construction process was to create a small cameo of a personal yet significant experience in the life of the participant specifically related to their experiences of and involvement in physical activity. While the authoring process varied from one individual to another in terms of the participant input and critique, attempt was made to capture the essence and 'lived' experience of a physical culture for the individual concerned. The resulting 'physical stories' serve to identify and illustrate the complex processes whereby young female bodies become active and physical as well as the processes whereby they are denied this power.

Generally the young women in this study gave evidence of multiple and changing bodily experiences or 'positions' regarding the relationship between the body, identity and physical activity. These bodily positions varied significantly and many participants moved fluidly between them depending on context, personal experiences and discourses available. However, in drawing on evidence from participant interviews and physical stories, a number of apparent, bodily experiences emerged regarding the relationship between the body, identity and physical activity. While it is artificial to separate these positions, as they shifted, overlapped and sometimes occurred simultaneously, they will be discussed independently in order to show both commonality and difference.

For this chapter I have drawn on interview data and physical stories to give evidence of three bodily positions. The 'Comfortable' body, the 'Bad' body and the 'Different' body have been selected for analysis as they most closely relate to connections between the body and identity construction. These positions also give evidence of the wide variation in 'lived' experiences of the young women within a physical culture. In the analysis that follows, an attempt has been made to identify the social and discursive practices that serve to inscribe bodies and impact on 'lived' bodily experiences. The physical stories give further evidence of these positions as well as illuminate the complexity and interconnectedness of an individual's subjectivity with regard to their body, gender and physical identity.

The Comfortable body

The term 'Comfortable' body was chosen to depict a bodily position derived from both acceptance of and satisfaction with the body. For those taking up this bodily position, the body was important and closely tied to self-identity in a positive way. Discourses around the need to be slim were clearly evident, as were those that perceived sport and physical activity as means to achieve a 'good' body. Thus in the context of this study the term 'comfortable' was attributable to individuals who were satisfied with their bodies *because* they complied with white, middle-class and Western conceptions of an acceptable female body.

Individuals indicated contentment about themselves, their gender and their body. Their physical experiences had usually been well supported in that there had had plenty of opportunities to develop motor skills and abilities that, in most cases tended to be 'appropriate' to their gender. Individuals were either committed to one form of physical activity or enjoyed participation in a number of different activities. Their statements often linked activity as a means to achieve a 'good' body with an unproblematic acceptance of the relationship between activity and health. They did not generally see a contradiction between being female and being muscular – as long as they weren't *too* big. However, it was certainly important for them not to be 'fat'. Whilst few could give a clear definition about what being 'fat' really meant, many were quick to comment that they were happy that they were not burdened with this 'problem'.

In the story that follows Lori positions her self within a comfortable body position, which impacts strongly on her personal identity, though she does move in and out of this position. The positive nature of her experiences in and around basketball contributes significantly to her self-identity. However, while she is very aware of her own 'good' body, she continues to survey herself and those around her.

Lori's Story: Basketball

My dad and family got me into sport. I was the youngest of three and I did everything my brother and sister did, and they did everything. Dad was pretty active too. I just kept playing basketball because I was good at it. It made me feel good about myself.

Basketball is great! It gives you energy and you feel good when you have done something good. You just feel like you are really healthy. After basketball you feel great cause you have cleaned your system out. It makes you feel strong, like you could play forever. Some of my best friends come from basketball. We do heaps together. My best memories were getting trophies. One year I won 'Best and fairest', it was such a big shock. After that I used to try even harder.

My idol is Michelle Timms. She is so fast on the court I think she is fantastic. She cuts her hair so short though and she's pretty muscly. I don't think that it's all that feminine, she probably can't help it though. She's still a great player. I used to think that if I played too much sport I would get too big but I don't think about it much now. It annoys me that some people can't help it and they get paid out [for being big].

There is so much pressure on girls to be thin. Guys do it. If you are not slim then you are not attractive. Girls do it too though; they can be unbelievably critical. Girls pick up on little things and they are so judgemental. I used to be really self-conscious but I do so much sport now that it keeps me in pretty good shape. I don't like my nose though. I'd like to look like Liz Hurley.

The nature and meaning of Lori's involvement in basketball has strongly impacted on her sense of self-identity. Lori's identity is tied to her sport and tied to discourses around activity and fitness, which are demonstrated, in the 'good body' that has resulted from lots of activity. She picks up on discourses around feeling good about herself and more confident through excelling in basketball. These rewards have motivated her continued participation.

She is generally comfortable with her body; however, having a body which is toned and devoid of fat is important to her. While being well aware of the pressures on women to be thin, Lori does not seem to appreciate that she perpetuates these discourses in her own surveillance of 'less suitable' bodies' like that of Michelle Timms. While her story expresses some frustration with traditional stereotypes that do not condone muscles for women, again she contributes to the perpetuation of these discourses with her comments on Michelle's looks not being 'all that feminine'. Somehow there is a need for Michelle to be both a great player and feminine, with feminine representing fairly limited characteristics or at least longer hair.

For individuals like Lori, being comfortable with their body seems to be a self-fulfilling cycle. By drawing on activity/fitness discourses they are able to feel 'OK' enough to present their bodies in the public sphere and to participate in regular physical activity. These individuals reap the rewards of participation on many levels. Socially, they are able to develop and enjoy their position within a group. Physically, they develop physical skills and competencies that give them greater bodily and physical confidence. Aesthetically, they develop a body that is toned, flexible and 'attractive', and emotionally, they develop a strong physical sense and acceptance of themselves. However, for the individual who does not experience the comfortable bodily position the associated rewards are definitely far less available.

The Bad body

The category of 'Bad' body was constructed to describe those participants who expressed dissatisfaction and a non-acceptance of their body. In taking up this position, self-identity was closely tied with attitudes and feelings toward the body and in most cases these feelings were negative. Discourses around the need for slimness were clearly evident and in many cases connected to social acceptance. Consistently, the young women taking up this position endured 'big body concerns' which impacted significantly on their sense of identity, social behaviour and involvement in physical activity.

These individuals were extremely conscious of their appearance and internalised a form of self-surveillance that focused on 'fat'. Whilst this is not surprising, given the number of social messages that condemn fat and value appearance as a sign of personal worth, at times their concern bordered on obsession and consequentially influenced their functioning in everyday affairs including their involvement in physical activity. These young women did not view themselves as physical or 'sporty' in any way. It seemed evident in their dialogue that they had had few opportunities to develop physical skills in an environment where they didn't feel watched and judged by others.

Dissatisfaction with their body was evident in their posture, their talk and their motion. As such they had embodied a damaged physical identity. Some seriously thought that their entire life experience would change and social transitions would be smoother if their body was different. By drawing on a discourse that severely curtailed their active participation in society, they believed that their whole life would be better if their body was 'thinner'.

Bartky (1988) suggests that a sense of female shame is related to the extent to which they have internalised patriarchal standards of bodily acceptability. Kerry's story speaks for itself in giving evidence of a sense of not measuring up to these standards. As a consequence her embodied identity is 'damaged' and her on-going engagement in a physical culture is severely compromised.

Kerry's Story: I feel awkward

The greatest pressure at the moment is schoolwork. I just don't have time for physical activity. I'm not really a sports person. During my time at school I haven't been involved in sport much at all. There is no real reason I just haven't. My family isn't really sporty and there is such a big age difference between my brothers and me. By the time I was to be involved in school sports my brothers were finished. I never really had anyone else to go with. In primary school I played netball for a bit but in high school I wasn't really interested except when we were forced to in PE. I sort of don't want to do it.

I didn't enjoy PE either. We had boys in the class and if you were on teams or getting picked and you weren't very good at sport then you would get put down and you would feel bad about that. They would just tell you that you were '[.] useless and that you can't play' or 'why is she on our team?' It was always said to the few of us who weren't any good at anything. From what they said I just accepted that I wasn't very good at anything. I felt pretty nervous if it was ever my turn especially when the team was depending on me. If you do bad then you will let them down again. They would say 'Ah good one'. I just felt rotten. It was the boys mainly because when we had an all girls' class there wasn't as much competitiveness and we all sort of supported each other. It was a lot better.

I hated softball where you have all the boys and girls picked into teams and you might miss your three strikes and everyone is looking at you. Everyone would just laugh. I didn't really bother with sport after that. Badminton was all right because I could do that and people didn't seem to be watching you all of the time.

In high school we had to change and because I was overweight I felt really bad because we had to wear like short netball skirts and t-shirts. I never felt comfortable. I would always prefer to wear long tracky pants, even in summer.

I don't really feel confident around all of the other skinny girls. Well, most of them are skinny and pretty. The boys like them. I was never that popular with the boys. My friends are good because my weight is not an issue for them, but I just feel like a bit of an outsider. Every commercial or magazine I see, I just think 'gosh I'm nothing like them'. They are beautiful and 'wow' they are skinny. It puts me off being involved in sports because I feel so out of place. I feel like people must say; 'Oh she's not fit' or 'She can't play because she is overweight' and stuff like that. It puts me off bothering.

Mum and Dad wanted me to get into some sort of sport so I did tennis for a while. It lasted about a month and a half. My coach sort of put me down because I was overweight. He told me I could do things better or that I wasn't trying or just comments. I was just really self-conscious about my body. I didn't like it if I knew he was watching. I would always mess up.

The PE teachers didn't really relate to me either. Most of the time I felt like I was invisible. They pay attention to the good kids. They would always ask them to go first. This was the perception I got anyway, maybe they didn't mean to. You didn't feel that they gave you much support. If you went up to do something, when your turn was over that was it. They wouldn't say anything. But if it was one of the good people who went up then they would pay a lot more attention.

Other people that are bigger like me I've noticed, like, some of us feel the same way. You know we're not the skinny mugs and we feel left out because of it. Because of my weight I don't feel confident. Like you don't know if people are looking at you or not but I just feel bad. If you have to go up in front of the class and give a speech or something, I'm not confident because you know that everyone is looking at you. I don't know but I know that I don't like being the centre of attention.

Just from the image you get of people doing sport you get the idea 'No I can't do that 'cause I'm not fit'. Whatever you see on TV is so far from where I'm at. It stops you from trying. There are probably a lot of things that you think that you might try if there wasn't that image that is presented to you of the beautiful and skinny person. I wouldn't even go to a gym – all those mirrors – Yuk. I'd definitely be happier if I were smaller. My whole life would be different.

There are many discourses identified in Kerry's story that impact on her physicality. The story provides a sad indictment on the institutions of physical education and sport in attempting to support her physical skills and develop a positive physical identity. Kerry partakes in a system of self-surveillance from which she continues to emerge as 'lacking'.

The dimensions of her involvement in physical activity generally have been severely hampered by her unfavourable perceptions of her body and lack of physical skills. Kerry has internalised that she is not 'sporty' and consequently is not 'good at anything'. These self-perceptions seem to have gone unquestioned or unchallenged by any of her experiences within physical education over twelve years, or within the few sporting activities her parents have encouraged her to try. Her experiences within these institutions if anything have perpetuated the very limiting self-perceptions and discourses she holds firmly 'that one needs to be slim to be seen' and 'you need to have skills before you attempt anything' in the presence of others.

Kerry's physical experiences are influenced considerably by a wider culture that celebrates thinness. The nature of physical activity itself often requires more revealing attire and thus emphasises an already body-focused activity. The nature and meaning of Kerry's involvement was more about a fear of being seen and judged rather than the physical demands of the activity.

Questions could be asked about what occurs in a physical education programme over ten years for an individual to emerge feeling that they are not 'good at anything'. Is it the nature of a sport-based programme, where notions of competition can serve to alienate individuals, or is it a teacher's focus on, and celebration of, students who are already talented? Either way, when an individual emerges from a system 'feeling ignored' it appears to have major ramifications on the development of a physical identity and continued enjoyment of a physical culture.

Kerry also acknowledges harassment from boys as contributing to negative physical experiences. It seems that gender has been constructed during her school experiences in ways that have made harassment behaviours more available as social discourses to boys whilst more supportive behaviours were more available to girls. This would only have exacerbated Kerry's anxiety in presenting herself within a physical activity setting. Clearly though, the most significant discourse that has inhibited the development of a sense of physicality for Kerry is the discourse around the need for thinness. It has impacted negatively on her sense of self and provides an enduring legacy in constraining the development of her physicality and physical identity.

The Different body

The 'Different' body position was constructed to represent individuals for whom the appearance of their body was less important to the construction of their self or physical identity. These young women were more likely to perceive themselves as different from the status quo and outside many of the existing discourses around the body, gender and physical activity. In contrast to the previous position though, individuals taking up a 'different' bodily position referred favourably to the 'lived' experience of their body.

Generally individuals in this position did not pick up on traditional discourses that centred on a visual identity. While their sense of self-identity was not necessarily tied to their body appearance, it was often tied to the experience of physical activity. Their narratives suggested that they enjoyed the sensuality and physicality of movement without feeling that their bodies were 'on show' or 'unworthy'. The nature and meaning of their involvement in activity revolved around sensation and empowerment rather than a focus on the body.

Some individuals indicated that they were frustrated with other girls who were 'caught up' with their looks and the appearance of the body. While they did not see themselves as drawing on these discourses to constitute their own identities at the time or having been influenced by these social pressures, they were not unaware of these discourses or their impact on people of their age. Vicky, for instance, said: 'I can see myself getting into the trap of saying why am I like this and why can't I be thinner and stuff but I think there's too many other things to enjoy' and from Tess, 'Well, I'm not going to starve myself to be skinny but it's just pumped into your brain'. In taking up this position participants talked about how women were portrayed in the media. Some felt that there were clear messages for women to 'be weak and stay weak' and spoke out on issues concerning gender inequality. Others expressed the view that health and functional fitness were more important to them than looks, thus picking up on notions of a medical model of health, which is no less body-based than discourses around appearance. However, their discussions exhibited an ability to seriously challenge taken-for-granted understandings around gender and the body, and at times they were successful in rejecting restrictive discourses to further their physical potential.

Marie's story gives an account of an individual who offers some resistance to traditional notions of femininity and the body. She presents a complex interplay of discourses seen to be traditionally feminine (creative) as well as discourses considered in a traditional sense to be more attention-seeking. In her story, Marie breaks boundaries of what women's bodies are supposed to 'be' as well as what young women are supposed to 'do' in terms of physical activity forms.

Marie's Story: I'm a bit different

People describe me as pretty creative. I play guitar, draw, and play on the computer. Probably, I'll move into something like multimedia or graphic design when I leave school, something in the creative field. I am a bit different and I like to be that way but I'm also a bit of an attention-seeker. You know, like to go over the edge. That can get to people sometimes because I say what I think and sometimes they don't like it. I've got to watch that. Sportwise, I'm more of a team person. I've tried almost every sport imaginable but I stuck with netball and football. Yes football, most people don't believe me, then they say 'I suppose that's typical of you Marie'. The social side of sport is what really attracts me. It's a good feeling being around others and doing things together.

When I was younger, if I didn't have someone to go with then I wouldn't go at all. Being an only child was pretty lonesome and I really liked it when my cousins were around. They were all boys and that's where I learnt to love football. My dad was a footballer too and I used to have lots of kicks with him and my cousins. They never left me out. We were really close. I was more a tomboy than a girl because I loved guy sports. Dresses were definitely out. My get up was jeans and gum-boots and getting wet. Probably that's why I prefer the company of guys to girls even now. Girls are really bitchy and guys are more down to earth and they don't say things like 'Oh! I've broken a nail'.

Some people think football is only for the boys. They didn't say it to my face but you could tell. There were a lot of girls who would have liked to do it too. But none of them could actually be bothered. They really missed out. They were too scared of what other people would think of them if they did it, you know, call them a lesbian and stuff. It happens too. When I talked to some of the guys at school and they found out that I played football they said 'Excuse me, girls don't play football'. I just thought 'you sexist pig' kind of thing but I said 'Well you are looking at one who does'. I really don't care what they think. I'm comfortable with my body and doing what I want to do. So if anyone says 'No you can't' then they can go and get stuffed.

I care about my appearance. I just don't fit into the feminine category all that well. And I'm not going to get caught up in all of this 'you must be thin' stuff. If I go out with a guy, he has to like my body or me for who I am, not necessarily what I look like. I'm just not going to be told how to act and I don't follow other people like sheep. People think that I am really confident and they try and intimidate me but they don't really know me at all. They think that I am really competitive too, and aggressive but that's not the case either. Sure I like to do well in the things that I know I'm good at. But I love to paint just as much as I like sport. People always try to put you into a little box and say 'Well you are like this'. They don't know at all. I'm happy being me but I'm lots of things.

I used to be a real wuss in primary school. I cried all the time, I don't know why. I knew what it was like not to be able to do something and having everyone laughing at you. I was sort of always on the outer. You know the last one to be picked in teams. It's amazing how things can change but I won't ever forget that. You get sort of affected by it and you start thinking that you really are a clux. My best memories are winning the premierships in both football and netball. In football once I actually kicked five goals and two points in ten minutes and I thought 'Wow I actually did that'. I felt really good inside myself. It's amazing how a good comment from someone or praise can make you feel so good about yourself and you feel really happy and accepted.

Marie's sporting pursuits give evidence of the way that she struggles to incorporate both masculine and feminine characteristics into her ways of being. Both netball and football offer attraction to her in terms of their social and competitive opportunities. In talking about these activities she draws on discourses around competition, playing well, scoring, extending herself and being a valuable team player. Both her father and her male cousins have accommodated her football participation and most significantly, made her feel included in their pursuits. This social situation allowed her to develop physical competence in a supportive and non-judgemental environment. She does however characterise herself as a 'tomboy', thereby suggesting that she also draws on dominant discourses of 'femininity' to explain her participation, that is, she accepts that it is not 'normal' female behaviour to play football, even if she has few investments in such notions of 'normality'.

Her childhood experiences have left her feeling comfortable in the company of males and she seems to reject traditional female discourses around body maintenance and over concern with bodily appearance.

Generally, Marie refuses to be positioned in terms of traditional discourses on gender. She doesn't like the idea that there should be gender rules which dictate how males and females should look, act, speak and play in a certain way and in certain activities. While she chooses to reject a male/female dualism along with some of its constitutive elements, in contradiction with this, she is reliant on this dualism for the maintenance of her position as 'different'. Her involvement in football has led her to experience or imagine animosity from those who do not consider it an appropriate female pastime. She feels that it is 'they' who have missed out on a fun pastime by internalising a gendered surveillance system. Marie, on the other hand, continues to play despite some strong barriers in the form of lesbian innuendo and total dismissal by male peers at school. Her strong physical identity and physical competence have enabled her to disregard those who criticise her football-playing.

Whilst her appearance is significant to her, Marie refuses to allow these discourses to completely consume her. She desires to be seen as an individual who is complete in herself. Marie's self-identity is less directly connected to her bodily appearance and more connected to her bodily skills and social confidence, both of which have taken time to develop. Childhood experiences have left her with a clear memory of being very much on the outer of the social group as well as the victim of harassment. Whilst Marie admits to being damaged by these experiences, she has developed a strong physical identity that allows her to resist many traditional notions of femininity and discourses around thinness. She also reaffirms the positive influence that personal praise has had on her physical achievements and sense of self.

Potential for change

In drawing on Giddens' (1991) theories on the body and self-identity, this chapter has attempted to investigate how young Australian women experience their body in contemporary culture and specifically in relation to a physical culture. While Foucault's theories on discourse, surveillance and technologies of the self have provided tools to analyse how meaning and control is created around the body, Shilling (1993) and Turner's (1991) notion of embodiment have allowed this analysis to be extended in order to consider how these meanings are given material form within a physical identity.

The bodily positions presented in this chapter give some evidence of the multiple ways in which young women experience their bodies and embody a physical identity. The young women in the study experienced themselves and their bodies in multiple and sometimes contradictory ways. Those young women, whom I have associated with a 'comfortable' position, demonstrated an embodied 'physicality' that enabled them to develop physical skills that in turn supported their on-going participation, social success and 'appropriate' body shape. Alternatively, this form of physicality was denied to those who had linked notions of a poor body with poor physical skills. It seems evident that for some young women, the development of a positive physical identity is compromised by experiences within a damaged female body. Whilst some of these issues are powerfully driven by a popular culture with vested economic interests in creating feelings of inadequacy, challenges and possibilities for the field of physical education can still be identified.

Young women are often trapped in this way by a vicious cycle where appearance is closely tied to self-worth and responsibility for the body is placed on the individual (Featherstone 1991). They also have to contend with an ideology that suggests they have choices and control over what sort of body they have. In drawing on discourses that link social standing to a slim body, Kerry gave evidence of a constrained body that she experienced as lacking in many ways and was definitely not comfortable being exposed in public. The need to challenge discourses that dictate what active bodies should be and should look like is clearly apparent.

Given that young women come to understand themselves in terms of their bodies, there is also a distinct need for them to have significant opportunities to critically examine their own lived experiences of their bodies. Presently, little attention is paid in schools to girls' increasing concern and even obsession with their bodies (Oliver and Lalik 2001). However, if the body were to become a focal topic in the school curriculum, attention could be drawn to the way social meanings are attached to the body, internalised and exert powerful influences on identity and behaviour. The capacity of a young woman to at least, partially recognise the role of the body in the constitution of the self is what makes resistance to dominant modes of subjectivity production possible. Perhaps then, through the construction of a more resilient female body can we see a way forward and a means by which young women can refuse discourses that restrict their personal and physical potential.

The notion of a physical identity developed in this chapter resonates with Young's (1997) concept of a woman's sense of physicality as a means by which young women can also begin to resist traditional notions of femininity and restrictive social discourses. Some young women recollected their bodily experiences in ways that extended beyond dominant appearance ideals. For those like Marie, physical activity and sport offered opportunities to experience their bodies in powerful and skilful ways. Her narratives indicate how a positive physical identity enabled her to refuse traditional gender positionings and experience herself as strong rather than fragile and less limited in choice of physical pursuits.

It seems that if physical education is to retain its cultural relevance and meaning to the lives of young people it must reflect on and actively challenge constructions of the body in popular culture that work against the development of a positive physical identity. Additionally, it is important to note that these identities are not only constructed discursively and materially but also dynamically in the relationships between males and females. Positive change for young women is therefore less likely to occur if issues of masculinity are not also addressed. Hence, physical education has major roles to play in challenging constructions of gender, both male and female, which serve to limit physical opportunities for any individual.

Young people need space, time and opportunities to develop and reflect on their physical potential. They need to develop competence and learn to be in control of their bodies in safe and supported environments. Many unresolved tensions and contradictions around gender, the body and physical activity still stand. By confronting these tensions physical education can assist young people to value physical activity as a pleasurable, sensual experience and an important part of life.

References

Amour, K. (1999) 'The case for a body-focus in education and physical education', *Sport, Education & Society* 4: 5–15.

Arthurs, J. and Grimshaw, J. (1999) 'Introduction', in J. Arthurs and J. Grimshaw (eds) *Women's Bodies: Discipline and Transgression*, London: Cassell.

Bartky, S. (1988) 'Foucault, femininity and the modernization of patriarchal power', in I. Diamond and L. Quinby (eds) *Feminism and Foucault: Rejections on Resistance*, Boston, MA: Northeastern University Press, 61–86.

Bordo, S. (1989) 'The body and the reproduction of femininity: a feminist appropriation of Foucault', in A. Jagger and S. Bordo (eds) *Gender/Body/Knowledge: Feminist Reconstructions of Being and Knowing*, London: Rutgers University Press.

Bordo, S. (1992) 'Postmodern subjects, postmodern bodies', *Feminist Studies* 18: 159–76.

Connell, R. (1995) *Masculinities*, St Leonards, NSW: Allen and Unwin.

Davies, B. (1993) *Shards of Glass: Children Reading and Writing Beyond Gendered Identities*, New Jersey: Hampton.

Fay, B. (1987) *Critical Social Science*, Ithaca: Cornell University Press.

Featherstone, M. (1991) 'The body in consumer culture', in M. Featherstone, M. Hepworth and B. Turner (eds) *The Body: Social Process and Cultural Theory*, London: Sage.

Foucault, M. (1979) *Discipline and Punish: The Birth of the Prison*, New York: Vintage Books.

Foucault, M. (1984) *The History of Sexuality: Part 1*, Harmondsworth: Penguin.

Foucault, M. (1988) 'Technologies of the self', in L. Martin, H. Gutman and P. Hutton (eds) *Technologies of the Self*, Amherst, MA: University of Massachusetts Press.

Frost, L. (2001) *Young Women and the Body*, Basingstoke: Palgrave.

Giddens, A. (1991) *Modernity and Self-Identity*, Cambridge: Polity Press.

Grosz, E.A. (1995) *Space, Time, and Perversion: The Politics of Bodies*, St Leonards, NSW: Allen and Unwin.

Hall, A. (1996) *Feminism and Sporting Bodies: Essays on Theory and Practice*, Champaign, IL: Human Kinetics.

Kirk, D. (1993) *The Body Schooling and Culture*, Geelong, Australia: Deakin University.

Kirk, D. and Wright, J. (1995) 'The construction of bodies: implications for health and physical education curriculum', *Unicorn* 21: 63–73.

McDermott, L. (2000) 'A qualitative assessment of the significance of body perception to women's physical activity experiences: revisiting discussions of physicalities', *Sociology of Sport Journal* 17: 331–63.

Oliver, K. and Lalik, R. (2001) 'The body as curriculum: learning with adolescent girls', *Journal of Curriculum Studies* 33: 303–33.

Shapiro, S. (1994) 'Re-membering the body in critical pedagogy', *Education and Society* 12: 61–79.

Shilling, C. (1993) *The Body and Social Theory*, London: Sage.

Theberge, N. (1987) 'Sport and women's empowerment', *Women's Studies International Forum* 10: 387–93.

Turner, B. (1991) 'Recent developments in the theory of the body', in M. Featherstone, M. Hepworth and B. Turner (eds) *The Body: Social Process and Cultural Theory*, London: Sage.

Whitson, D. (1994) 'The embodiment of gender: discipline, domination and empowerment', in S. Birrell and C. Cole (eds) *Women, Sport, and Culture*, Champaign, IL: Human Kinetics.

Wright, J. (1998) *Gender, the State and Education: Images of the Body*, Geelong, Vic.: Deakin Centre for Education and Change Faculty of Education Deakin University.

Young, I. (1980) 'Throwing like a girl: a phenomenology of feminine comportment, motility and spatiality', *Human Studies* 3: 137–56.

Young, K. (1997) 'Women, sport and physicality', *International Review for the Sociology of Sport* 32: 297–306.

11 From performance to impairment

A patchwork of embodied memories

Andrew C. Sparkes

Introduction

Our lives in and as bodies profoundly shape our sense of identity. As Jackson (1990) states:

> Even though my body seems the most private and hidden part of me, I carry my life history in my body, almost like the way the age rings of a sawn tree trunk reveal the process through time. My personal history of social practices and relationships is physically embodied in the customary ways I hold my body, imagine its size and shape, and in its daily movements and interactions.
>
> (Jackson 1990: 48)

The body, therefore, as Smith and Watson (2001) suggest, is a site of autobiographical knowledge, as well as a textual surface upon which a person's life is inscribed. For them, the body is a site of autobiographical knowledge because 'memory itself is embodied. And the life narrative is a site of embodied knowledge because autobiographical narrators are embodied subjects' (p. 37). Memories serve particular personal and social functions within the stories we tell ourselves, and others, to explain who we are, what we are, and where we are in life at a particular time and place. As Antoniou (2003) notes:

> Through telling/writing our memories, we piece together our embodied identities. We construct a sense of our bodies/selves. And we do this via a 'patchwork' process. We sew together scraps. Of physical sensation, emotion, images, words . . . Of messages from outside ourselves. And from inside ourselves. To create seemingly coherent – but inevitably patchworked – accounts of past events. And seemingly coherent – but inevitably patchworked – bodies/selves.
>
> (Antoniou 2003: 148–9)

Of course, as Smith and Sparkes (2002) remind us, storytellers *do* coherence through *artful* practices. They recognise the essential reflexivity of coherence and the manner in which this is a negotiated achievement among the participants involved in the telling and listening to a story. Memory, therefore, refers to the *retelling* of the past from the experience of the present. They are active practices that involve current thoughts, wishes and motivations. Therefore, memories are not the 'truth' of the past. Nor are they 'facts'. According to Stanley and Morgan (1993), like all autobiographical acts they are works of artifice and fabrication. They are a partial, selective, weaving together of events, persons and feelings which are not necessarily connected to one another within the life as it was actually lived.

Furthermore, in considering the relationship between narrative and reality, Neisser (1994) provides four controversial categories with regard to autobiographical memory:

> (1) actual past events and the *historical self* who participated in them; (2) those events as they were experienced, including the individual's own *perceived self* at the time; (3) the *remembering self*, that is, the individual in the act of recalling those events on some later occasion; and (4) the *remembered self* constructed on that occasion.
>
> (Neisser 1994: 2)

Neisser (1994) also speaks of the *oblivious self*, and warns that autobiographical memory is best taken with a grain of salt. This is because, for him, 'The self that is remembered today is not the historical self of yesterday, but only a reconstructed version. A different version – a new remembered self – may be reconstructed tomorrow' (p. 8).

With the above points in mind, in this chapter I construct an autoethnographic tale (Sparkes 2002a) to provide a partial, selective, somewhat ragged, and loosely stitched patchwork of memories that relate to my transition from a performing body to an impaired body, and the identity dilemmas this has instigated for me. Importantly, as Ellis and Bochner (2000: 739) emphasise, autoethnography is an autobiographical genre of writing and research that 'displays multiple layers of consciousness, connecting the personal to the cultural'. Thus, writing about my own experiences, rather than an act of self-indulgence, becomes a form of social analysis (see Sparkes 2000, 2002b). This is because culture circulates through all of us, the self is a social phenomenon, all identity is relational, and my subjective experience is part of the world I (we) inhabit.

In what follows, there are impressions of memories as recalled by me, and also impressions made by others that I do not recall but remain connected to me in stories told about me. For example, I do not remember an elite, non-problematic, performing body I inhabited in my youth, and so I have called upon what was written publicly about this body. Other memories of impairment and pain are more immediate (but none the less constructed) and I explore these in various genres. In the process, I stage the text by calling upon different voices. Thus, following Tsang (2000), in the stories told there is my *experiential* voice through which different identities and bodies announce and foreground themselves while others regress. Formal *academic* voices are also incorporated that I call upon without direct explanation in order to hint to the reader some of the multiple interpretations that might exist regarding my experiential stories. My hope is that by adopting this strategy, various voices mingle in a multi-layered text that draws the reader in, allowing them to construct their own meanings from their current position in relation to mine.

As part of this process, a number of issues are raised for discussion regarding the complexities of embodiment and gendered self-identity (de/re)construction via sport and physical activity (for further reflections, see Sparkes 1996, 2003; Sparkes and Silvennoinen 1999). For example, following Antoniou (2003), I (we) might ask the following questions as the text unfolds. What is the relationship between my memories and my body, then, now, and in the future? How are my memories experienced in embodied ways? What do my memories tell me about the social, historical and political location(s) of my body? What do they reveal about the socialisation of my body? What role do my memories play in my knowledge-making practices. You as the reader are invited to ask these same questions of yourself, and to add others of your own.

Academic voice(s)

The lived body is not just a thing in the world but a way *in* which the world comes to be. (Leder 1990: 25)

Bodies, in their own right as bodies, do matter. They age, get sick, enjoy, engender, give birth. There is an irreducible bodily dimension in experience and practice; the sweat cannot be excluded . . . Bodily experiences are often central in memories of our lives, and thus our understanding of who and what we are. (Connell 1995: 51–3)

The human body, for all its resilience, is fragile; breakdown is built into it. Bodily predictability, if not the exception, should be regarded as exceptional; contingency ought to be accepted as normative. (Frank 1995: 49)

Watching a script unfold

Standing back from the other parents, not shouting, I watch.

Short blond hair shines. A body moves. Gracefully into spaces not available to others. Balance shifts. Drifting. Blending elements together.
The ball is his. A playmaker.

Standing back from the other parents, not shouting, I watch.

Crescendo. The game is won. Hands shake. Water pours into dry throats.
'Alexander, you were brilliant today. *Brilliant!*' declares the coach with a smile.
Bemused, the boy asks 'Why?'

Standing back from the other parents, not shouting, I watch.

A son. My son. Eight years old. Talented, skilful, fast, strong.

Performer. Identity construction in process.
Love and pride infuse the tears that swell in my eyes.

Standing back from the other parents, not shouting, I watch.

Embodied memories connect my flesh to him.
In shared movement, in sinews, masculinities crystallise.
Him-I-he-me-we, touching trajectories in time and space.

Standing back from the other parents, not shouting, I watch.

A ghost brushes against me.
My skin shivers.
This script has been lived before.

My father, standing back from the other parents, not shouting, watching me.

Academic voice(s)

Children are always episodes in someone else's narratives. (Steedman 1986: 122)

It is in boys' relationships with fathers that we may find many of the keys to the emotional salience of sport in the development of masculine identity . . . The fact that boys' introduction to organized sport is often made by fathers who might otherwise be absent or emotionally distant adds a powerful charge to these early experiences. (Messner 1992: 27–8)

A performing body: public statements of a me I do not remember

1968. Autumn term. Age 12. Member of unbeaten U13 Rugby XV. First public announcement about an emerging elite body. School magazine states, 'This has been a very successful season in many ways . . . Sparkes has been outstanding in the centre.'
    1968. Summer term. Age 12. School magazine states:

> The outstanding athlete this term, however, has been a junior, A.C. Sparkes. In the School Sports he set new records in the 220 yards, Discus, Shot and Javelin, and in the last event he went on to come first in the North East Somerset Junior Atheltics Meeting in Radstock with a throw of 122 ft 6 ins. This beat the existing record by over 20 ft.

1969. Age 13. Win South West of England Championships in the Javelin. Compete in the English Schools Athletic Championships. Achieve 6th place in the country.
    1970. Age 14. Captain of unbeaten U15 Rugby XV. Coach comments in school magazine:

What a truly magnificent season this has been. Unbeaten after twelve games, this has been without question the finest team I have ever had the privilege of coaching. From the start we knew we had in Sparkes a player of outstanding ability and potential. But although the side was clearly built around his skills, our success has been based entirely on teamwork . . . This allowed Sparkes at stand-off the chance to display the full range of his skills. He delighted us with his strong, penetrating runs, his 32 tries, his crunching tackles, his touch-line conversions and his long relieving kicks out of defence. In addition, he has now learned to vary his play and feed the rest of the line . . . the remarkable team spirit and the superb captaincy of Sparkes have all been factors in this season's success story.

1972. Age 16. Captain of 1st XV. Most successful season ever. Coach comments in school magazine:

Without doubt the success of the side has stemmed from his inspiring leadership. His changes of speed, combined with swerve or side-step, have made him a most dangerous attacking player. He has carried out his duties as captain with real efficiency, insisting on a high standard of fitness, and keeping a firm hold on the tactical situation.

1973. Age 17. Debut in first class Rugby for Bath 1st XV against arch West Country rivals Gloucester at their home ground. Newspaper reports state the following:

King Edward's School Captain, followed in the illustrious footsteps of Geoff Frankom [a former England International] when he made his debut at Gloucester last week. And a very encouraging start it was too, for this well-built 17-year-old in front of what is notoriously one of the most partisan crowds in the country . . . Sparkes not only gave a competent all-round display, but scored half of Bath's points by kicking two penalties and a conversion.

It was a memorable debut for the young Bath centre, Sparkes, who is not yet 18. He distinguished himself by converting one of Bath's two tries and adding two penalty goals.

Bath's 17-year-old kicker, Sparkes, made a superb debut.

1974. Gain place at Loughborough Colleges, an elite, all-male institution specialising in the training of PE teachers. Gain immediate place in the Rugby 1st XV, a rare event. Programme for one of the games against our major rivals states the following.

Wing/Centre. Age 18. Height 6ft. Weight 13st 4lb. The only freshman to play in the back division this year. The youngest of the squad, he played for Bath, and Somerset U19 before entering college. First year PE and Biology. Home Club: Bath.

Academic voice(s)

In becoming a member of a new group, such as a sports team, two complementary processes must occur – identity construction and identity confirmation. One cannot become a full participant in a new sport without both. It should be noted that these processes seem to take place without much notice when sports are started at a young age. (Donnelly and Young 1999: 68)

There is often an exhilarating energy in school sport for many boys . . . Boys learn about the necessity of hardening their bodies, accepting violent confrontations as a 'normal' way of life and splitting themselves off from their feelings . . . In order to achieve this fantasy of heroic virility, boys have to learn to go for aggressive performance, success, superiority over women, emotional stoicism, physical strength and goal-directedness in their sporting activities. However, they often learn to do this at the expense of their capacity to act as human beings. Their abilities to relate to other people, to feel for others, to trust, cooperate, to link together their bodies with their hearts, are all damaged and severely limited by such sporting practices. (Salisbury and Jackson 1996: 204–5).

The disciplined body – Defines itself primarily in actions of self-regimentation that make itself *predictable*. Most important action problems are about control and experiences its most serious crisis in loss of control. Other-relatedness is *monadic*. In terms of self-relatedness is *dissociated* from itself.

The dominating body – Defines itself in *force*. Tend to be male bodies. Characterised by a sense of lack, anxiety, and fear. Thus, this body's response to its sense of its own contingency, its *dissociated* self-relatedness, and its *dyadic* other-relatedness, are all configured by lack. Although dyadic in its other-relatedness, it is *against* others rather than *for* others. (Mixture of Frank 1991 and 1995)

Fateful moment: summer 1974

Back and chest done. Pecs and lats flushed, warm, pumped. Vest sticks to skin, soaked. Sweat beads run down my face. Drip off my nose, my chin. Feeling bigger than an hour ago. Glance at my right bicep. See the thick, swollen vein running over its curve. Blood swimming in chemicals. Muscle fibres broken ready for repair. 20 minutes left. Time for legs. This will hurt. It always does. Move to leg-press machine. Adjust seat location. Pin in at stack 5. Ease muscles in. 25 reps. Sweat slips into my mouth. Tastes salty. Pin in at stack 7. Do 20 reps. Quadriceps begin to burn. Sinews tight, hard. Pin to stack 10. Tougher now. Hamstrings like ropes. Last set. Legs full of blood. Sensual. Like walking on air. Stack 12. Thrust, tension, power explodes. The weights elevated. Suspended by my flesh, my will. But then, quietly. Oh so quietly. In a whisper. My body speaks. A *click* in my lumbar spine. I just about hear it. But feel it. Conversation begins. A story. A pain-full story unfolds.

Academic voice(s)

Insofar as the body tends to disappear when functioning unproblematically, it often seizes our attention most strongly at times of dysfunction; we then experience the body as the very *absence* of a desired or ordinary state, and a force that stands opposed to the self. (Leder 1990: 4)

Disempowered masculinity . . . Compromised health often confounds injured male athletes who are often dependent for their self-identity on physical power and fitness . . . Athletes are forced to recognise, perhaps for the first time, that the physical body and its talents are integrally tied to self and relationships. For men who conceive of sport in a principally gendered fashion, then, injury has consequences for the masculine self. (White *et al.* 1995: 173)

The medical gaze: inside of me

CT scan of lumbar spine
Date: November 1988

> *Report*: consecutive images between L3 and S1 were recorded. The striking initial feature is a developmental spinal stenosis.
>
> At L3/4 there is evidence of disc degeneration with a broad-based annular bulge extending back into the neural canal. This is of significant proportion and extends across to the right and dips below the upper plate of L4. Facet joints are broadened with minor osteophytosis.
>
> At L4/5 similar features are shown. The disc is narrowed with a broad-based bulge extending back into the neural canal. This is probably a partial extrusion of part of the disc, best appreciated on scan 16. Again there are broadened facet joints with thickening of the Ligamenta Flava.
>
> At L5/S1 there is some evidence of degenerative disc disease; however, there is a high termination to the sacral sac, and no convincing evidence of nerve root or thecal sac compression is seen. Facet joint osteoarthritis is present.
>
> *Summary*: The most striking feature is developmental stenosis with significant acquired stenotic features due to disc disease at L3/L4 and L4/L5.

Them

Osteopaths
Chiropractors
Physiotherapists
Occupational therapists
Orthopaedic surgeons
Neurosurgeons
Push
Pull
Stretch
Twist
Manipulate
Inject
Cut
Extract

Suture
Repair
Rehabilitate
Return me
Once again
To the world
In a different
Body

Memory jars

Three small jars. The contents are not visible unless turned upside down. The sides are surrounded by a white seal with 'official' writing on it: 'specimen for histology', a name – Andrew C. Sparkes, gender – M, DOB – 2–7–55, dates – 1988, 1994, 2000, and a note detailing the disc levels operated on – L3/L4, L4/L5 (right side), L4/L5, L5/S1 (left side).

I pick them up in turn and hold each one just above eye level so I can see the debris (disc material, bone shavings and other gristle), in the bottom of the jar. Swishing them around, they move slowly in the formalin that preserves them, long after they should have rotted outside of my body. The bits of me from 1988 and 1994 look blanched and pale, slightly ragged, flaky. The debris from 2000, has more substance, it looks fresher, moves and sinks faster to the bottom. There is a red tinge to the formalin. I suddenly get the urge to smell these remains. The lids come off. I inhale. I inhale memories.

I'm 17. The forwards win the ball, quick ball, good. I check where my opposite number is and drop back deeper. The outside half has the ball. He hears the call, flings a long pass out in front of me. I stretch, fingertips touch, then caress the ball as I hit the line at an angle. I cut air, feeling speed oozing through my lean, sinewy body as it arcs to the right, swerving away from the flailing hands of the tackler. I hear his body crumple to the ground. The crowd roars me on. Lightning strides. Moving so fast the world turns molten, melting in wavy space around me. Detached, floating, I watch myself in slow motion. Every fibre focused on this fluid moment of being, untouchable, balanced, harmonious, running fast, running so fast. A state of grace. Touchdown.

I'm 26. Period 1. Athletics. 'OK, so slide your fingers down the javelin till they touch the cord'. The group of 12 year-olds oblige. 'That's called the horse-shoe grip.' They nod and twiggle their fingers. Michael, one of my favourite pupils, shouts, 'Go on Sir, show us a throw. A long one.' I demonstrate. Short run up, cross over step, and launch the javelin. It flies. I feel its long arc tingle down into my arm and into my spine. Pupils gasp in admiration. Good PE teachers 'do' it. Show don't tell.

I'm 26. Period 4. Athletics. Back in spasm. Torso twisting to the right. Body rebelling. Locking me in. Putting rust in my veins. Hobbling. Hurting. Muscular frame distorted by an invisible hand. No obvious signs of injury. Nothing broken. Pupils bemused. Unsure of what to say. Triple jump. No demonstration. No gasps. No confirmation of me. Good PE teachers 'do' it. Show don't tell. Shit! Where does that leave me? Time to go.

I'm 33. The departmental secretary has already taken my box of handouts for the undergraduate students over to the lecture room. It hurts me to carry them. I've asked her to go ahead because I can't keep up with her walking pace. She's 20 years older than me. I will get there in my own time, a slow time. Get the lift from my office on the first floor to the ground floor. Stairs are difficult for me. Once outside, the walking journey to my destination is about 250 metres.

Inhaling, I unfold my collapsible walking stick and begin to hobble. As my left foot hits the ground a searing, slashing pain, arcs from my lower back into my left buttock, left thigh, left calf muscle, and finally, into my foot. Right step – fine. Left step – stab. Right step – fine. Left step – stab. Left, left, left – stab, stab, stab . . . Stand still, lift left foot off the ground. Stand still, take all the weight on the right foot. Lean on my walking stick. Relief. Stand still. Move. Left step – stab. The world, my world, collapsing, into the left side of my lower body. I am my left limb. I am the space between pain and no pain. I stand still. I cannot take one more step. This is a world of stillness, slowness, impairment, disability, of otherness.

Some male students on their way to my lecture pass by me with consummate ease, unthinking, unaware of their bodies in motion. Their leisurely pace accentuates my slowness. I feel my slowness. One of them turns and says, 'You look in a bad way.' I joke about the dilemmas of ageing. They laugh. I laugh. They move on. Watching them, I resent their youth, their muscularity, their well-toned, tanned legs in their baggy shorts. I resent my own body for what it makes me look like, and feel, in front of them. Their pace of movement offends me, reminding me of the distance I have travelled from the self I used to be in performance terms. I recognise my alienation from my own body and the body of others. Two of them glance back, as if they want to return and say something, to offer help. But they don't. They feel awkward and unsure. My strange gait transgresses the norms of their culture. Looking at me makes them feel uncomfortable, threatened. Perhaps, I remind them of what might be on the horizon for them. Right now, they are afraid of me. I <u>scare</u> them.

I'm 39. I have walked down this hospital corridor many times before. The navy blue carpet is familiar as are the hand rails on either side. Determined not to use these for support I hobble slowly down an imaginary centre line. It's hot and I'm sweating. I'm crying and afraid. Here, in 1988 I had surgery on my lumbar spine. I have the feeling this hospital is soon going to swallow me up again. I want it to, I want this pain to be taken away.

Stopping for a rest I turn towards Kitty, my partner, 6 months pregnant. 'Déjà vu', I say to her, 'It's happening again.' The tears well up in her eyes. We hold each other close in the corridor. I kiss the tears on her cheeks. I kiss her eyes, I want to drown and be saved in the blueness of those eyes. As the roundness of her stomach presses against me a wave of guilt washes over me. Kitty is pregnant, so tired, caring for Jessica our three-year-old, now having to worry and cope with the stress of me and my body failure. My uselessness makes me angry with my body. At that moment I hate it intensely.

An elderly woman is coming out of the shop. She is limping in a similar pattern to me. We cross trajectories like some infirm ballet dancers. We do not acknowledge each other. I feel embarrassed at our similarities in gait and our differences in age. People looking at me, but as I catch their eyes they avert their gaze.

I'm 45. Feeling the ice injected into the vein of my right arm. It spreads. Time slipping, sliding, so gently away. Drifting now. Count to ten. One , two, three, four, five, six, seven. . . . Is this like dying?

  Shivering, shaking. Cold so cold. Teeth chatter uncontrollably. Body twitching. In the distance. 'Andrew . . . Andrew . . . Can you hear me?'
  Closer now. Holding my arm. 'Andrew. Can you hear me?'
  'Ye, ye, ye, yeesss.'
  'Everything's fine. You're in the post-op room. How are you feeling?'
  'C,c,cold.'
  'He's cold. Let's get some heat on him.'
  'Andrew, are you in pain?'
  'Y,y,y, yes.'
  'On a scale of 1 to 5, where are you? Five is a lot.'
  'Four.'
  'This is morphine I'm giving you. It will help with the pain.'
  Cotton wool. Cocooned. Warm. Undulating. Pain slips out of my body as silently as it crept in.

Still 45. I feel the tug of the wound and the stitches in my back as I shift my knees to see him better. He sits in a chair at the end of my bed. I look at him. My gaze envelopes him, holding his image in my brain. Sitting, doing nothing, just talking, does not come easy to my 76-year-old Dad. Eternally shy and self-conscious, he normally hides behind a newspaper. But now, with me lying once again in hospital bed, he talks. He tells me stories. Stories about his own youth, growing up fatherless from the age of two, growing up working class, but most of all growing up poor. Stories of the armed forces and National Service. Stories of labouring as a shoe cutter in a factory, dreaming of escape from the daily grind, the drudgery, and the brain-numbing boredom. Stories of breaking away, of his dreams and aspirations, his successes and disappointments. But mostly the stories are about sport. It's woven into the tapestry of my Dad's life. He tells me stories of performing bodies, his, mine, my brother's, sportsmen he remembers. All told in the past tense. He tells me stories because he feels my pain, my bewilderment, my confusion about my body, about who I am and who I might become. It's his way of coping, of helping. It's his way of telling me he loves me.

Maybe when I was younger he would have held me in his muscular arms, as I have held my own young son and daughter. Perhaps my childish soft cheeks would have felt the pressure of his chest. I would have smelt him, a young man, a young father, and just perhaps, I might have even heard his heartbeat, as he made the pain, the demons, and the fear go away. Will my own children, Jessica and Alexander, remember me by my smell, will they remember hearing my heart beat when I held them in troubled times and wiped away their tears?

Maybe, I held him tight to me then, hugging him, and feeling my own growing strength in relation to his. Today, I know for sure I want to hold him close and tell him just how much I love him. How, I want him to live forever, to always be there when I fall. I want to squeeze away the anxieties, depressions, and insecurities that have haunted him throughout his life. I want to tell him that whatever mistakes he made, how many things he felt he got wrong, whatever guilt he feels, he is still <u>my</u> Dad and I'm proud of him. And, whatever else I am, or become, I am still <u>his</u> son. Our stories, our lives, forever entangled.

But I don't. I can't. He is a father, a man, of his time, of his history. It would embarrass him, make him feel uneasy. The words remain unspoken.

This morning the Australian nurse told me I was not allowed out of bed. But my Dad is allowed in, allowed into my room, into a space, a landscape, where once again he can tell stories to his son. I cherish the moment. His stories soak into my bones.

I'm 47. First time back in my old school since I left 29 years ago. Again, feeling strange, out of place, not belonging. All the old working-class insecurities come flooding back. One thing, one person only, draws me once more to this place – my old PE teacher, Lang, retiring after 45 years of teaching in the same school. A surprise 'This Is Your Life' has been organised by his colleagues for an invited audience of around 200 people. I am one of the twelve 'secret guests' moved out of sight into the main hall, where we remain hidden backstage until it our turn to make a surprise appearance. I am the eleventh to go on stage.

Behind the curtain, I am given the microphone to say a few lines out of sight, 'Hi Lang. Do you remember the rough little kid from the transport café who threw the javelin a long way and scored lots of tries for you?' I then walk on to the stage, blinded by the lights as the presenter announces, 'Yes, Lang, it's Andrew Sparkes. Now Professor Andrew Sparkes at the University of Exeter.' Big applause as Lang and I meet in the middle of the stage and hug each other. I tell two funny stories about my experiences in school athletics and rugby to illustrate my relationship with this important man in my life. The crowd laugh at each story. I'm good at this. It's what they want to hear. I know the script.

I also thank Lang for getting me through school and for all the help and support he gave me. And I sincerely mean it. More applause. As I go to sit down with the other guests on the stage, Lang takes the microphone from the presenter and faces the audience. This is what he tells them:

Andrew Sparkes is without doubt the finest rugby player this school has <u>ever</u> produced. He was <u>awesome</u>. Chosen to play for Bath against Gloucester when he was in the lower sixth, only 17. He scored 22 points and Bath won the game. He then went to Loughborough College and went straight into the 1st

XV in the centre. Tragically, he damaged his back and never played again. If he had, there is no doubt that he would have played for England.

Thunderous, prolonged applause erupts. First, I nod at Lang, then at the audience. I watch their hands beat together in unison and feel waves of air as they hit my ears. They are celebrating a me I don't remember. A me I don't recall. Their applause is for a historical self, a ghost. Someone who was a 'me' long ago. Things have changed. My body has changed. I have changed. Or have I? Have I really changed that much? Who is the 'me' on the stage accepting their applause? Where am 'I' in the web of stories others tell about me, and I tell about myself? How will I (re)story the events of this evening?

Memories subside.

Now, looking down on the debris, I do something I have never done before. The little finger of my right hands creeps in and touches it. I am surprised at how rough and hard 2000 feels under the pressure of my fingertip. I had expected more give, something smoother, softer, like octopus flesh. Fragments of 1994 and 1988 are softer, but still resistant to my touch. My dead flesh offers no caress.

Suddenly I feel repulsed and ill at ease, like a grave robber disturbed in the early hours of the morning. Knowing I'm desecrating Holy ground, sensing someone watching me. I put the lids back on and sit very still for a few minutes.

Standing, back aching, I place the jars gently on the shelf. Silently apologising to my various bodies and selves that have just been invaded once again by my insensitive prodding. It will be a while before I look at them again. They will not be disturbed.

Later that day, Alexander, my eight-year-old son inquires, 'Dad, can you run now?'

Academic voice(s)

But pain strikes one alone . . . pain is marked by an interiority that another cannot share . . . pain tends to induce self-reflection and isolation. It effects a *spatiotemporal constriction* . . . The disruption and constriction of one's habitual world thus corresponds with a new relation to one's body. In pain, the body, or a certain part of the body emerges as an *alien presence*. The sensory insistence of pain draws the corporeal out of self-concealment, rendering it thematic. No event more radically and inescapably reminds us of our bodily presence. Yet at the same time pain effects a certain alienation . . . The painful body is often experienced as something foreign to the self. (Leder 1990: 74–6)

Disability is experienced in, on and through the body, just as impairment is experienced in terms of the personal and cultural narratives that help to constitute its meaning . . . Most importantly, the (impaired) body is not just experienced: It is also the very basis of experience . . . Disability is, therefore, experienced from the perspective of impairment. One's body is one's window on the world. (Hughes and Paterson 1997: 334–5)

Many of us are ill-equipped to cope with the problems of illness and disability, having had no opportunity to learn. Cultural silence about pain, limitation, suffering, and dying also increases our fear of them, and thus contributes to our need to believe that we can control our bodies. (Wendell 1996: 109)

Others resent [us] for this reason . . . the disabled serve as constant, visible reminders to the able-bodied that the society they live in is shot through with inequity and suffering, that they live in a counterfeit paradise, that they too are vulnerable. We represent a fearsome possibility. (Murphy 1987: 116–17)

Reflections

The patchwork of embodied memories I have provided, like all such retellings by a 'remembering self' (Neisser 1994), are embedded within and framed by a series of dominant scripts or 'master' narratives made available to me throughout my life in relation to age, gender, able/impaired/disabled bodies, social class, race, ethnicity and sexuality. Some of these, such as gender and impairment, have been highlighted more than others in the stories I have chosen to tell in this chapter. The question remains as to what we might learn from them.

If nothing else, the patchwork confirms the immense power that 'master' narratives associated with, for example, hegemonic masculinity have to shape the experiences and identities of boys and men via physical education and sport. The power of these narratives is that they offer people a way of identifying what is assumed to be a normative experience. For Andrews (2002: 1),

such storylines act as a blueprint for all stories; they become the vehicle through which we comprehend not only the stories of others, but crucially of ourselves as well. For ultimately, the power of master narratives derives from their internalization.

These narratives that infuse the flesh and soak into our sense of self, draw on models of identity provided by the cultures we inhabit. Importantly, some of these models and narratives are life-enhancing, some are not.

We might, therefore, wish to ask a number of questions regarding the dominant narratives that circulate in physical education classes and physical education teacher education (PETE) along with the manner these become internalised (Sparkes 1999). For example, what are the processes that lead some narratives within PE to be privileged, foregrounded, and institutionalised (e.g. the myth of the perfect and perfectible, performing, controlled, dominating and disciplined body) while others (e.g. the impaired or disabled body) are suppressed, devalued, marginalised, abnormalised, or silenced? Following on from this, we might ask how can the dominant narratives in PE that reflect cultural trends and shape the repertoire of life story possibilities be challenged and changed? What strategies enable different stories to be told and how are spaces created for them? How can alternative, counter-narratives, be introduced, and circulated in ways that empower individuals and groups to alter the trajectories of their lives, infusing the individual's history with new meaning and complexity so as to enhance not only *their* experiences, but also the experiences of *others*, as they inhabit different bodies throughout their lives?

In short, within the context of PE in school and PETE, I suggest we need to expand the cultural repertoire of narratives that are available for synthesis into personal stories, and widen the access people have to this repertoire. If this could be accomplished, then over the life course people may develop greater sophistication in their potential for telling a variety of life stories and may develop the capacity to reconstrue their lives in ways that enhance their present situations, relationships and needs. Here, communicative bodies, as opposed to disciplined and dominating bodies, have the opportunity to be foregrounded. The communicative body, according to Frank (1995) is an *idealised* body in the process of *creating itself*. The body's contingency is no longer its problem but its possibility. That is, the communicative body accepts contingency as part of the fundamental contingency of life. In its relationship with others it is *dyadic*, and with regard to self-relatedness it is *associated* with itself.

Of course, as my own patchwork of embodied memories indicates, transcending one's narrative resources, reconstructing body-self relationships, and foregrounding a communicative body when appropriate, is no easy task (also see Sparkes 1996, 2003; Sparkes and Smith 2002). I continue to struggle on a daily basis. The domains that I have inhabited, and continue to inhabit (e.g. a university environment dominated by a 'publish or perish' work ethic and the constant measurement and monitoring of research output) are not awash with counter-narratives on which to build alternative identities, notions of self, and forms of embodiment that recognise and acknowledge, among other things, issues of vulnerability, fragility, impairment and disability. Indeed, work conditions in schools and higher education seem to actively cultivate and celebrate disciplined and dominating bodies at the expense of communicative bodies. Against this backdrop, therefore, the stories I have told in this chapter provide a moment of resistance against the dominant narratives that surround me and many of my colleagues. Furthermore, as Frank (1995: 25) points out, 'One road to the achievement of the communicative body is through storytelling'.

According to Frank (1995), bodies are not just represented but realised and created in the stories they tell. For him, this realisation can and should be reflexive. That is, by telling certain stories, ethical choices are made, and these choices, in turn, generate stories. As such, just as people have some responsibility for their stories and their bodies, there is also the possibility of exercising that responsibility *through* stories.

Frank (1995) also emphasises the need to think *with* stories, of allowing one's own thoughts to adopt the story's immanent logic, its temporality, and its tensions and contradictions. When we think with stories, we should not immediately move on once the story has been heard, but continue to live in the story, *becoming* in it, reflecting on who one is becoming, and gradually modifying the story. Again, this is no easy task. It is very difficult to truly listen to one's own story, and equally as difficult to truly listen to the stories of others. However, as Frank points out, thinking with stories is the basis of *narrative ethics*.

> The moral imperative of narrative ethics is perpetual self-reflection on the sort of person that one's story is shaping one into, entailing the requirement to change that self-story if the wrong self is being shaped. Narrative ethics is an ethics of commitment to shaping oneself as a human being.
>
> (Frank 1995: 158)

Clearly, narrative ethics and the need to expand narrative resources presents a number of important challenges to those involved in PE and sport at all levels. I hope these challenges will be taken up in the future. For the moment, a useful starting point is to become aware of the general type of narrative one is telling or responding to, and then to see where this takes us.

References

Andrews, M. (2002) 'Introduction: counter narratives and the power to oppose', *Narrative Inquiry* 12(1): 1–6.

Antoniou, M. (2003) 'Writing my body: exploring methods of embodiment', unpublished Ph.D. thesis, University of Manchester.

Connell, R. (1995) *Masculinities*, Cambridge: Polity Press.

Donnelly, P. and Young, K. (1999) 'Rock climbers and rugby players: identity construction and confirmation', in J. Coakley and P. Donnelly (eds) *Inside Sports*, London: Routledge.

Ellis, C. and Bochner, A. (2000) 'Autoethnography, personal narrative, reflexivity: researcher as subject', in N. Denzin and Y. Lincoln (eds) *Handbook of Qualitative Research*, second edition, London: Sage.

Frank, A. (1991) 'For a sociology of the body: an analytical review', in M. Featherstone, M. Hepworth and B. Turner (eds) *The Body: Social Process and Cultural Theory*, London: Sage.

Frank, A. (1995) *The Wounded Storyteller*, Chicago: University of Chicago Press.

Hughes, B. and Paterson, K. (1997) 'The social model of disability and the disappearing body: toward a sociology of impairment', *Disability and Society* 12(3): 325–40.

Jackson, D. (1990) *Unmasking Masculinity*, London: Unwin Hyman.

Leder, D. (1990) *The Absent Body*, Chicago: University of Chicago Press.

Messner, M. (1992) *Power at Play*, Boston: Beacon Press.

Murphy, R. (1987) *The Body Silent*, New York: Henry Holt.

Neisser, U. (1994) ' Self-narratives: true and false', in U. Neisser and R. Fivush (eds) *The Remembering Self*, Cambridge: Cambridge University Press.

Salisbury, J. and Jackson, D. (1996) *Challenging Macho Values*, London: Falmer Press.

Smith, B. and Sparkes, A. (2002) 'Men, sport, spinal cord injury, and the construction of coherence: narrative practice in action', *Qualitative Research* 2(2): 143–71.

Smith, S. and Watson, J. (2001) *Reading Autobiography*, Minneapolis: University of Minnesota Press.

Sparkes, A. (1996) 'The fatal flaw: a narrative of the fragile body-self', *Qualitative Inquiry* 2(4): 463–95.

Sparkes, A. (1999) 'Exploring body narratives', *Sport, Education and Society* 4(1): 17–30.

Sparkes, A. (2000) 'Autoethnography and narratives of self: reflections on criteria in action', *Sociology of Sport Journal* 17(1): 21–43.

Sparkes, A. (2002a) *Telling Tales in Sport and Physical Activity: A Qualitative Journey*, Champaign, IL: Human Kinetics Press.

Sparkes, A. (2002b) 'Autoethnography: self-indulgence or something more?', in A. Bochner and C. Ellis (eds) *Ethnographically Speaking: Autoethnography, Literature, and Aesthetics*, London: Altamira Press.

Sparkes, A. (2003) 'Bodies, identities, selves: autoethnographic fragments and reflections', in J. Denison and P. Markula (eds) *'Moving Writing': Crafting Movement and Sport Research*, New York: Peter Lang.

Sparkes, A. and Silvennoinen, M. (1999) (eds) *Talking Bodies: Men's Narratives of the Body and Sport*, Jyvaskyla, Finland: SoPhi.

Sparkes, A. and Smith, B. (2002) 'Sport, spinal cord injuries, embodied masculinities and the dilemmas of narrative identity', *Men and Masculinities* 4(3): 258–85.

Stanley, L. and Morgan, D. (1993) 'Editorial introduction', *Sociology* 27(1): 1–4.

Steedman, C. (1986) *Landscape for a Good Woman: A Story of Two Lives*, Brunswick, NJ: Rutgers University Press.

Tsang, T. (2000) 'Let me tell you a story: a narrative exploration of identity in high-performance sport', *Sociology of Sport Journal* 17(10): 44–59.

Wendell, S. (1996) *The Rejected Body*, London: Routledge.

White, P., Young, K. and McTeer, W. (1995) 'Sport, masculinity, and the injured body', in D. Sabo and F. Gordon (eds) *Men's Health and Illness*, London: Sage.

12 'Hungry to be noticed'

Young women, anorexia and schooling

Emma Rich, Rachel Holroyd and John Evans

Introduction

> I don't think that school caused my anorexia because there were a lot of issues at home and things, but I think it probably contributed to it because of the things that happened there.
>
> (Karen, 17 years)

Despite the volume of popular and mainstream sociological interest in 'the body' in recent years, very little attention has been given either in the sociology of education or the literature on pedagogy as to how processes of schooling may be implicated in the aetiology and development of eating disorders. In this chapter, therefore, we draw upon the voices of a number of young women (aged 14–17) suffering from anorexia nervosa, in order to better understand the ways in which some complex, immediate and negative effects of informal and formal education inherent in the form, organisation, content of schooling may erode young women's sense of competence, responsibility and control, propelling some towards disordered eating and serious ill-health.

Anorexia nervosa, like all other eating disorders, is an extremely complex condition variously understood and much debated across the disciplines of psychiatry, medicine, psychology, biology, sociology, epidemiology. We have no wish here to understate the sophistication of the perspectives that abound within these fields (see Lask and Bryant-Waugh 2000). However, 'anorectic' behaviours and experiences have tended to be viewed both in the popular media and much of the mainstream academic press as pathological conditions distinctly different from 'normal' and 'healthy' experiences and practices of non-anorexic women and girls (Malson 1998). Malson goes on to assert that as such they become separated from their social context and from the everyday experiences of 'ordinary' women and girls, and the mainstream object of enquiry is often essentially 'the disorder' anorexia, not the varied, complex and socially conceptualised experiences of individual girls and women who have been diagnosed as 'anorexic'. This chapter departs from these more traditional pathological perspectives to reveal an emerging theoretical position on narratives of anorectics in relation to education. The data presented prompt us to reconsider the interplay between 'the body', power, knowledge and (ill-)health within schools in relation to the aetiology ('causes') and development of eating disorders, in this case anorexia nervosa.

We have no wish either to suggest that formal education and schooling in particular, '*cause*' eating disorders, or lay the blame for such 'conditions' on the doorsteps of teachers or others in schools. The 'aetiology' of anorexia and other eating disorders is extremely complex, multi-determined (Lask 2000) and layered and their origins and connections with schooling have yet to be adequately explored (Evans *et al.* 2002). However, we take the view that health and health-relevant behaviours are too often studied in isolation of the social contexts in which they are embedded and given meaning (Backett-Milburn 2000), including those constructed by formal education and schools. As researchers and teachers we therefore need to develop better understandings of how and why health problems arise in particular social settings and spaces, in order to identify ways in which we might better prevent destructive influences impacting upon young people's lives (Oliver and Lalik 2000). We share Hepworth's (1999) view that eating disorders need to be understood as a public issue or process rather than an individual problem. Education, which at its best should help young people avoid illness, disease and oppression, whatever form these take, is part of this public process.

Methods

In presenting this framework we draw on the narratives of a number of young women involved in an on-going qualitative study of the relationships between disordered eating and formal education, set in a leading centre in the UK for the treatment of eating disorders. The centre caters for both males and females between the ages of 11 and 18. However, reflecting broader patterns in the social spread of eating disorders (see Doyle and Bryant-Waugh 2000), at the time of study only one of the 25 young people attending was male and could not be included in the first phase of research. Bearing in mind the multi-dimensional nature of both young people's lives and of eating disorders, the project has attempted to understand and highlight the relationships between formal education and wider social practices, including those occurring within the family, among peers and in relation to leisure and employment, with reference to the aetiology and development of eating disorders (Brettschneider 1992; Holroyd 2003; Evans *et al.* 2002). The research has employed a qualitative methodology using a variety of techniques designed to allow for an examination of the issues central to the investigation. In line with a growing trend in youth studies, we have focused on the active involvement of the research participants in the generation of data (e.g. Alderson 1995; Christensen and James 2000; Oliver and Lalik 2000). Within the overall research design various activity based tasks such as memory writing (Lupton 1996), journal keeping (Oliver and Lalik 2000) and drawing (Holroyd 2003) have been combined with semi-structured interviews, focus groups discussions and life history work (Sparkes 1995). These provide a means by which key issues can be generated and deliberated over. Moreover, the use of both group and individual activities reflects an awareness of the deep sensitivities of the issues under investigation for the young people concerned. Every stage of the project has progressed in consultation with those far more experienced than ourselves, medically, in working with young people with eating disorders. The various informal and formal methods used have provided a means of identifying prevailing attitudes and practices relating to food, diet, physical activity, education and much else, that have had bearing on the attitudes of these young women towards their bodies and selves. The data generated have been analysed following the principles of grounded theory (Glaser and Strauss 1967), an on-going process of recording, coding and analysis providing continuing direction for subsequent phases of the research. The young women whose voices are heard in this paper are aged between 11 and 17, come from 'middle-class families', and all have attended what might be described as 'high status' comprehensive, grammar or private, secondary schools. All are experiencing anorexia nervosa at different stages of 'illness' or recovery but each is suffering in sufficient severity to warrant residential treatment and care.

Beyond the 'cult of slenderness'

Anorexia nervosa and bulimia nervosa are relatively rare in comparison to other affective disorders, and although debate continues to surround the nature and extent of their epidemiological 'spread' (Doyle and Bryant-Waugh 2000). However, there seems to be agreement that 'the sub threshold components, for example, negative body image, fear of fat, feeling powerless and insecure, are prevalent enough among girls and women in many countries to be considered normative and an epidemic', and that this 'horrible state of affairs, coupled with the astounding gender differences in eating disorder and the risk periods in early and late adolescence, points to the need to think about what "eating problems" mean in the lives of girls and women' (Levine and Piran 1999: 321) and increasingly, of young men. In the UK the Eating Disorders Association estimate that about 165,000 people have eating disorders and this condition is responsible for the highest number of deaths from psychiatric illness (*BBC News Online: Health: Medical notes* 2000). It is hardly surprising, then, that the rise of eating disorders in the US and Western Europe has been described by some (though not without contestation, see Palmer 2001) as a modern epidemic, one which now is extending to areas with which they were once thought to be culturally incompatible, including China, India, Mexico and Brazil (Gordon 2001).

Although myriad assumptions circulate around the aetiology of eating disorders, at the core of these discussions is the enduring and powerful notion of body control through the marketing of a slender, or thin, ideal and its spread within and beyond the Western world. 'Our' (Western) culture, it is argued, has been 'swept up in a web of peculiar and distorted beliefs about health, virtue, eating and appetite'; an ethic, or a 'cult of slenderness', pervades societies and the cultures of schools (Kirk 1999). Viewing eating disorders as a Western 'culture-bound syndrome' or 'ethnic disorder' (Gordon 2000) 'rooted in Western cultural values and conflict' (Prince 1985: 300), bound up in a focus on thinness, however, presents a number of problems (see Katzman and Sing Lee 1997: 387–8). In criticising this approach,

Bray (1994, 1996) refers to anorexia as a 'reading disorder', related to the common assumption that anorexia is a pathology brought about by women's uncritical consumption of media images of thin femininity (1996: 413). The emphasis on body image, on 'slenderness' acting as a contemporary metaphor for desire and the management of female sexuality, while useful in emphasising the importance of the image/media in the development of eating disorders, neither explicates fully the complex relationships between the image and eating practices, nor those between young women, men and other elements of their lives. Bodily dissatisfaction may be necessary (Emmons 1994) but it is certainly not a sufficient condition for the development of eating disorders. Indeed, although within popular discourse the tendency of the imagery of body depiction towards thinness is ubiquitous, the majority of young people may engage and reflect on these but do not develop long-term disordered eating or 'dysfunctional' behavioural patterns (Phelps *et al.* 2000).

We take the view that 'the image of eating disorders as a transitory, self inflicted problem developed by young women lost in their world of fashion and calorie restricting can be a belittling stereotype that may mask women's real worries' (Katzman and Sing Lee 1997: 389) and we also believe it may hide more immediate and complex concerns including those emanating from within formal education and schools. As we will see, locating eating disorders only in a 'cult of slenderness' does not allow for an understanding of the complexities of gendered, embodied experiences, or the ways in which power is enacted in social relations, or the sense of distinction that can be derived from such 'deviant' posturing as an 'anorexic'.

Accepting these caveats, we none the less need to consider how this imagery finds its way into the socio-cultural fabric of schools and into specific subject areas, as well as to other cultural terrain (Evans *et al.* 2002). At the same time, whilst acknowledging that these educational/cultural conditions may be constructing and legitimising particular body images, other, deeper, more complex multiple emerging conditions of schooling within high modernity may also have seriously deleterious effects on young people's lives about which we know relatively little in terms of their embodiment, and these also need to be brought to the fore. We require a clearer understanding of how these processes may generate alienating and isolating tendencies propelling some towards disordered eating and other forms of ill-health.

We have found Warin's (2002) somewhat abstract notion of '*practices of relatedness*', developed in her study of the everyday experiences of eating disorders, useful in explicating these dynamics. Warin uses the term to articulate the relationships between the social and the biological, applying this to the *multiple* elements of relatedness of eating disorders, 'which are themselves not necessarily bounded entities but may overflow or contain parts of each other or take new forms' (p. 4). If relatedness, in all its forms, is central to people's practices and experiences of anorexia and perhaps other disorders we might ask how formal education in conjunction with other social settings is implicated in the processes, struggles and strategies that propel some young people towards them. We share the view that these conditions are embedded in a series of interconnected spaces (Good 1994) and processes, a perspective that allows for a consideration of the role of formal education in the articulation and practices of these conditions. Schools may be regarded as having as much potential to connect and transform people as they have to dislocate and constrain them. The places where 'relatedness' is central yet problematic in the narratives of anorectic young women are evident in Warin's (2002) and our research.

The eating disorders literature and research has alluded, in some places, to education and its effects on young people. Dyer and Tiggeman (1996) suggest that girls in single-sex schools associated professional success with the thin figure. Such schools overly encourage high achievement in girls and are also likely to produce achievement striving in the domain of the body, which, in our society, is the pursuit of a thin body ideal. Such environments may then also be conducive to the extremes of such behaviours resulting in eating disorders (p. 137). Similarly, Silverstein *et al.* (1986) suggest that the shifting standard of bodily attractiveness towards a slimmer and less curvaceous ideal is related to women's increasing concern about intelligence and professional competence. Indeed, the fat body is construed as embodying a number of 'moral aberrations' in Western society, such as laziness, greediness and even low intelligence (Lupton 1996). These analyses, which offer valuable insights into education and eating disorders, rarely get beyond highlighting the potentially deleterious effects of a heightened achievement orientation/ competition on some young women, especially in contexts where this is both paramount and combined with a focus on body improvement and control (e.g. ballet schools, private schools and in health and PE). The concepts of competition and high achievement are an under-explicated shorthand in much of this literature, disguising the material conditions of the curriculum, assessment and the dynamics of the pedagogical relationships that prevail within schools. As a result of a raft of education policies in recent years in the UK, these have greatly 'intensified' the work of teachers and students, leading, for some, to heightened pressure, intense stress, isolation and alienation (Woods and Carlyle 2002) not only from further academic engagement but, in the case of some children, from their bodies, or at least the version of the body (strong, fit, healthy, feminine) which society celebrates and industry putatively needs.

As the focus for this particular chapter is essentially on the culture of 'healthism' within schools, we do not have space here to explore the growing emphasis on performance codes and modalities within them. It is worth reiterating, however, that the intensification of school work, that is to say, the increasing pressures wrought by examinations, assessment, expectations for achieving high grades at 'learning', was a pressing concern for all the girls in our study.

> They're [schools] very hard on you, and they're always talking about what you're going to get in your GCSEs or what you're going to get in your A Levels. They never actually really encourage you, they just say 'oh if you don't do that you're not going to pass your A Levels or your GCSEs' and then you just worry the whole time. There's such a lot of pressure on you.
>
> (Mia, 16 years)

> I was starved when I took my GCSEs. I wasn't eating and I wasn't drinking, I was sitting there and I couldn't concentrate. I was really dizzy.

Int: Did your teachers know you were ill?

> Yeah, but it was important that I sat the GCSEs and got the grades

(Karen, 17 years)

Locating eating disorders in these tensions, constraints and pressures arising in schools and between them and other social spheres, e.g. the family, leisure and work (Holroyd 2003) is a necessary precursor to understanding not just disordered eating, but also other forms of 'deviancy', success and failure in schools. All the girls in our study suggested that schooling played a central role in the development of their eating disorder, highlighting, to various extents, problematic experiences with competition, between individuals for grades, achievement, status, sporting recognition, popularity, bullying, 'cliques', groups, stereotyping and lack of individual recognition.

> I just know that most of my problems at school were caused by anxieties about my relationships with other people . . .
>
> What anorexia has got to do with school is that most anorexic cases are established in school, they ruin people's lives, and gifted and talented kids get destroyed.

(Lauren)

In the remainder of the chapter we explore two main areas of interest: the influence of the culture of 'healthism' on the aetiology of eating disorders and young people's health; and the discourses through which anorexia is understood, set against a backcloth of the intensified conditions of schooling and cultures now dominated and driven by performance modalities and codes (see Evans and Danes, Chapter 14).

'Healthism' and social hierarchies of the body in schools

Research illustrated in this book and elsewhere has suggested that new 'ortho-doxies' are emerging in physical education and health in schools relating to the body, health and self. Evidence suggests that teachers and policy-makers in the UK and elsewhere remain wrapped in an ideology of 'healthism' orientated, amongst other things, to making young people active, 'fit' and thin (Gard and Wright 2001 and Chapter 5). Within this discourse individuals are deemed largely responsible for their own health and for 'making healthy choices'; its individualism constructs the 'person' as an entity relatively independent of the structural constraints and cultures that prevail throughout Western societies (Henriques *et al.* 1984) that bear upon individuals 'opportunity' to achieve the healthy behaviours desired and prescribed. Critiques of this perspective have paid particular attention to the emergence and centrality of an 'obesity discourse' within healthism; a discourse which points to the health risks putatively born of sedentary high-tech society lifestyles and concomitantly the need for governments to ensure that schools and other health care agencies take action to help people become more active, fit and 'thin'. Evidence suggests that an unquestioning acceptance of this discourse in physical education and health curriculum may help construct anxieties about the body that are ironically detrimental to students' health (Evans *et al.* 2002). Whilst few of the young women in our study talked specifically about contexts of physical education and health, all alluded to this narrow perception of 'health' as a corporeal condition – that is to say, as an achieved outcome of eating 'the right' foods, 'being active' and achieving the 'right size' – that had emerged from, or at least been reinforced and endorsed in schools.

> And exercising is another thing, you get manic about exercise and it's like . . . because schools promote exercise as *such* a good thing.
>   . . . that was at school. She [teacher] picked out this girl who was literally like this thick [pointing to a pole in the room] and she said 'now this looks like a girl who is the right weight'. That really upset me because I just thought I have to get [my weight] down quick, so yeah that probably had a big effect on me.
>
> (Lydia, 15 years)

Moreover, their narratives not only describe a 'cultural toxin' that had pervaded all levels and many sites of schooling, from the formal curriculum to more informal aspects and spaces of school life (playgrounds and peer group cultures), they also reveal the emergence of hierarchies of the body relating to size, shape and weight (Evans *et al.* 2002). As Ritenbaugh (1982: 352) has pointed out, in the USA the terms 'obesity' and 'overweight' have become 'the biomedical gloss for the moral failings of gluttony and sloth', a tendency equally apparent in the UK and elsewhere. In the 'blame the victim' culture which this nurtures, fat is thus interpreted as an outward sign of neglect of one's corporeal self; a condition considered either as shameful as being dirty or irresponsibly ill [*sic*] in effect, reproducing and institutionalising moral value beliefs about the body and citizens.

We emphasise that we have no wish here to suggest that 'self-starvation' is driven by a 'fear of fatness'; nor is it our intent to attempt to define some absolute catalyst or cause of an eating disorder such as anorexia nervosa. However, the voices of these young women about their anorexia highlight the powerful ways in which a culture of 'healthism', if recontextualised as a discourse of certainty about exercise, food and diet, may be taken up within the more informal cultures of school life and have a powerful bearing on an individual's developing sense of well-being and self. Consequently, in the lives of these young women particular body shapes are recognised as being of high status and value so that some were unable to recognise themselves as having a body and 'self' of any value at all.

> I had hassle when I was fat. You know, I wouldn't get asked out by boys . . . every time I walked past a mirror I would *hide* myself.
> There's a lot of bitchiness, and of course there's a lot of 'oh, I look so fat'.

> You know there's a lot of that going around. You know, you have to look perfect or you're not going to look good, and the popular girls [in schools] are just going to look at you and go (derisive noise) and you know you don't really want that. There's a lot of pressure . . .
>
> (Lydia)

The pressure to obtain the right body size/shape is not simply about being healthy but carries moral characterisations of the obese/overweight as lazy, self-indulgent and greedy (Gordon 2000). The corollary of this is that control, virtue and goodness are to be found in slenderness and the processes of becoming thin. The central point here is the placing of moral responsibility on the individual to achieve correct diet and involvement in physical activity. These are strong features of the narratives of all these girls, contributing towards the development of particular (often negative) identities, relations, attitudes and practices towards the body and health. The message these young women are hearing is that *they* are to *take control* of their health by making 'healthy choices', particularly in relation to diet, where schools were teaching them what was 'good' (i.e. fruit and veg) and 'bad' (i.e. fat):

> You learn that some things are good and some things are bad and should be avoided.
>
> (Carrie, 17 years)

> You see fat and sugar and that's 'bad'.
>
> (Lydia)

Similarly, Carrie commented that she 'honestly thought' that she 'was just being healthy by cutting out fats entirely' and noted that this was how her 'eating disorder started'. Given the social sanctions that go with this discourse – the bullying, stigma and labelling these girls talk of in association with being defined by their peers as 'fat' – are these really 'choices'? In this representational discourse health is constructed either as a personal attribute, an achievement, or as an individual problem to be addressed. Notably, some girls reported that particular foods were utilised as either a reward or punishment in this endeavour:

> Another thing I think is really important is the use of food as a reward or punishment. People don't talk about it much, but especially in schools food is often used as a reward or treat and it's just not very helpful. It just creates negative relationships with food, because you think I don't deserve that food, I shouldn't eat it . . .
>
> (Carrie)

Of course, this alone may not 'cause' an eating disorder. At worst it may contribute to, at best do little to challenge, the ways in which anorectics and others experience their bodies and bodily processes as 'dirty' (Warin 2002) or 'unworthy' with regard to any 'pleasurable' relationship with foods. A strong Puritan tradition pervades the discourse, giving it all the hallmarks of a religious practice, masked as the 'epitome of secular rationalism' (Gordon 2000: 152). Once more, these are pervasive themes in the anorectics' narratives, which are far more complex than some desire for the 'thin slender body'.

> Yeah, and it's like I want to go somewhere [a school] where there's a pressure to eat, because there there's a pressure to not eat, because if anyone sees you eating then it's wrong.
>
> (Lauren)

As the above comment demonstrates, the cultures of school are perceived to endorse resistance to eating rather than construct it as a routine pleasurable exercise. As a consequence, for most participants, 'not feeling at home in one's own body was an unwelcome and powerful source of displacement' (Warin 2002: 120). Far from empowering individuals, or contributing to health and well-being, social practices such as those described thus leave some feeling powerless, labelled and alienated from their bodies, believing that they have less rather than more control over essential elements of their lives.

We have no wish to contest the commitment of teachers or schools who focus on health education or attempting to enhance the lifestyles of the young people in their care. Our point is simply that, although the aim to eradicate risks in people's lives on the surface appears value-neutral the actions implied in the above narratives suggest that they are not. Rather they are manifestly practices defined and constituted by the major themes implicit in wider discourses of obesity and health. In these cases, power is exercised not just through the 'panopticon of the curriculum', a technology of regulation and surveillance impinging on all aspects of daily life in school, but, as we shall see, through the informal structures, including peer cultures and networks in schools.

'Hungry to be noticed': achieving self-determination within the cultural demands of school

One of the strongest aspects of these girls' stories is a powerful feeling of lack of recognition of their individuality and 'agency' at school; a damaging condition leaving some to claim that they had simply felt 'like a number'.

> I've found that the teachers in this school were like, they're very cold and they never talk to you personally like you're a person, they'll talk to you like you're a number to them and that's all it is basically.
>
> (Mia)

> I think that one thing that schools could do is start to look more at the individual.
>
> (Lauren)

Ellie (11 years) mentioned that her headmaster 'didn't really seem to care about his students', Carrie commented that she just felt that they weren't 'treated as individuals' within school but just stereotyped or categorised in relation to abilities. Their stories indicated a lack of care about their broader spiritual, mental and emotional health and development. For many of the girls, the thought of returning to 'normal' school presented a great deal of distress:

> I've been to several different schools, since I've become ill this is, trying to get away from the illness at school . . . I have actually just been sitting with [the clinic's head teacher] trying to find alternatives to go back to because I know I can't go back to that school for my health, if you know what I mean . . . But in terms of whether school actually started the illness, I really don't know whether it did. All I know was that before I became ill I was immensely, immensely depressed, and I think the depression came from the school.
>
> *Int*: Because of the environment?
>
> Mmm . . . and because I've always been a very insecure person and school provided me with no security whatsoever.
>
> (Lauren)

We reiterate that these conditions of schooling do not *cause* eating disorders, but the following analysis suggests that these girls saw food and diet as a 'resource' to cope with the cultural demands placed on them in these environments by teachers and their peers. This raises some particularly alarming questions about the ways in which the body is used by children and young people in the power relations that are played out in schools. What is so interesting and perhaps unique about eating disorders is that research suggests that many sufferers come to see this as a horrifying yet desired practice, which, if drawn on over time, becomes deeply sedimented as a habitual way of thinking and acting (a form of 'habitus'). Indeed Warin (2002) suggests that the 'power of anorexia' comes from people's immersion in a habitus that promotes a particular 'representation of the "female body" as desirable and valuable', a commodity in the weight-conscious culture (Lynch 1987: 128). Lydia for example, commented:

> And that's something that goes on quite a lot, 'fat=bullying' (reading from her poster) You feel that if you're fat you get bullied, and you want people to notice you as well. So you want to be *noticed* as the stunning, skinny people.
>
> (Lydia)

> I competed with my friend to see who could lose the most weight.
>
> (Mia)

In effect, as Featherstone (1991) and Bordo (1993) highlight, the body has become the outward marker of 'value' in a consumer culture reflected in schools. The slim body signifies 'romantic femininity', associated with a variety of positive psychological characteristics (Wilkinson 1986) and self-control, status and 'worth' (Malson 1998).

> I always used to look at my friends and think that I wanted to be as good, or as pretty, or as clever as them. So I decided that not eating was a way that I could maybe achieve that.
>
> (Hayley, 15 years)

But again, to read this as simply a response to the ideals of slenderness would be naïve in the extreme. These clearly are deeply influential ideas but we need a more sophisticated understanding of multiple body perspectives that acknowledges the complexity of the conditions that these young women experience. Just as anorexia cannot be said to be about one issue, so the thin/'anorexic body' also sustains a multiplicity of meanings (see Moore 1998). For some of these girls it was a way of demonstrating self-control, autonomy, individuality, and achieving recognition by peers and others, the end product of disciplined dietary restraint.

> It's like what I've found at school is that, well as I've put on my poster, I was just *branded*, that was just who I was. And I just found that in some cases I could get away with things because I was anorexic and because I wasn't as capable as other people, and I don't know, that was awful really because I want to succeed at life because I'm talented not because people feel sorry for me.
>
> *Int*: So it was a label that you didn't want?
>
> Mmm, but in some respects I did want it because it made me feel special, it made me feel that I was more important than everybody else, and I think in some ways that was why I couldn't get rid of it at school . . . Because you have the dominants, the leaders, the thinkers, I was just the anorexic, that was who I was. And when this other girl at the school became anorexic, I felt that I had been pushed out of my place and I was furious . . . it [anorexia] shows that you have a strength that they don't, because let's face it, not many people have the ability to starve themselves to death.
>
> (Lauren)

Some young women who 'self-starve', therefore, quite understandably perceive anorexia as a positive resource, signifying success and control (Malson 1998). Self-starvation may, thus, come to represent a personal solution to broader social problems, amongst them a lack of order, control (Eckerman 1997) and recognition within schools. As Turner (1992) comments:

The anorexic avoids the shameful world of eating, while simultaneously achieving personal power and a sense of moral superiority through the emaciated body. Their attempt at disembodiment through negation becomes the symbol of their moral empowerment.

(Turner 1992: 221)

For Lauren, for example, anorexia is constructed as a way of differentiating herself from others at school, providing her with an identity. Her eating disorder might not have started either with that intent or realisation in mind, but the casting of anorexia (and extreme slenderness) as positive in terms of achieving some symbolic status and power in school, should raise alarm bells about what young people believe to be *valued* and appropriate 'body work' in these contexts. Clearly the achievement of this 'condition' is a double-edged sword. Whilst anorexia functions to produce an identity, it also indicates a 'concomitant negative construction of "the self" as otherwise lacking identity' (Malson 1998). It simultaneously signals not only that one has an anorexic identity, but that without anorexia, one has no identity at all.

'School didn't have a clue about what it's all about'

A large part of the conversations with the young women in our study centred on how schools dealt with and understood their illness. Asking 'how or through which discourses the desire to be thin is understood within schools?' presented further insights into the ways in which the body, (ill-)health and identity were being constructed in the educational contexts each had experienced. It also further illustrates the potentially damaging effects of a culture of healthism within schools.

Interestingly many of the girls in the study suggested that there were clear narratives they wished to convey about the social orders of schools which had helped propel them towards their eating disorder, but which they had been unable to express to medical professionals, teachers, family or friends:

> It was nice to actually get in a group and talk about it, and I felt that I would kind of like to record it myself so my mum could have heard what it's like and how hard it is. Because, you know, when you're one on one with your mum and dad you just lose all knowledge of being anorexic, you can't think of what to say and your mind goes blank.
>
> (Lydia)

Schools were not considered a place where problems could be voiced. On the contrary, they were deemed part of the problem. Similarly Lauren felt that others' narratives or understandings of her 'illness', body and self would be very different to her own:

> You could talk to friends of anorexics in school, and friends of people with eating disorders. Because it's like saying this is how I feel, that people have branded me as anorexic, but one of my friends could say something completely different. It would be worth while, and maybe going to teachers to see what they have to say . . .

There was a general sense amongst these young women of their illnesses being 'hushed up' as Karen put it; it was not 'something that was talked about':

> They [teachers] could have told people about it, and informed them about what it meant. Because I used to get bullied for being anorexic, and I knew that people must be talking about it because people I didn't even know used to look at me really strangely and talk about me behind my back.

Indeed Karen had to 'try and hide the fact that she was ill when she returned to school', and commented that when she had been in hospital she had 'to think of different reasons for why she had bandages on her hands where the drips had been . . . as if having anorexia was not an acceptable illness'. Such statements allude to the discursive struggles over the interpretations of self and anorexia, and the types of health and illness narratives that are accepted and legitimised within schools. The work of Weingarten (2001) who applies Chatman's (1978) narrative theory, in particular, concepts of narrative coherence, narrative closure and narrative interdependence, to the context of illness narratives is particularly useful here. According to Chatman (1978), 'narrative coherence' is established by the inter-relationships between plot, character roles and themes or values. In an illness narrative the patient, the patient's family and medical personnel all play parts, and often a plot sequence unfolds according to fixed and known responses.

These illness/eating disorder narratives were not well understood in schools (nor, it must be said, by friends, doctors, family and friends, in the perspective of the young women). Moreover, these environments were seen to reinforce the conditions that propelled them towards their illness, in part because the significance of any event in these narratives *is* unknown, and the plot unfolds chaotically. Nor is it clear who the relevant players are – should they see a doctor? psychiatrist? the school counsellor? How should family, school friends, teachers feel about this? Is this an illness? A condition? Should they be putting on weight? How quickly? There is wisdom but few certainties to be found in this field.

The second useful concept here is 'narrative closure'. The more familiar people are with the situation described the higher the cultural resonance will be and the more likely that others will be able to participate with the person whose narrative it is in a way that supports, endorses and elaborates the story that the person has to tell. As stated above, it is clear that the contemporary health discourse which constructs the relationship between exercise, weight and health as an *individual responsibility* is dominant in education. Within this discourse a 'restitution narrative' (Frank 1995) is much easier to engage with than others and is seen as the preferred illness story in Western cultures (Weingarten 2001). Within this narrative the individual tells the story from the perspective of the diagnosis and treatment: all that has been done, is being done and will be done if treatment fails. Unsurprisingly, then, few people in schools knew how to respond when faced with the 'chaotic', 'regressive' and 'rebellious' narratives of these 'anorectic' girls. Hence, as the participants describe, there is a lack of *relatedness* between the stories they wish to convey about their illness and the discourses of others around them used to understand them. We therefore see what Weingarten (2001) describes as 'micro-processes of withdrawal' from others around them as they fail to follow the prescribed restitution narrative or refuse to package their illness narratives in an appropriate form. As a result they are found deficient and may be marginalised along with attention to their illness.

> My friends didn't seem to understand just how much was going on in my head, they thought, I don't know, that I was being stupid or trying to get attention or something.
>
> (Carrie)

Carrie points towards the identity 'options' made available to her. Being anorexic comes to signify a pathologised subject position but, at the same time, a rebellious one. Anorexia is thus being 'discursively produced as both too thin and rebelliously individualistic' (Malson 1998). Such interpretations of eating disorders within the discourse of individualism and healthism which currently preside in schools may have a number of problematic implications. First, this approach constructs the desire to be thin as opposing rather than conforming to social pressures. We end up with depoliticised explanations of the desire to be thin, undermining the disciplinary power of discourses in schools which promote thinness and negatively constructs the subject who is interpellated and ultimately damaged by such discourses. Within the humanistic discourse of healthism these girls are likely to be positioned still as self-determining, as losing weight because of *internal individual* reasons, not as something connected to external social conditions, including those featuring in schools. Concomitantly, such pathology is then 'inevitably' deemed to be treatable through progression in health choices: the expectation that since the individual is governed by an internal self rather than by society, they are able and expected to make the choice to return to 'normal' health, which meant 'to gain weight':

> One of my teachers came up to me and said 'oh how have things been' and I said 'Oh not too well, I think they're thinking of putting me back in a unit' and he goes 'well you don't look too thin', and I was like (sighs) 'but you don't understand, there is more to it than just being thin' . . . And also when I came back to the sixth form, the same teacher saw me in a corridor and the first thing he said to me was 'are you putting on weight'. He *shouted* it across the *whole* corridor. He saw me and it obviously triggered in his head 'oh weight issue, are you putting on weight?' and I was like 'Oh my God!'
>
> (Lauren)

There is clearly no consideration by these teachers that the focus on the body, on weight and image may be the very precursor to the problem of gaining weight. In focusing solely on the visual spectacle of anorexia and in such a public way, the female body continues to be 'positioned and reproduced as public, as an object to be examined, beholden and always visible' (Warin 2002: 13).

The stories of these girls begin to point towards the pathological way in which their illness was perceived by others, not only damaging to their own identities, but pointing towards a healthist school culture that does little to consider its role in the aetiology and development of these conditions. Of course our arguments may be read as overly critical of a condition which is extremely complex and difficult for anyone to deal with. However, whilst a teacher's desire that their anorexic students put on weight appears laudable, it also deflects attention from narratives about who is responsible, how this is to be achieved and how and why anorexia arises. We might expect the presentation of the 'starved body' to prompt schools to look critically at the negative aspects of healthism in schools. The situations described here, however, suggest that school cultures do little to challenge the patriarchal discourses which present experiences around eating and body weight as a problem of individual pathology rather than as at least a partial consequence of the social environments (Malson 1998). In effect they depoliticise the promotion of the slim ideal and disguise the political and moral overtones of 'health' promotion within schools.

Conclusion

Eating disorders are complex conditions which could well develop even if one did not attend school. As one of the young women in our study succinctly comments: 'Anorexia is just like a person pulling you back from something.' However, the narratives of these young women highlight a school culture which builds pressure for perfection and performance, often in forms which are undesirable or impossible to achieve. We remain concerned by the social injustice of placing such moral obligation and blame on individuals for their health/problems and in ways which, as illustrated, depoliticise the roles that schools and other social influences play in peoples lives. Moreover we remain critical of the notion that eating disorders are a 'culture-bound syndrome', tied to media imagery and the cult of slenderness, nor can it be seen to be only about the process of regaining order and 'control'.

We need a clearer understanding of how the various 'medical', 'social' and 'spiritual' understandings of the body, and the emaciated body, are appropriated, fused and legitimated within schooling. What is clear from the stories of the young people is that the complexity of social interaction in schools belies any simple notion of gender socialisation, or reform strategy (for example, critical literacy) geared towards the treatment of a single factor bearing on their lives. If nothing else the data presented here should warrant a fundamental critique of any discourse that reduces the practice of education to the trivium of food (diet), exercise and weight, or generates social practices in which the child/young person is reduced to a 'body' rather than a person whose circumstances need to be understood if their health and educational requirements are to be met.

Acknowledgements

We are extremely grateful for the support and assistance offered by the management, staff and young people of the clinic in which our data was generated. Most of all, however, we offer our sincere thanks to the girls whose voices are heard within this text, for without their willingness to so openly and generously share their life experiences our research would be much the poorer

References

Alderson, P. (1995) *Listening to Children, Ethics and Social Research*, Ilford: Barnados.

Backett-Milburn, K. (2000) 'Parents, children and the construction of the healthy body in middle-class families', in A. Prout (ed.) *The Body, Childhood and Society*, Basingstoke: Palgrave Macmillan.

Bordo, S. (1993) *Unbearable Weight: Feminism, Western Culture and the Body*, Berkeley: University of California Press.

Bray, A. (1994) 'The edible woman: reading/eating disorders and femininity', *Media Information Australia* 72: 4–10.

Bray, A. (1996) 'The anorexic body: reading disorders', *Cultural Studies* 10(3): 413–30.

Brettschneider, W.D. (1992) 'Adolescents, leisure, sport and lifestyle', in T. Williams, L. Almond and A. Sparkes (eds) *Sport and Physical Activity: Moving Towards Excellence: The Proceedings of the AIESEP World Convention*, London: Spon.

Chatman, S. (1978) *Story and Discourse*, Ithaca, NY: Cornell University Press.

Christensen, P. and James, A. (eds) (2000) *Research with Children: Perspectives and Practices*, London: Falmer Press.

Doyle, J. and Bryant-Waugh, R. (2000) 'Epidemiology', in B. Lask and R. Bryant Waugh (eds) *Anorexia Nervosa and Related Eating Disorders in Childhood and Adolescence*, Hove: Psychology Press, Taylor & Francis.

Dyer, G. and Tiggemann, M. (1996) 'The effect of school environment on body concerns in adolescent women', *Sex Roles* 34: 127–38.

Eckerman, T. (1997) *Foucault, Self-Starvation and Gendered Subjectivities*, in A. Petersen and R. Bunton (eds) *Foucault, Health and Medicine*, London: Routledge.

Emmons, L. (1994) 'Predisposing factors differentiating adolescent dieters and non-dieters', *Journal of American Dieticians Association* 94: 725–31.

Evans, J., Evans, B. and Rich, E. (2002) 'Eating disorders and comprehensive ideals', *Forum for Promoting 3–19 Comprehensive Education* 44(2): 59–65.

Featherstone, M. (1991) 'The body in consumer culture', in M. Featherstone, M. Hepworth and B.Turner (eds) *The Body: Social Processes and Cultural Theory*, London: Sage.

Frank, A. (1995) *The Wounded Storyteller*, Chicago: University of Chicago Press.

Gard, M. and Wright, J. (2001) 'Managing uncertainty: obesity discourses and physical education in a risk society', *Studies in Philosophy and Education* 20: 535–49.

Glaser, B.G. and Strauss, A.L. (1967) *The Discovery of Grounded Theory: Strategies for Qualitative Research*, New York: Aldine de Gruyter.

Good, B. (1994) *Medicine, Rationality and Experience: An Anthropological Perspective*, Cambridge: Cambridge University Press.

Gordon, R.A. (2000) *Eating Disorders: Anatomy of a Social Epidemic*, Oxford: Blackwell Publishers.

Gordon, R.A. (2001) 'Eating disorders East and West: a culture bound syndrome unbound', in A. Nasser, M.A. Katzman and R.A. Gordon (eds) *Eating Disorders and Cultures in Transition*, Hove: Brunner-Routledge.

Henriques, J., Hollway, W., Urwin, C., Venn, C. and Walkerdine, V. (1984) *Changing the Subject: Psychology, Social Regulation and Identity*, London: Methuen.

Hepworth, J. (1999) *The Social Construction of Anorexia*, London: Sage.

Holroyd, R. (2003) 'Fields of experience: young people's constructions of embodied identities', unpublished Ph.D. thesis, Loughborough University.

Katzman, M. and Sing Lee (1997) 'Beyond body image: the integration of feminist and transcultural theories in the understanding of self-starvation', *International Journal of Eating Disorders* 22: 385–94.

Kirk, D. (1999) 'Physical culture, physical education and relational analysis', *Sport, Education and Society* 4(1): 63–73.

Lask, B. (2000) 'Aetiology', in B. Lask and R. Bryant-Waugh (eds) *Anorexia Nervosa and Related Eating Disorders in Childhood and Adolescence*, London: Taylor & Francis.

Lask, B. and Bryant-Waugh, R. (2000) *Anorexia Nervosa and Related Eating Disorders in Childhood and Adolescence*, Hove: Psychology Press, Taylor & Francis.

Levine, M. and Piran, N. (1999) 'Reflections, conclusion, future directions', in N. Piran, M. Levine and C. Steiner-Adair (eds) *Preventing Eating Disorders: A Handbook of Intervention and Special Challenges*, Philadelphia: Brunner/Mazel (Taylor & Francis Group).

Lupton, D. (1996) *Food, the Body and the Self*, London: Sage.

Lynch, M. (1987) The body: thin is beautiful', *Arena* 79: 128–45.

Malson, H. (1998) *The Thin Woman: Feminism, Poststructuralism and the Social Psychology of Anorexia Nervosa*, London: Routledge.

Moore, K. (1998) 'Anorexics' narratives on recovery', unpublished M.A. in Medical Sociology, University of East Anglia.

Oliver, K.L., and Lalik, R. (2000) *Bodily Knowledge: Learning about Equity and Justice with Adolescent Girls*, New York: Peter Lang.

Palmer, B. (2001) 'Commentary 1', in A. Nasser, M.A. Katzman, R.A. Gordon (eds) *Helping People with Eating Disorders: A Clinical Guide to Assessment and Treatment*, Ontario: Wiley Canada, pp. 17–19.

Phelps, L., Sapia, J., Nathanson, D. and Nelson, L. (2000) 'An empirically supported eating disorder prevention programme', *Psychology in the Schools* 37(5): 443–51.

Prince, R. (1985) 'The concept of culture bound syndrome: anorexia nervosa and brain-fag', *Social Science Medicine* 21: 197–203.

Ritenbaugh, C. (1982) 'Obesity as a culture bound syndrome', *Culture, Medicine and Psychiatry* 6: 348–61.

Silverstein, B., Perdue, L., Petersen, B., Vogel, L. and Fantini, D.A. (1986) 'Possible causes of the thin standard of bodily attractiveness for women', *International Journal of Eating Disorders* 5: 907–16.

Sparkes, A.C. (1995) 'Living our stories, storying our lives, and the spaces in between: life history research as a force for change', in A.C. Sparkes (ed.) *Research in Physical Education and Sport: Exploring Alternative Visions*, Lewes: Falmer Press.

Turner, B.S. (1992) *Regulating Bodies: Essays in Medical Sociology*, London: Routledge.

Warin, M. (2002) *Becoming and Unbecoming: Abject Relations in Anorexia*, unpublished Ph.D. thesis, Adelaide University, Adelaide.

Weingarten, K. (2001) *Making Sense of Illness Narratives: Braiding Theory, Practice and Embodied Life. Working with the Stories of Women's Lives*, Adelaide: Dulwich Centre Publications.

Wilkinson, S. (ed.) (1986) *Feminist Social Psychology: Developing Theory and Practice*, Milton Keynes: Open University Press.

Woods, P. and Carlyle, D. (2002) 'Teacher identity under stress: the emotions of separation and renewal', *International Studies in Sociology of Education* 12(2): 169–91.

13 Threatening space

(Physical) education and homophobic body work

Gill Clarke

Introduction

This chapter explores how space(s) shape pupils' and teachers' sexual identities in physical education. In doing so it reveals how spaces are not neutral, but shot through with power such that bodies are schooled along narrow and often homophobic lines. Spaces thus are also gendered, racialised, sexed and (hetero)-sexualised such that some locations become hostile places for lesbian women and gay men. Although queer activists[1] have begun to reclaim the largely heterosexual landscape and to extend the boundaries of sexual citizenship, schools in England and Wales largely remain sites of compulsory heterosexuality, where few have dared to cross the (hetero)sexual boundaries.

As Bell and Valentine (1995: 8) comment: 'A whole body of work is emerging in geography that explores the performance of sexual identities and the way that they are inscribed on the body and the landscape.' With few exceptions this approach has yet to extend into the educative context in general and physical education specifically. This chapter seeks to address this by revealing the significance that space, be it the gymnasium or the locale of the class/staff room, has for the construction and contestation of sexual identities. In particular attention is drawn to the ways in which pupils and teachers learn to negotiate and pass through these different territories. The costs however may be high; accordingly consideration is given to the impact of such strategies on mental health and to an examination of (hetero)sexualised bullying in schools. In seeking to illustrate these claims qualitative data generated from biographical research with lesbian physical education teachers in England is employed.

The sexualisation of space

In conceptualising 'space' as more than mere terrain I write not as a geographer but as a lesbian feminist educator who is interested in how spaces impact on (and for some of us, define) our sexual identities and how subsequently we come to express ourselves and the places we 'choose' (or are permitted) to visit and/or inhabit. For me, space is not static, rather it is dynamic, fluid and liable to destabilise. So, whilst space (and places) may influence and shape who we are, we too can act back on space.

In examining the sexualisation of space it is important to understand how and why space(s) is/are inhabited and used and by whom. The use of space is closely allied to the *control* of space and it could be argued that the more a particular group colonises a space the more others' use of that space is restricted. However, to suggest that any one group has absolute power over a space would be misleading and it is perhaps therefore more useful to conceive of 'groups', such as hetero-sexuals, as having hegemonic control of space. Such a view recognises that there is 'space' for alternative usage/occupation and contestation of the space.

Spaces become sexualised through a variety of strategies, for example by how they are physically and socially organised (Valentine 1993a) and by how people perform in those spaces (Valentine 1996). The (pre)dominance of heterosexual performances marks out many public places as being heterosexual spaces, i.e. spaces where lesbians and gay men do not feel free to perform their sexuality (see Clarke 1998a). Thus, it is to the public world of schooling and the struggles over educational spaces that I now turn.

The educational landscape and the (hetero)sexual politics of schooling

Schools and physical education departments are sites of moral and sexual regula-tion wherein docile and useful bodies are produced and identities are constructed, normalised and negotiated on a daily basis. This identity construction operates within what Butler (1990: 151) has termed the heterosexual matrix, by this she means that 'grid of cultural intelligibility through which bodies, genders, and desires are naturalized'. It is this naturalisation and taken-for-grantedness of heterosexuality that is so pervasive and damaging to both teachers and pupils. Further, the assumption of heterosexuality contributes to the marginalising of ways of being male or female and to the elevation of traditional forms of masculinity and femininity. Moreover, it leads to an invisibility, which contributes to the 'naturalisation of heterosexuality [and thus] provides an *absent centre* in relation to the curriculum' (Kehily 2002: 57). Hence, we can also see how policy documents and the formal/official curriculum in particular contribute to the maintenance and supremacy of heterosexuality (see Nutt and Clarke 2002). Thus, there are few places in the curriculum where 'other' sexualities might be discussed.

Nevertheless, it is not only *what* goes on in schools that governs ways of being, the often very 'rigid' architectural structures and layouts and the spaces of and between buildings and playgrounds embody and demarcate ways of being, for school is clearly more than just a place for transmission and reception of the National Curriculum. As Shilling (1991: 23) states: 'Space is no longer seen merely as an environment in which interaction takes place, but is itself deeply implicated in the production of individual identities and social inequalities.' Some of these inequalities relate to the ways in which boys use and dominate space and academic resources.

The playground is one highly visible site where this gender dominance has been well documented (see Mahony 1985 and Thorne 1993). Indeed, Swain (2000: 95) has shown how boys participating in playground football not only actively exclude and displace girls but also how 'some of the boys in the subordinated group who become feminised by their lack of skill and competence, and are subjected to homophobic abuse, as the hegemonic group acts within the "cultural imperative of heterosexuality"'. This leads to those excluded being driven to occupy less desirable and often smaller environments on the margins (see Sibley 1997).

This occupation of space is clearly gender-differentiated and as has been illustrated boys tend to vie for and use more space more confidently, although this is not to deny within-group differences (see Gordon *et al.* 2000). Further, girls are traditionally 'expected to move and speak out less, to take up less space, to sit in stillness and silence' (ibid.: 190).

In addition, school rules, rituals and sanctions become embedded within the structures of the institution and govern *how* spaces are used and entered into. Thus movement in corridors and other spaces is regulated and dictated by the timetable, which permits ordered and controlled movement between classrooms at certain times of the day only. These masculinising practices are as Connell (1996: 206) reveals 'concentrated at certain sites: curriculum divisions, discipline systems, and sports [and within physical education].'

This conception of physical and social space whilst helpful neglects the presence and significance of mental spaces (see Gordon and Lahelma 1996 and Gordon *et al.* 2000). For some this may be the only space they have power and control over, thus this may be an important and safe space for the self away from the surveillance and intrusion of others, be they teachers or other pupils. And as will be illustrated in the following section it is particularly difficult for lesbian and gay youth to find safe spaces to be themselves since all pupils are largely deprived of private spaces, though for the heterosexual majority it might be contended that this is somewhat less of an issue of personal safety.

Sexual bullying: policing the mind and body

> I'm 15, still at school and it's a living hell. People trip me up and call me names and there's no one I can tell. My parents hate gays. I told my RE teacher, but he treats me like I'm ill. I feel like I'm a stranger at school, like in a freak show. Why can't I be treated normally?
>
> (Chris, 15, Hillingdon, *Attitude* 2000)

> I have four teachers on my side but the rest aren't. A huge problem is that most of them won't accept I'm gay – they say it's a phase that everyone goes through. Well, I've known since I was 5 years old – long phase! The only thing that keeps me going is knowing that one day I will be happy and in love.
>
> (Michael, 14, *Attitude* 2000)

> I'm very depressed and very alone . . . I used to be a perfect pupil getting high credit marks, but because of the bullying my marks have fallen to a foundation

level. I can't tell anyone. I wish I was dead – just to have some peace. I am so tired of this so-called life. . . .

(17, anon., *Attitude* 2000)

Life in school as these letters from the 'Gay Youth' special edition of the magazine *Attitude* show in a compelling way how schools are highly sexualised and for some harmful spaces. These harrowing experiences for lesbian and gay youth would appear to be not uncommon. Rivers' (1995, 1996) on-going research vividly demonstrates the widespread extent of bullying in schools of lesbian and gay pupils and those perceived to be so. His study of the long-term effects of homophobic bullying on the mental and social development of his eighty respondents who were subjected to such abuse revealed the following experiences.

- Name calling (80 per cent)
- Open ridicule by pupils and occasionally teachers (69 per cent)
- Being hit or kicked (59 per cent)
- Having rumours and stories spread about them (55 per cent)
- Being teased (49 per cent)
- Being sent to Coventry [ignored/not spoken to] (23 per cent)
- Being sexually assaulted (8 per cent)

(Cited in Douglas *et al*. 1997: 13)

Further, the research for the report *Playing it Safe* (1997) commissioned by the Terence Higgins Trust[2] and Stonewall[3] and undertaken by Douglas *et al*. found from a questionnaire survey and telephone interviews with teachers that over 80 per cent were aware of homophobic bullying in their schools. In making sense of their findings Douglas *et al*. used the following definition of bullying which they rightly acknowledge is fairly narrow, but as they point out they wanted to distinguish between other forms of bullying and the type of bullying which their study was concerned with. Thus, for them,

Homophobic bullying takes place where general bullying behaviours such as verbal and physical abuse and intimidation is accompanied by or consists of the use of the terms such as gay, lesbian, queer or lezzie by perpetrators.

(Douglas *et al*. 1997: 12)

The use of these and other pervasive and derogatory terms warrant close attention, given, as Wallace (2001: 9) notes: 'The word gay has suddenly become the ultimate putdown in schools – even nursery children are using it to insult each other.' Such situations are particularly disturbing as language transmits the moral and heterosexual order and further language acts are, as Unks (1995: 110) states, 'acts of power'. These insults are directed at those who are different and don't conform to socially sanctioned and publicly approved ways of being masculine and feminine. Physical education is one distinct site where traditionally there have been and continue to be rigid ways of being physically and emotionally literate, hence for those who fail or who step out of these boundaries homophobic and heterosexist insults abound, albeit not always well documented (see, for example, Clarke 2002; Parker 1996; Swain 2000). Such insults are powerful and effective ways of ensuring that sexual difference remains policed and largely invisible; visibility for some is simply too dangerous to countenance.

The consequences of such bullying can be devastating and especially so for lesbian and gay youth. Indeed, Charter (2000: 12) reports that 'children who are intimidated at school about being homosexual are more likely to leave at 16 . . . Four out of ten children bullied about their sexuality attempted suicide or harmed themselves . . . '. It is clear that schools in general and teachers specifically are in the main failing to deal with homophobic bullying despite the DfEE Circular on *Social Inclusion: Pupil Support* (10/99), which advised that:

> The emotional distress caused by bullying in whatever form – be it racial, or as a result of a child's appearance, behaviour or special educational needs, or related to sexual orientation – can prejudice school achievement, lead to lateness, or truancy and, in extreme case, end in suicide . . . Pupils should be encouraged to report any bullying . . . Low report rates should not of themselves be taken as proof that bullying is not occurring.
>
> Head teachers have a legal duty to take measures to prevent all forms of bullying among pupils. All teaching and non-teaching staff . . . should be alert to signs of bullying and act promptly and firmly. Pupils may see failure to respond to incidents or allegations as tolerating bullying.

The research of Warwick, Aggleton and Douglas (2001) confirms the failure of teachers to address the needs of lesbian and gay pupils. Further, given as they point out 'the concern around promoting mental health . . . the elevated rates of suicide among these groups . . . it is worrying that little concrete action has been taken to foster the emotional and physical safety of lesbian and gay youth in schools' (p. 131).[4]

Undoubtedly physical education and sport is a site of homophobic bullying and heterosexist harassment not only for pupils but also for teachers (see, for instance, Clarke 1996, 1997, 2002). Rivers' (1995: 37) research confirms this *vis-à-vis* pupils and while stating that 'The school yard was the most likely place for bullying to occur, followed by school corridors . . .', he points out that 'roughly equivalent levels of bullying occurred in . . . the changing rooms . . .'. Much remains to be done if these are to be safe locations for all.

Having considered the experiences of pupils the sections that follow focus on the experiences of lesbian physical education teachers and how they deal with the various locations they inhabit whilst at school, home or out and about.

The government of location: border crossings

As I have previously claimed, spaces are not neutral, they provide terrains for the development of power relationships, such that some locations, be they public or private,[5] become hostile places for lesbians. Indeed, Section 28 of the Local Government Act of England and Wales,[6] which was passed in 1988 by the Conservative government under the then Prime Minister Margaret Thatcher, stated:

(1)   A local authority shall not –
    (a)   intentionally promote homosexuality or publish material with the intention of promoting homosexuality;
    (b)   promote the teaching in any maintained school of the acceptability of homosexuality as a pretended family relationship.
(2)   Nothing in subsection (1) above shall be taken to prohibit the doing of anything for the purpose of treating or preventing the spread of disease.

Section 28 was arguably designed to maintain cultural and spatial conformity in schools whilst at the same time defining, regulating, policing and enforcing sexual borders.

Sexual borders necessitate crossing and negotiation, for some this is a matter of ease, but for those on the margins the 'right' heterosexual credentials may be missing. As Anzaldua (1987: 3–4) incisively claims:

Borders are set up to define the places that are safe and unsafe, to distinguish *us* from *them*. A border is a dividing line, a narrow strip along a steep edge. A borderland is a vague and undetermined place created by the emotional residue of an unnatural boundary. . . . The prohibited and forbidden are its inhabitants.

Knowing how to read the borders and practices of educational institutions is a strategy that many lesbian (and gay) teachers develop in order to conceal their sexual identity so as to guard against possible harassment (Griffin 1991; Sparkes 1996; Squirrell 1989). Consequently, many engage in the performance of a pseudo-heterosexual identity.

Bernstein's concepts of classification and framing are helpful to make sense of these issues insofar as his ideas have acted as something of a catalyst in my attempts to map the borders and terrain of sexual identities, hence I use his notions of classification and framing like Atkinson *et al.* (1986: 152) 'as heuristic sensitising devices rather than as definitive concepts'. Classification here refers to the strength of the boundary/border between the lesbian and gay and heterosexual worlds from the point of view of officially prescribed sanctions (e.g. Section 28). Framing here refers to the strength of the boundary between lesbian and heterosexual interactions within the formal setting of schools, between, (1) teachers and teachers, (2) pupils and teachers and (3) pupils and pupils. Inasmuch as I draw on Bernstein's concepts it is worth noting that in spite of his more recent work around the formation of identities and in particular that of 'prospective identities' his work continues to be in the main silent about issues of sexual identity (see Bernstein 1996). It is the first of these interactions that I next focus on in the domain of the staff room.

The locale of the staff room and the framing of sexual identities

The staff room has traditionally been regarded as something of a place of sanctuary and a locale where teachers can relax and be themselves away from the demands and view of pupils. However, as I have earlier claimed, such sites are not neutral environments for they are clearly implicated in the construction and in some cases contestation of identities (see Shilling 1991). Further, they are environments where relations of power, privilege, domination and social control are established.

None of the lesbian teachers in my research[7] were completely open about their sexuality: for most their sexual identity was carefully concealed from all but a small number of 'trusted' colleagues, for some their 'true' identity was known to no one within the school. Indeed, lesbian teachers often promote strong negative framing to ensure that they are not perceived to be weakening the strong, officially sanctioned, boundary between lesbian and heterosexual worlds. All feared that should their lesbian identity be discovered colleagues and pupils would view them differently and in a non-positive light and ultimately they would lose their jobs. To avoid this they constructed sometimes quite complex boundaries around themselves in order to deflect suspicion. Thus, they were constantly vigilant about the public persona they presented in school and in particular in the staff room; hence they felt the need to live two lives and to endure the stress and strain that this entailed.[8] These two lives were the school life and the home life: the former required portrayal of a pseudo-heterosexual lifestyle. This was accomplished via strict self-censorship and surveillance through, for instance, the avoidance of talking about home life and partners; in some cases introducing mythical males into conversations; and for those who had been married, the retaining of the 'Mrs' title provided some evidence of a heterosexual identity.[9] Having briefly considered one particular aspect of school life that is the staff room I want now to consider the home life and how this too is framed in some instances by hegemonic discourses of heterosexuality.

Home life: a place of sanctuary or another site of surveillance?

As Ingram *et al.* (1997: 32) rightly contend 'Where we live and our passages across space are central to our identities, outlooks . . .'. Consequently, the importance of where lives are lived and located should not be underestimated (see Clarke 1998a). The home should be a place to be yourself and a site that is free from the surveillance of others (Johnston and Valentine 1995). This freedom may not always extend to members of the teaching profession (and specifically lesbian teachers). Most of the teachers in my study worried about living close to the school where they taught for fear of the gaze and scrutiny of their pupils. Hence, they preferred to live outside of the catchment area of their schools. Further, while in school they often felt anxious when pupils asked where and with whom they lived. Such questions were steered to safer topics or answered somewhat ambiguously so as to deflect suspicion.

While heterosexual teachers may also seek to live away from the immediate environment of the work-place and avoid answering questions about their private lives, the pressures are not the same since there are sharp differences in how hetero-sexuality and homosexuality are viewed and valued. Given that homosexuality is often defined as a stigmatised, abnormal and marginal identity that is socially threatening, it is heterosexuality that takes on the privileged position, hence the pressures to be seen to be 'normal' in schools, that is heterosexual. For lesbian teachers who work within the domain of physical education the situation is compounded due to the subject matter of physical education, that is the centrality and physicality of the body, which creates additional anxieties and pressures for these teachers.

Out and about: the fear of being seen

These teachers also worried when they were out that they would be seen in the company of their lesbian partner or other lesbian friends, and that their carefully concealed lesbian identity would be 'sussed'. In connection with these worries it is pertinent to note that smaller, rural-type communities can often pose particular problems for lesbians (and gay men) who want to feel at home but do not want to stand out as being markedly different from those round about them. Castells (cited in Adler and Brenner 1992) and others (Grosz 1995; Valentine 1995) have noted a tendency for lesbians (and gay men) to gravitate towards urban areas in search of a certain degree of anonymity and/or critical mass of lesbians (and gay men).

In schools and everyday life the notion of compulsory heterosexuality and its attendant assumptions prevails, except in those, largely urban, areas where lesbians and gay men have created what they perceive to be 'havens' for alternative perfor-mances (Myshick 1996). These 'havens' may also be construed as being 'ghettos' within which lesbians and gay men come to be cut off from the sexual mainstream; 'havens' where they may also live, work and/or enjoy their leisure. However, not all lesbian teachers are able to live in such 'havens', but for some entering urban areas does offer the possibility of leisure spaces to be openly lesbian, that is, within the locale of lesbian and gay clubs.

Nevertheless, Valentine (1993b) has argued that not all lesbians seek out club life: she claims some are rather wary, not knowing quite what to expect but having to 'take the risk' because they are so limited in terms of spaces where they can be assured of meeting other lesbians. Deb for instance admitted that when she first thought about going to a lesbian club she 'didn't know what to expect inside'. Further, when she did actually go to a club, she acknowledged that she

> was so nervous about going in that . . . [she] waited outside and this gay chap came down and I told him I was nervous to go down and I'd never been in one before and he said 'I'll take you in' and the both of us went down.

Some support for Valentine's claim is also provided by Caroline's admission that she used to visit clubs 'all the time when . . . [she] was single', as she saw it 'as the only place that you ever met anybody', in other words 'she took the risk'. Now that Caroline is in a long-standing relationship she is less frequently involved in the club scene. However, it is worth noting that Caroline's Head of Department, who was also a lesbian, had expressed her concerns about her going to gay clubs and pubs and told her to be careful and discrete in terms of how she lived her life.

Lucy described how the 'club scene' didn't appeal to her so she never found out where clubs existed; she revealed that 'perhaps more importantly I didn't want to run the risk of being recognised by parent, pupil or governor and it compromising my job – which I enjoyed doing'. Few of these teachers therefore had any interest in going 'clubbing'; indeed, Ethel said 'I don't think it does our cause any good to have separate clubs'.

The extent to which these places are actually experienced as 'safe' seems to depend on whether you are lesbian or gay. Assaults on gay men are more frequently reported to have occurred in the vicinity of gay clubs or well-known gay districts, while lesbians are more likely to be attacked in heterosexual spaces (Mason and Palmer 1996). Safe spaces for gay men and lesbians may well mean different things, particularly as lesbians are not only vulnerable to attack as lesbians, but also as women. For this reason, some lesbians are reluctant to seek out alternative spaces such as clubs and bars because often they are located in more run-down parts of cities.

Having the freedom to portray and perform your homosexuality openly therefore carries a number of risks and so heterosexual hegemony leads gay men and lesbians to either ignoring the risks, self-censoring their performances or finding 'safe' spaces where their performances are not threatened or challenged. What is 'safe' needs to be understood within a particular context, for example being lesbian or gay, whilst not illegal, carries a certain degree of 'risk' for those in education. Ignoring the threat of sanctions may expose the individual to 'risk' while self-censorship can lead to lesbians and gay men passing as heterosexual and therefore able to work and/or engage in leisure in some safety. However, passing as a strategy is not always successful, as the heterosexual mask may slip and there may be personal and political costs to be borne in the process of concealing a lesbian or gay identity (see Clarke 1998a). As Valentine (1993a: 410) argues:

> By concealing their identity in this way, lesbians become invisible in everyday environments. This fear of disclosure feeds the spatial supremacy of hetero-sexuality in three ways. First, it masks the number of lesbians present and so reinforces the heterosexual identity of environments. Second, it facilitates the perpetuation of negative stereotypes about what lesbians are like. Third, it ghettoises gay sexuality by making it difficult for lesbians to identify and meet other lesbians except in gay-defined spaces.

The spaces for lesbian (physical education) teachers to be themselves are severely restricted and contained: for these women their safe spaces are largely confined to the margins. Their sexual identity 'choices' are severely constrained by a complexity of forces that operate within both the wider social and political world and the microcosm of the school.

Concluding remarks

In this chapter I have sought to demonstrate how educational landscapes impact upon the identities of pupils and teachers. In doing so it has been shown that the impact is often damaging since identities are not free-floating but limited and policed by the heterosexual borders of schooling. There is clearly a need to challenge and dismantle these hegemonic heterosexual borders. For as Connell (1996: 224) points out:

> Education [and physical education] is a moral trade, and a good education must embody social justice. If we are not pursuing gender [and sexual] justice in the schools, then we are offering boys [and girls] a degraded education – even though society may be offering them [boys] long-term privilege.

The pursuit of social justice requires teachers, teacher educators and policy-makers to look critically at the content of the formal (and informal) curriculum and the ways in which it is delivered. We need a curriculum and teaching resources that tell of diverse experiences and linked to this is a need for more inclusive pedagogies which will allow all to realise fully their potential to learn.

Schools[10] and higher education institutions should be safe, respectful and inclusive spaces for all. Indeed, much could be learned from the *Safe Zone* programme as developed and utilised in some states in America. This programme in essence seeks to 'increase the visible presence of student and adult allies who can help to shape a school culture that is accepting of all people regardless of sexual orientation, gender identity/expression, or any other difference' (GLSEN 2003: 1).

Finally, we need to ensure that all educational establishments welcome pupils and teachers regardless of who they are or how they identify; in that way schools might begin to become truly representative of the diverse communities that they represent.

Notes

1   I use the term queer activists to refer to groups who have begun to fight back through direct (in your face) action and through the formation of such oppositional groups as OutRage in London and Queer Nation in New York. These and other groups have staged various challenges to the assumed heterosexuality of places; spatial pushes in London have included, for instance, a mass KISS-IN in Piccadilly Circus and a Queer Wedding in Trafalgar Square, both of which were organised by OutRage (see Clarke 1998a; Bell 1995). Being queer involves reclaiming an identity and label that was pejorative. It is to be visible, to be playful, to engage in parody and performance; to be queer is to be inclusive, to recognise diversity and to blur the sexual boundaries. It is also the rejection of sexual and gender binaries, labels and 'normative' moralities. However, it needs to be asked if queer politics are hostile/oblivious to lesbian feminist politics, and whether

the agenda is too narrow and based on a particular 'brand of gay male politics?' (Jeffreys 1994: 175). For a more detailed discussion, see Clarke 1998b.

2   The Terence Higgins Trust is a national HIV and AIDS charity based in London.

3   Stonewall is a national civil rights group working for legal equality and social justice for lesbians, gay men and bisexuals; it too is based in London.

4   The organisation SCHOOLS'OUT NATIONAL! has produced a useful leaflet 'Legislation and DfEE Guidance on Tackling Homophobia in Schools' which clarifies the position *vis-à-vis* Section 28, available at http://www.schools-out.org.uk/legislation. html

5   For a discussion of 'Public and (partially) private spaces', see Clarke 1998a.

6   The new Local Government Bill which includes a cross-party amendment to scrap Section 28 in England and Wales was passed in the House of Commons by 356 votes to 127 on March 10 2003. The Bill will now move to the House of Lords for consideration.

7   In seeking to illustrate these claims I draw on qualitative data generated from in-depth interviews with eighteen lesbian physical education teachers who were white, able-bodied and aged between 23 and 47. Some were single, some had been married, some were currently in long-standing lesbian relationships, and none had children. At the time of the research they had been teaching for just over one year to twenty-five years. All taught pupils aged between 11 and 18, some worked in mixed state schools, others in girls' schools, church schools or private schools located in inner cities, urban or rural areas.

8   Ferfolja (1998) describes the homophobic harassment of lesbian teachers in Australia and how three of the six she interviewed took stress leave.

9   For further details of the strategies they employed to pass as heterosexual, see in particular Clarke 1995 and 1996.

10 In Clarke 2002 I have outlined the ways in which schools might challenge homophobia and heterosexism.

References

Adler, S. and Brenner, J. (1992) 'Gender and space: lesbians and gay men in the city', *International Journal of Urban and Regional Research* 16: 24–34.

Anzaldua, G. (1987) *Borderlands: The New Mestiza = La Frontera*, San Francisco: Aunt Lute Book Company.

Atkinson, P., Dickinson, H. and Erben, M. (1986) 'The classification and control of vocational training for young people', in S. Walker and L. Barton (eds) *Youth, Unemployment and Schooling*, Milton Keynes: Open University Press.

Bell, D. (1995) 'Pleasure and danger: the paradoxical spaces of sexual citizenship', *Political Geography* 14(2): 139–53.

Bell, D. and Valentine, G. (eds) (1995) *Mapping Desire: Geographies of Sexualities*, London: Routledge.

Bernstein, B. (1996) *Pedagogy, Symbolic Control and Identity: Theory, Research and Critique*, London: Taylor & Francis.

Butler, J. (1990) *Gender Trouble: Feminism and the Subversion of Identity*, London: Routledge.

Charter, D. (2000) 'Victims of gay bullying "drop out of school"', *The Times*, July 18: 12.

Clarke, G. (1995) 'Outlaws in sport and education? Exploring the sporting and education experiences of lesbian physical education teachers', in L. Lawrence, E. Murdoch and S. Parker (eds) *Professional and Development Issues in Leisure, Sport and Education*, Eastbourne: Leisure Studies Association.

Clarke, G. (1996) 'Conforming and contesting with (a) difference: how lesbian students and teachers manage their identities', *International Studies in Sociology of Education* 6(2): 191–209.

Clarke, G. (1997) 'Playing a part: the lives of lesbian physical education teachers', in G. Clarke and B. Humberstone (eds) *Researching Women and Sport*, London: Macmillan.

Clarke, G. (1998a) 'Working out: lesbian teachers and the politics of (dis)location', *Journal of Lesbian Studies* 2(4): 85–99.

Clarke, G. (1998b) 'Voices from the margins: lesbian teachers in physical education', unpublished Ph.D. thesis, Leeds Metropolitan University.

Clarke, G. (2002) 'Difference matters: sexuality and physical education', in D. Penney (ed.) *Gender and Physical Education: Contemporary Issues and Future Directions*, London: Routledge.

Connell, R.W. (1996) 'Teaching the boys: new research on masculinity, and gender strategies for schools', *Teachers College Record* 98(2): 206–35.

DfEE (1999) *Social Inclusion: Pupil Support*, Circular 10/99, London: DfEE.

Douglas, N., Warwick, I., Kemp, S. and Whitty, G. (1997) *Playing it Safe: Responses of Secondary School Teachers to Lesbian, Gay and Bisexual Pupils, Bullying, HIV and AIDS Education and Section 28*, Health and Education Research Unit, Institute of Education, University of London: Terence Higgins Trust and Stonewall.

Ferfolja, T. (1998) 'Australian lesbian teachers – a reflection of homophobic harasment of high school teachers in New South Wales government schools', *Gender and Education* 10(4): 401–15.

GLSEN (2003) *Safe Zone Programs*. Available HTTP: http://www. glsen.org/templates/resources/record.html?section=18&record=1520 (12 March 2003).

Gordon, T. and Lahelma, E. (1996) '"School is like an ant's nest": spatiality and embodiment in schools', *Gender and Education* 8(3): 301–10.

Gordon, T., Holland, J. and Lahelma, E. (2000) *Making Spaces: Citizenship and Difference in Schools*, Basingstoke: Macmillan.

Griffin, P. (1991) 'Identity management strategies among lesbian and gay educators', *Qualitative Studies in Education* 4(3): 189–202.

Grosz, E. (1995) *Space, Time and Perversion: Essays on the Politics of Bodies*, London: Routledge.

Ingram, G.B., Bouthillette, A.M. and Retter, Y. (eds) (1997) *Queers in Space: Communities/Public Spaces/Sites of Resistance*, Seattle: Bay Press.

Jeffreys, S. (1994) *The Lesbian Heresy: A Feminist Perspective on the Lesbian Sexual Revolution*, London: The Women's Press.

Johnston, L. and Valentine, G. (1995) 'Wherever I lay my girlfriend, that's my home; the performance and surveillance of lesbian identities in domestic environments', in D. Bell and G. Valentine (eds) *Mapping Desire: Geographies of Sexualities*, London: Routledge.

Kehily, M. (2002) *Sexuality, Gender and Schooling: Shifting Agendas in Social Learning*, London: Routledge Falmer.

Mahony, P. (1985) *Schools for the Boys? Co-education Reassessed*, London: Hutchinson.

Mason, A. and Palmer, A. (1996) *Queer Bashing: A National Survey of Hate Crimes Against Lesbians and Gay Men*, London: Stonewall.

Myshick, N.D. (1996) 'Renegotiating the social/sexual identities of places: gay communities as safe havens or sites of resistance?', in N. Duncan (ed.) *BodySpace: Destabilizing Geographies of Gender and Sexuality*, London: Routledge.

Nutt, G. and Clarke, G. (2002) 'The hidden curriculum and the changing nature of teachers' work', in A. Laker (ed.) *The Sociology of Sport and Physical Education: An Introductory Reader*, London: Routledge Falmer.

Parker, A. (1996) 'The construction of masculinity within boys' physical education', *Gender and Education* 8(2): 141–57.

Rivers, I. (1995) 'The victimisation of gay teenagers in schools: homophobia in education', *Pastoral Care*, March: 35–41.

Rivers, I. (1996) 'Young, gay, bullied', *Young People Now*, January: 18–19.

Shilling, C. (1991) 'Social space, gender inequalities and educational differentiation', *British Journal of Sociology of Education* 12(1): 23–44.

Sibley, D. (1997) *Geographies of Exclusion: Society and Difference in the West*, London: Routledge.

Sparkes, A. (1996) 'Physical education teachers and the search for self: two cases of structured denial', in N. Armstrong (ed.) *New Directions in Physical Education: Change and Innovation*, London: Cassell.

Squirrell, G. (1989) 'In passing . . . teachers and sexual orientation', in S. Acker (ed.) *Teachers, Gender and Careers*, Lewes: Falmer Press.

Swain, J. (2000) '"The money's good, the fame's good, the girls are good": the role of playground football in the construction of young boys' masculinity in a junior school', *British Journal of the Sociology of Education* 21(1): 95–109.

Thorne, B. (1993) *Gender Play: Girls and Boys in Schools*, Buckingham: Open University Press.

Unks, G. (ed.) (1995) *The Gay Teen: Educational Practice and Theory for Lesbian, Gay and Bisexual Adolescents*, London: Routledge.

Valentine, G. (1993a) '(Hetero)sexing space: lesbian perceptions and experiences of everyday spaces', *Environment and Planning: Society and Space* 11: 395–413.

Valentine, G. (1993b) 'Desperately seeking Susan: a geography of lesbian friendships', *Area* 25(2): 109–16.

Valentine, G. (1995) 'Out and about: geographies of lesbian landscapes', *International Journal of Urban and Regional Research* 19: 96–111.

Valentine, G. (1996) '(Re)negotiating the "heterosexual street": lesbian productions of space', in N. Duncan (ed.) *BodySpace: Destabilizing Geographies of Gender and Sexuality*, London: Routledge.

Wallace, W. (2001) 'Is this table gay? Anatomy of a classroom insult', *Times Educational Supplement*, January 19: 9–10.

Warwick, I., Aggleton, P. and Douglas, N. (2001) 'Playing it safe: addressing the emotional and physical health of lesbian and gay pupils in the UK', *Journal of Adolescence* 24: 129–40.

Part IV

Future directions

Research and development in PEH

14 Endnote: the embodiment of consciousness

Bernstein, health and schooling

John Evans and Brian Davies

Coding consciousness: from performance and competency to perfection

Post-structural theories invite us to consider the possibility that power resides in knowledge, that discourse can be reproduced or contested in a multiplicity of sites and is not held centrally by the state or a conspiratorial group (Skelton 1997). But how are particular forms of knowledge and discourse encoded and translated into pedagogical practices and with what consequences for identity and consciousness? We share Bernstein's view that Foucault's analysis of power, knowledge and discourse is a mighty attempt to show the new forms of the discursive positioning of subjects. Yet there is no substantive analysis of the complex of agencies, agents, social relations through which power, knowledge and discourse are brought into play as regulative devices; nor any discussion of modalities of control. It is a discourse without social relations. Further, Foucault ignores almost completely any systematic analysis of the common denominator of all discourses, education and the modalities of its transmission (Bernstein 1996). Here, then, we ask, how are wider social forces, economic interests and trends such as those mentioned throughout this book embedded and encoded in the practices of schooling, and ultimately internalised as distinctive forms of embodied consciousness? In pursuing this question we move from Foucault to the work of Bernstein, and elaborate on one of the major themes that has run throughout this and other chapters, that physical education and health (PEH) curricula are now increasingly dominated by pedagogic modalities expressing body *perfection* and *performance* codes.

Our use of the term code is drawn explicitly from the work of Bernstein (1996, 2000; see Davies 1994; Hasan 2002) and we use it, as he does, to explore how the distribution of power and principles of control in society translate into pedagogic codes and pedagogic modalities in schools; and, thereafter, how these codes and their modalities are acquired, shape pedagogic consciousness and, in our terms, are 'embodied'. In this way the concepts of code and modality allow us to make connections between macro structures of power and control and micro processes. Other researchers in physical education, preoccupied with a similar problematic, have sometimes used other elements of Bernstein's work and/or other social theory to make links of this kind (see Kirk 1998; Gard and Wright 2001; Pronger 2002).

It is worth reminding ourselves, however, of the questions that lie at the heart of Bernstein's project.

> First, how does a dominating distribution of power and principles of control generate, distribute, reproduce and legitimate dominating and dominated principles of communication?
>
> Second, how does such a distribution of principles of communication regulate relations within and between social groups?
>
> Third, how do these principles of communication produce a distribution of forms of pedagogic consciousness?
>
> In summary, how does power and control translate into principles of communication, and how do these principles of communication differentially regulate forms of consciousness with respect to their reproduction and the possibility of change?
>
> (Bernstein 2000: 4)

In Bernstein's view, *power* always operates on the relationships between categories (agencies, agents, discourses, practices, spaces, etc.) and establishes legitimate relations of order (both externally and internally). By contrast, *control* establishes legitimate forms of communication appropriate to the different categories. It carries the boundary relations of power and socialises individuals into these relationships. Importantly, Bernstein then defines two concepts to help us interrogate these processes: for the translation of power, or power relations, *classification*, for the translation of control relations, *framing*; with both expressed as having different strengths and given, for example, as C+F+ or C–F– in pedagogical contexts of various forms. If the insulation between categories changes, the principles of the social division of labour also change. Armed with these concepts, we can ask, amongst other things, what preserves the insulation, for example, between the disciplines or activities that constitute PE, or between PE and other subjects on the curriculum? What preserves the space between categories? What preserves the regions of silence, the insulations of power? The concepts 'classification' and 'frame' are of enormous analytic value, allowing us to explore how the distribution of power and principles of control translate into pedagogic codes and their modalities and how these codes are then acquired and shape consciousness (Evans *et al.* 1987). They offer a conceptual scheme par excellence for tracing the relationships between social structures and consciousness, cultural production and reproduction, agency and change in society and schools. More specifically, in Bernstein's (2000) terms, code refers to the

> regulative principles which select and integrate relevant meanings (classifications), forms of their realisation (framings) and their evoking contexts. The values (strong/weak) and functions (classifications/framings) carry the code potential. How this potential is actualised is a function of the struggle to construct and distribute code modalities which regulate pedagogic relations, communication and context management. Conflict is endemic within and

between the arenas in the struggle to dominate modalities and in the relation
between local pedagogic modalities and official modalities

(Bernstein 2002: 202)

But what are the regulative principles to which Bernstein alludes, in contexts of
formal education and PEH? What are the social and historical bases, the logic and
grammar of the codes and pedagogies by which pedagogic messages are relayed?
Following Bernstein, we need think of pedagogic practice as wider than the
classroom relationships between teachers and taught in schools, to include, for
example, relationships between parent/guardians and child, doctor and patient,
counsellor and client, coach and player. Codes are embedded in formal and
informal structures, so that within school, for example, lunch-time practices and
playground behaviours that may not at first sight be considered embodiments of
the pedagogic device, may be of great relevance. In all cases, pedagogic practice
constitutes the social context through which cultural production and reproduction
take place. All invoke power relations and are contexts in which, we claim,
'difference from', 'similarities to', and 'relations of' the body come to the fore and
are embodied. The project then becomes that of analysing how a pedagogic text
has been put together, 'the rules of its construction, circulation, contextualisation,
acquisition and change' (ibid.: 30). Any such analysis would need to be informed
by an historical perspective on curriculum and pedagogical developments, such as
that in PEH of David Kirk (1992). Such analysis would also concern itself
especially with the ways in which knowledge in the wider social system (e.g. by
research and scholarship) is recontextualised (selected and reconfigured) in what
Bernstein calls the official recontextualising fields (ORFs; for example, government
agencies responsible for policy on education and health) and pedagogic recontextualising fields (PRFs; for example, institutions of higher education, publishing
companies) and made available for reproduction (and may be some further degree
of recontextualisation) by teachers in schools and colleges.

Competency, performance and perfection in PEH

Bernstein (2000) proposed two models of pedagogic discourse to encompass
the recent history of formal education in the UK and elsewhere, which he labelled
competency and *performance*, each referring to specific procedures for engaging
with and constructing the world. Each has a social logic, that is to say, an implicit
model of communication, interaction and the subject. Perhaps underplaying
the longer historical legacy of these concepts, he pictured the intellectual bases
of the first as arising from a conceptual convergence of quite disparate disciplines
within the social and psychological sciences in the 1960s around the concept of
'competence'; 'in linguistics, in the notion of "linguistic competency" (Chomsky);
in psychology, "cognitive competency" (Piaget); in socio-linguistics, "communicative competence" (Dell Hymes); and in sociology "cultural competency"
(Levi-Strauss)' (ibid.: 42). Bernstein argued that, although quite disparate in intellectual origin, in all these cases 'competences' were viewed as 'internally creative

and tacitly acquired in informal interactions'. They are practical accomplishments. Their internal logic implies 'a universal democracy of acquisition' where everyone is considered inherently competent; there are no deficits and the subject is active and creative in the construction of a valid world of meaning and practice. In this perspective, there are *differences between* people but not deficits, subjects are self-regulating, sceptical of hierarchical relations and the focus of analysis is upon the 'present tense', on what can be achieved in the here and now (ibid.: 43). Such 'recontextualised competence', based on ideas and knowledge generated in the primary research fields, received, 'read' and reconfigured by policy-makers and educationalists, constructed a specific pedagogical practice found predominantly in primary and pre-schools. It was reflected most obviously in the UK in the Plowden Report in 1969 that was greatly influential in the legitimation of British child-centred education in primary schools. It also found expression in the development of educational gymnastics, teaching games for understanding (TGFU) and recent emphases on student-centred situated learning in PEH and sport education.

In contrast to competency modalities Bernstein saw *performance* pedagogical modes arising from quite different fields of discourse and theories of learning of a behaviourist kind which had quite different epistemological leanings, origins and implications. These place emphasis upon the specific outputs of acquirers, upon particular texts they are expected to construct and upon the specialised skills necessary to the production of the specific outputs, texts or products. For Bernstein, this modality was clearly expressed by the selective grammar schools in the UK and their discursive organisers, 'codes of singulars' (knowledge structures whose creators have appropriated a space to give themselves a unique name and special-ised discrete discourse; see Bernstein 2000: 52) and strongly classified collection codes. He discusses both models with reference to the features which they share. Whereas competency modes (CM) focus on procedural commonalities shared within a social class, ethnic or other relevant category, performance modes (PM) focus on something that the acquirers do not possess, upon an absence, as a consequence placing emphasis on the text to be acquired and upon the transmission (ibid.: 57). Whereas competency modes are predicated on '*similar to*' relations (what people have in common), performance modes are based on '*different from*' relations (what sets them apart); in competency modes differences are viewed as complementary, in performance modes as hierarchically distinct. Performance modes are more directly related towards the interests of the economy than the systems of symbolic control to which competency modes are primarily oriented and are, argues Bernstein, pervasive and empirically normal across all levels of formal education (ibid.: 52), including physical education (see Tinning 1992, 1997). Which discourse is appropriated depends on the dominant ideology in the official recontextualising field and upon the relative autonomy of the pedagogic recontextualising field. There was a shift in formal education from performance to competency modes in the 1960s, with a reverse shift from competency to performance modes in the 1970s and 1980s as a result of state intervention in the official recontextualising field and a weakening of the PRF, reflected most clearly in the UK in the Thatcher years but endorsed and sharpened under the New Labour governments of Tony Blair ever since.

Bernstein stressed that although these models and modes can be considered discrete and give rise to distinct forms of pedagogy, mixes take place on what he neatly refers to as a 'pedagogic palette'. Moreover, it is quite possible to map and interrogate curriculum development in PEH in these terms. For example, 'traditional' games teaching and the post-1988 Education Reform Act emphasis in the UK on a sport-dominated curriculum, were expressions, *par excellence*, of performance modes. In contrast, educational gymnastics and the more recent post Piagetian/Vygotskyan emphasis on situated learning in PE which foregrounds the active acquirer in a situated pedagogic relation may be taken as examples of competency modes. At the same time, we might interpret the emergence of health-based physical education in schools during the late 1970s and 1980s in the UK, Australia, New Zealand and elsewhere, as an example of the pedagogic palette at work, involving a convergence of performance and competency modes, a coming together of the scientific functionalist concerns for physical fitness (PM) and educational gymnastics (CM) concerns for the individual learner and locating exercise and health within the context of the pupil's total lifestyle (Kirk 1992: 166).

However, unlike Durkheim (see Shilling, Foreword to this book), Bernstein was not particularly concerned to interrogate how social relations are 'embodied' and his characterisation of two contrasting modes as models for heuristic purposes, adapted insensitively, could obfuscate both the presence and the significance of other codes and their modalities that have their social and intellectual origins outside the social, psychological and behavioural sciences. Some have their social bases outside formal education, for example, in the economic interests of business, industry and the media and the medical and health fields and they centre, unlike performance and competency, on the dynamic between body and nature, and biology and culture, on what we refer to as *'relations of'* 'the body' rather than 'relations to' or 'differences from' individuals and agencies *out-with* 'the self'. If we were using a more Foucauldian language we would, no doubt, here refer to 'relations to one's embodied self'. In this respect, for reasons which we will endeavour to make clear below, we suggest that they are best characterised as body-centred perfection codes. Furthermore, in our view, the changes that have occurred in PEH since the 1970s represent not only a mixing of modes but rather a *paradigmatic shift* in the social bases, logic and coding of PEH knowledge and, concomitantly, of pedagogic modalities and consciousness in schools. It represents a shift from explicit pedagogies of *order* (featuring hierarchy, positional relations and imposed discipline) to implicit pedagogies of social *control* (featuring personal relations, horizontal hierarchies and the self-regulation of individuals and by extension, of populations via a focus on 'the body'); in effect, a shift from a concern with repairing the 'physical body' to protecting/preserving the unfinished body by reconfiguring body, mind and soul through intervention which is everyone's concern. This notion would appear to have a great deal in common with one of Bernstein's (2001) last ideas where he saw Prime Minister Blair's Britain as the emergent 'Totally Pedagogised Society' (TPS) where every teenager is to have access to a counsellor to enable the adolescent to map an appropriate career . . . [and is] positioned in flexible time which translates as being able to be repositioned whenever or wherever external change requires. Family units, whatever form they take, are new sites for parenting skill. So another pedagogic transition is possible, family units become parenting skills. The world of work translates pedagogically into Life Long Learning and this is both the key and the legitimator of T.P.S.

(Bernstein 2001: 365)

This, then, is a social order 'shaped, animated and maintained through the discursive principles of pedagogy as embodied in new educational technologies, life long learning policies and a fluid, highly credentialised work force' (Tyler 2001). This is a society in which cognitive and 'social processes are to be especially developed in the actor for a pedagogical future' of socially empty 'trainability' (Bernstein 2001: 366), 'empty' because it is 'a mere shell for the expansion of consumption, electronic communications and the circulation of the images of global capital culture' (Tyler 2001: 5). In this context, identities nurtured, monitored and regulated over many different sites (e.g. in families, work and leisure) are recognised through consumption, displayed through the 'right' embodied capacities, and managed by a strong state 'through processes of centralised decentralisation' (ibid.: 367). Significantly, the main force of the pedagogic relation becomes

its invisible normalising effects through an apparatus of symbolic control which valorises trainability, a capacity for endless forming and reforming of individual desire. This society depends on the workers' capacity to find meaning – not in coherent or stable social relations, commitment or careers but rather in the gratifications of consumerism.

(Tyler 2001: 5)

Tyler sees this information-centred modality as another stage beyond its precursors, Bernstein's subject and student-centred modalities (characterised as performance and competency). We see it as the social context in which perfection codes and modalities must be located. As such we should view them, at least in part, as reflections of consumerism and global capitalism's capacity not only to 'manufacture' and manipulate desire and emotion but also define embodied 'trained' and 'trainable' 'qualities' as just what industry and commerce requires and the nation state needs.

The social bases of perfection codes

We cannot yet provide further detailed analysis of the social bases of perfection codes. However, it is important to note that these codes have their origin outside formal education in the trends alluded to above. The massive proliferation of interest in 'the body' in Western cultures contexted in an era of 'flexible capitalism' is endorsed and supported in the health and media industries in the UK, for example, where it is estimated that around £1.5 billion a year is now spent on 'gyms', while the health supplements industries are now worth £350 million a year (*The Times Magazine* 2002). It also reflects developments that have occurred in primary research in the fields of medicine and health over the last fifty years. As Le Fanu (1999) points out, by the early 1970s, the main pillars of post-war medical achievement through clinical science, medical chemistry and technical innovation were in deep trouble. There remained a vast ocean of ignorance at the centre of medicine, for example, on conditions like multiple sclerosis and Parkinsons. The search for the 'causes' of ill-health became the dominant medical paradigm from the 1980s onwards, driven by very different specialities. Genetics, or rather 'the new genetics', opened up the possibility of identifying abnormal genes in social disease. Epidemiology, with its 'social theory', insisted that the most common diseases such as cancer, heart disease and strokes are caused by social factors connected to unhealthy lifestyle and are preventable by switching diet and reducing exposure to risk factors. Such discourses provided the basis of a radical departure from *therapeutic* measures to *intervention*, for example, in the form of getting people to change diet and controlling populations to eradicate poverty, or the management of faulty genes. The project was substantially reoriented towards prevention and health promotion around three major lifestyle planks: pollution; poverty; and food. In Le Fanu's view, both developments filled medicine's intellectual vacuum, while proving, in their own ways, to be blind alleys, quite unable to deliver on their promises. Their failure, reflected in the fall of modern medicine, may also mark the end of some versions of PEH (see Gard, Chapter 5).

These changes have been, at least in part, reflected in the curriculum of PE in the UK and elsewhere. Kirk (1992, 1998) notes that the calculated use of PE as a means of contributing to the health of school children stretches back to 1800s. Though ever present discursively, not until the late 1970s did 'health' become a significant, pervasive and accepted presence in the school curriculum, ideologically and intentionally influencing and constructing pedagogic modes. Briefly, again following Kirk (1996), we can trace three phases in the development of health codes in PE and their reflected pedagogical modes. Initially embedded in a medico-health rationale, they were expressed in the elementary schools as an emphasis on hygiene, wholesome diet and physical activity (essentially through Swedish gymnastics), their focus upon *correcting* the physical defects born of poverty, poor physical environment, diet and nutrition amongst the mass of working-class children newly found in city schools. In bourgeois girls' schools, their focus was on correcting aberrations from norms of posture, elegance and poise and preparing for motherhood (women's work at home). In such strongly gendered discourse, 'the body' was positioned as in deficit and in need of correction or *compensation* for the pathological failings of social class, family and home and never taken seriously in boys' public schools. In the second phase, in the 1950s, we witness the emergence of 'scientific PE' offering new insights derived from experimental science and new knowledge of skill acquisition, body mechanics and physiological responses to exercise and health. The development of strength, endurance and fitness, found congenial to boys' PE, were now discursively (if not as thoroughly in practice) to define relationships between PE and health (see Kirk 1998). The 'scientific functionalism' of the 1950s and 1960s, informed by clinical science, led to the systematic pursuit of fitness, strength and endurance through pedagogic practice focused upon circuit training and sport, adding kudos and impetus to these relationships. In this phase, the health work of PE was essentially *therapeutic*, concerned with how the body could be physically ameliorated and improved through systematic involvement in exercise, physical activity, sport and good living (including non drinking and smoking). Fitness and health, however, were largely seen as the functional by-products of physical activity – health is caught incidentally or accidentally rather than taught formally through specific PE curriculum. By the late 1960s, however, as Kirk (1992) points out, a discourse, driven by 'new' knowledge, was beginning to highlight the degenerative effects of modern living bringing, by the early 1980s, a new emphasis on education and PE as 'intervention, prevention and health promotion', generating new pedagogic modes as the full legitimating force of epidemiology (and especially 'obesity research') has taken hold.

The distinctive features of perfection modes

Just as there are three forms of performance and competency modes (see Bernstein 2000) so too there are three forms of perfection modes (PFM). The first, predicated on residual features of medico-health discourse is *corrective*; its focus is the body in deficit and in need of treatment and repair through compensatory intervention (e.g. via better hygiene, diet and healthy exercise). The second, informed by the discourses of scientific functionalism and the clinical and physical sciences, *is ameliorative and therapeutic*, focused on improving the body through systems of fitness training and exercise for health. Both invoke a dualism that centres 'the physical body' in need of attention and care. The third, representing a radical departure from the preceding, predicated on the 'new' discourses of social theory (epidemiology) and genetics, is focused on *prevention* through health promotion and intervention that is self-referential, dedicated to mind-set and lifestyle changes to diet, exercise and the avoidance of the 'risk factors' of modern society. Again, although there are tensions between the variety of health discourses and modalities now found in schools, all, in one way or another, focus on the body as *imperfect* (whether through circumstances of ones class and poverty, or self neglect), *unfinished* and to be ameliorated through physical therapy (circuit training, fitness through sport and a better diet), *threatened* (by the risks of modernity/lifestyles of food, overeating, inactivity) and, therefore, in need of care and being *changed*.

The first two variants of perfection modes that were recontextualised and formed between the 1950s and 1970s largely by influential elements in the pedagogic recontextualising fields (for example, the specialist PE wing colleges and their in-house text book writers). The third, prevention, as suggested above, has been shaped largely outside and independently of these in the official recontextualising fields, for example, by agencies such as the World Health Organization and, in the UK, the British Heart Foundation. All three variants are produced by an analysis of what are taken to be the underlying features necessary for the achievement of health (physical, psychological, social, intellectual). They share features of both perfection and competency modes. As in performance modes, the body is seen as in deficit, unfinished, or at risk and, therefore, in need of rescue from conditions over which individuals or populations have increasingly less control. The focus is directed to outside school experience, work and lifestyle generally, the perspective is on the future, on what could or is to be achieved if one develops the 'right' embodied capacities. Its influence is pervasive in primary and secondary schools. As in competency modes, the focus is on what 'is present in the acquirer's product' (Bernstein 1996: 59) (actions/behaviours/attitudes) because this reveals their cognitive, affective or social development. The emphasis is on the possible, the attainable and what the 'self' can achieve. Whereas performance modes are linked primarily to the economy and competency to symbolic control, perfection modes are truly Janus-faced, turned both to systems of symbolic (the pursuit of correct/fashionable body size, shape, avoidance behaviours) and economic ('fit' and having the embodied capacities for paid work) control. They invoke multiple relationships with agents, individuals, languages and signs. Critically, however, whereas competences are predicated on 'similar to' relations and performance on 'different from' relations, where the reference point for both are objects, individuals or agencies out-with the (disembodied) 'self', perfection modes are predicated on 'relations of' the body defined reflexively as a dynamic between body and nature, the social and the biological, with reference to signs, signifiers, languages of symbolic and economic control. Thus, although perfection modes share features of performance and competency modes and, for this reason, can be seen as 'products' of the pedagogic palette, their dedicated concern with enactment on and regulation of 'the body' lead us to view them as distinctive pedagogic modes characterising our emergent TPS in new contemporary Western situations devoted to body-centred concerns, within wider discourses of 'trainability' and 'health'.

Again we emphasise that all pedagogical relations are power relations. There is no instruction without regulation, no pedagogy divorced of control. Perfection codes and modes are no exception to this rule. Indeed we might consider the 'ethic' embedded in perfection codes as particularly virulent (and explicit) due to their enactment directly on body consciousness. The code determines what bodily acts are permitted and forbidden, the positive and the negative values of different possible behaviours of and on the body. It determines and defines simultaneously what 'the body' is and ideally ought to be.

Classroom codes and contexts

We can, finally, ask how 'performance' ('differences from') 'perfection' ('relations of') and 'competency ('relations to') are encoded through classification and framing and given form as distinctive modalities of PEH, and how they are recontextualised and their subsequent modalities shape pedagogical consciousness in primary, secondary and other sectors of formal education. What is distinctive and special about each mode? We can analyse and discuss these codes and their modalities with reference to features which they share. Following Bernstein, this is to consider how they variously construct *categories of space, time and discourse* (whether weakly or strongly classified); their *evaluative orientation* (whether their focus is on presences or absences); their *forms of control* (implicit or explicit); their *pedagogic text* (focus on the acquirer or performance); the *autonomy* they afford (high or low/high) and their '*economy*' (high cost or low cost) (see Bernstein 2000: 45). Perhaps, more importantly, we can also consider how these codes and their modalities intertwine, for example, the 'new' perfection modes expressed through health-related education in the UK, and enduring performance (sport-centred) modes in contexts of PEH. To what conflicts of identity, consciousness and corporeality do such intersection give rise? With what consequences for a student's 'ability' or health? (see Chapter 12). Of each context we can consider how interactional practices (IP)[1] are constructed, coded and formed through principles of classification and framing and how they impact on the pedagogic consciousness of teachers and pupils. We need to know how: children learn in each context, socially, intellectually, affectively and corporeally; 'childhood', 'health', 'ability' are constructed discursively in contexts where there is harmony and homogenisation of pedagogic codes and modes and where there is a 'pedagogic palette'; pupils are positioned relationally to knowledge, self and others in such contexts; and what 'relations to', 'differences from' and 'relations of' the body are formed and managed within and between pedagogical modes.

Asking such questions may lead to a greater understanding of how the distribution of power and principles of control in society, so usefully articulated by Foucault and Bernstein, translate into principles of communication, differentially regulating forms of embodied consciousness and the possibilities for change. Awareness of how the bias and focus of various interactional practices construct in teachers and students particular forms of moral disposition, motivation, aspiration and orientation towards 'the body' would be research agenda enough, we suggest, for forthcoming years. We must pursue it in the fullest awareness of the relationships between teachers, teaching and the public discursive practices relating to public health, elite sport, popular culture, government, and social class, 'race', 'ability' and gender among others, in which they are embedded and which they help reproduce.

Note

1   Interactional practice (IP) is defined by classification and framing procedures. These act selectively on the recognition rules (rules defined by C+Fs that determine what the context demands and enables the 'reading' of the context) and the realisation rules (that allow the acquires to 'speak' the expected legitimate text) (Bernstein 2000:17). Recognition and realisation rules, at the level of the acquirer, enable that enquirer to construct the expected legitimate text. In short, children may 'recognise the rule' but

not be able to realise it. They may know they have been taught but also that they have not learned. The text that is constructed may be no more than how one sits or how one moves. In this system the text is anything that attracts evaluation. Thus 'evaluation condenses into itself the pedagogic code and its classification and framing procedures, and the relationships of power and control that have produced these procedures' (ibid.: 18).

References

Bernstein, B. (1996) *Pedagogy, Symbolic Control and Identity: Theory, Research and Critique*, London: Taylor & Francis.

Bernstein, B. (2000) *Pedagogy, Symbolic Control and Identity: Theory, Research and Critique*, revised edition, London: Rowman & Littlefield.

Bernstein, B. (2001) 'From pedagogies to knowledges', in A. Morais, I. Neves, B. Davies and H. Daniels (eds) *Towards a Sociology of Pedagogy*, New York: Peter Lang, pp. 363–8.

Davies, B. (1994) 'Durkheim and the sociology of education in Britain', *British Journal of Sociology of Education* 15(1): 3–25.

Gard, M. and Wright, J. (2001) 'Managing uncertainty: obesity discourses and physical education in a risk society', *Studies in the Philosophy of Education* 20: 535–49.

Hasan, R. (2002) 'Ways of meaning, ways of learning: code as an explanatory concept', *British Journal of Sociology of Education* 23(4): 537–49.

Kirk, D. (1992) *Defining Physical Education: The Social Construction of a School Subject in Post War Britain*, London: Falmer Press.

Kirk, D. (1998) *Schooling Bodies: School Practice and Public Discourse 1880–1950*, Leicester: Leicester University Press.

Le Fanu, J. (1999) *The Rise and Fall of Modern Medicine*, London: Abacus.

Pronger, B. (2002) *Body Fascism. Salvation in the Technology of Physical Fitness*, London: University of Toronto.

Skelton, A. (1997) 'Studying hidden curricula: developing a perspective in the light of post modern insights', *Curriculum Studies* 5(2): 177–95.

The Times Magazine (2002) 'Fit', 19 October 2002: 15–18.

Tinning, R. (1992) 'Teacher education pedagogy: dominant discourses and the process of problem-setting, in T. Williams, L. Almond and A. Sparkes (eds) *Sport and Physical Activity, Moving Towards Excellence*, London: E&FN Spon.

Tinning, R. (1997) 'Performance and participation discourses in human movement: towards a socially critical physical education', in J.-M. Fernandez-Balboa (ed.) *Critical Postmodernism in Human Movement, Physical Education and Sport*, New York: SUNY.

Tyler, W. (2001) 'Silent, invisible, total: pedagogic discourse and the age of information', revised version of paper presented to the Bernstein Symposium of AARE Conference, Fremantle, Western Australia, 3–7 December 2001.

15 Conclusion

Ruminations on body knowledge and control and the spaces for hope and happening[1]

Richard Tinning

And the culture comes down[2]

(A line from a song by Australian singer Ruth Aplet)

Introduction

Making sense of body knowledge, education, health and physical culture is a complex task. Collectively, the authors of the chapters in this book provide a sophisticated response to the task. In particular they have interrogated how the processes of schooling have been, and continue to be, implicated discursively and pedagogically in the social construction and control of the body and the implications for this on identity, well-being and health of young people.

They have discussed conceptual and methodological issues in researching body knowledge; the discursive production of childhood, identity and health; and the pedagogies of identity particularly related to sexuality, gender, homophobia, and ill-health. Each chapter makes connections with the issues and discourses that form the focus of other chapters. In this sense they all engage in a form of 'relational analysis' (see Kirk 1999) or what Naomi Klein (2000) calls 'connecting the dots' to map something of this complexity. We know a good deal more about how pedagogical work on the body is done both through formal institutionalised educational practices and through physical culture as a result of their collective work. Certainly we can find out more. There is much more to know.

I have enjoyed reading the contributing chapters to this book. The authors have reinforced many of my particular opinions, understandings and perspectives on matters relating to body knowledge, education, health and physical culture. This book, I would argue, does 'good' pedagogical work in helping to explore, analyse and develop an increasingly sophisticated critical sociology of the body. But of course I would say this because I am a 'believer' of the discourse of the social construction of the body. Indeed I even have investments in this discourse (like being invited to write a chapter for this very book!). In my professional work however, on a daily basis I am confronted with the hegemony of a particular view of knowledge, the body and health that marginalises (albeit pleasantly and amicably) the social. I am surrounded by 'true believers' of the obesity crisis discourse, of the importance of the 'new public health' discourses, and of the significant role that physical activity can and should play in the making of healthy citizens. They too have investments in their beliefs and their particular embodied identities are reflexively influential in reinforcing them. Accordingly, my thoughts for this chapter are located in that context and I find I constantly wrestle with the tensions between hope and happening. My ruminations on the contributions to this book are embodied. They are not only solely (or even largely) intellectual, they are also corporeal and emotional. For that I make no apology.

Chapter organisation

For this concluding chapter the editors asked me to 'reflect on the major themes of the book highlighting their implications for research, teaching and curriculum development in the globalised conditions of a fast changing world.' So I too must attempt to 'connect some dots'. After presenting a brief cautionary preface I will first argue that schools are moving further from models of, or spaces for, 'effective democracy' in which young people can be active participants. Moreover, the power of schooling to influence the hearts and minds of young people has diminished and this is particularly so in relation to issues of bodily knowledge and health. Second, I suggest that curriculum development offers opportunity for more demo- cratic practices but all too often the pedagogical work done in schools fails to capitalise on these possibilities for complex reasons, often connected with teachers' embodied identities. Third, I report a reform to initial teacher education as part of the strategy to counter this trend. Finally I offer some thoughts on research as one dimension in the constant and never-ending process of making better educational practice.

A cautionary preface

Let me begin by making the claim that for all our theorising on the body IN culture, the practices and discursive productions of meaning that are part of the social processes of post-modern culture have continued to increase the importance of the body in the struggle for cultural capital (Bourdieu 1991). In other words, notwith- standing what we know as a result of our theorising and research about how certain cultural practices contribute to limited, restricted or oppressive bodily practices, we have seen little significant systemic change in such practices. While acknow- ledging that some young people have positive and healthful attitudes to their bodies, many young people still graduate from our schools oppressed by the tyranny of the cult of the body (Petersen and Lupton 1996). Anxiety regarding our bodies (what we put in them, what we do and can do with them, what they look like, what they 'should' look like) continues to be endemic. 'The fears and panics around the body that fill the news impel a continuous series of fads, diets and exercises . . .' (Shapiro 2002: 14). Indeed, according to Bauman (2000), the social production of the body is the primal scene of post-modern ambivalence and neuroticism. Importantly, as many of the chapters in this book attest, the fields of health and physical education and health promotion must share some responsibility for this state of affairs since the discourses underpinning their professional missions inform, advocate and reinforce risk avoidance, prudent living and preventative and ameliorative physical activity.

But what can be done? Is the future hopeless as greater power is yielded to the pedagogical work done by the 'corporate curriculum' (Kenway and Bullen 2001) and 'cultural players' beyond the school gates? What are the spaces for curricula and pedagogies that can begin to reverse these trends? In reading this chapter you should be aware that I remain somewhat circumspect with respect to the impact that our work can have on the problems of post-modern ambivalence and neuroticism that are generated through the contemporary social production of the body. What I know about the problematic role of expertise in the process of reflexive modernisation (see Kelly *et al.* 2000) makes me cautious as to where to move, what to do. But move I must. What follows is offered more as the unrefined ruminations of a thoughtful educator than the sophisticated expositions of a sociologist.

The contributors to this collection in various ways are all seeking to understand something of the relationships between body knowledge, education and physical culture. In seeking understanding much will depend on where we look and through what lenses we make our viewing. Importantly however, many authors seek more than to merely understand – they seek to make an effect, to *make a difference* (see Evans and Davies, for example, Chapter 1). However, as Lundgren (1983) informed us, there is always a tension between hope and happening and in this case it is likely that some practitioners and policy-makers may not even read this book since it will be on the library shelves outside their discursive field.

Notwithstanding this possibility, in seeking to make a difference we need to be cautious of a possible implicit assumption that might be lurking in the back of our consciousness. Some time ago Evans and Davies (1986) claimed that physical education makes friends and enemies of pupils. This continues to be the case. Evans and Davies (Chapter 1) recognise that schools (and HPE) 'can never hope to please or touch the interests of every young person in their care, no matter how innovative or progressive they are, or how hard they try' (p. 10). Yet the assumption (implicit or otherwise), or perhaps the hope, that this new 'body of knowledge' about the body in physical culture might somehow *enable* a better curriculum to be developed, a better pedagogy to be enacted, a better educative experience for all girls and boys in and through the school system, though laudable, is an unrealistic ambition. PE and health cannot make friends of *all* young people and enemies of none.

Schooling in the contemporary context

In their introductory chapter Evans and Davies suggest that education has (or rather should have) a crucial role in creating tomorrow's optimism in the context of today's pessimism. They suggest that, in a context in which teachers and researchers are increasingly 'steered by the barren managerial mantras of liberal individualism – achievement, assessment and accountability', higher, worthier principles could drive the curriculum in its pursuits of social, educational and moral ideals (p. 10).

Following Bernstein (2000) they suggest that these worthier principles are 'those that provide for the conditions of an effective democracy' (p. 10). One of the conditions that must be met to develop such effective democracies within schools is that parents and students and, I would add, teachers 'must feel they have a stake in it [the effective democracy] and confidence that its arrangements will realise or enhance this stake' (p. 10).

I agree. This is an admirable aspiration. However, I am also chastened by Kenway and Bullen's (2001) analysis of the nature of contemporary schooling in Australia where the introduction of neo-liberal market discourses and practices into the education system has meant that students would seem to getting *further removed* from having a legitimate stake in schooling. They argue that there has been a 'hybridisation of entertainment, education and advertising and the commodification of children's education and school life' (Kenway and Bullen 2001: 82) and '[a]ddressing these complex issues . . . requires schools to reconsider their pedagogies, indeed their *raison d'être*' (p. 89). As many government schools increasingly look towards the market (in competition for students and other resources) they move *further away* from meeting the needs of young people. This represents a serious challenge for educators who might, like Evans and Davies, desire to create the opportunities for effective democracy within schools.

Commenting on the results of their research Kenway and Bullen (2001) state:

> We have shown that when schools put themselves on the market they are pitching to anxious Stress Generation parents who want to protect their young from the present, the future and themselves. They are also pitching to Stress Generation teachers who are nostalgic for traditional authority relations between teacher and student. Educational fundamentalism is comforting. It provides apparent certainty in an age of uncertainty. It talks of the future in terms of the past and offers adults a sense of control when they feel their lives and their young are out of control.
>
> (Kenway and Bullen 2001: 149)

This feeling of 'life out of control' is rather common in the context of post-modern or 'new times'. According to Kenway (1998: 2) 'Everywhere across the many landscapes of our lives we hear stories of dramatic, life-altering, and confusing change. But is difficult to pin down exactly what is happening and how all the changes come together'. We have learned elsewhere (see for example McLaren 1986; Kirk 1993) that control over one's body through exercise and diet regimes is, for some individuals, a response to this very situation. However, partly as a direct result of globalisation we now see the emergence of a post-traditional social order that results from the challenge to traditional ways of doing things, organising our lives, and interacting with nature – including our own bodies. The loss of much of what we knew as tradition has resulted in 'a runaway world of dislocation and uncertainty' and to live in a such a world has 'the feeling of riding a juggernaut' (Giddens 1991: 28).

For many teachers and teacher educators whose task it is to prepare young people for the twenty-first century, the challenge to traditional ways of doing things represents a significant threat to their own ontological security. As Giddens (1994) has argued, the post-traditional social order has brought a crisis of legitimation both in terms of knowledge and the institutions of authority. In this contemporary context, many people see conservatism and even fundamentalism as reassuring, as a check on the juggernaut, as a little certainty in an increasingly uncertain world. Penney and Harris (Chapter 7 of this volume) recognise a similar concern when they reported on how 'teachers themselves actively (re)created notably narrow but also very gendered understandings and images of fitness, health and participation in physical activity'. They 'are left questioning why the ongoing conservatism and what part developments in pedagogy can play in beginning to challenge such a sustained status quo' (p. 109).

Whether or not we find uncertainty threatening or stimulating, or perhaps even a non-issue, there seems little doubt that we must to learn to live with uncertainty. As Giddens (1991), Beck (1992), Bauman (2001), Evans and Davies (Chapter 3) and many others argue, certainty *is* illusory in contemporary times. But it's not just that certainty is illusory, the actual quest *for* certainty can be highly problematic. Sociologist John Law (1994) is forthright in condemning the holy grail of certainty as a feature of modernity that leads to 'hideous purity'.

> Many of us have learned to cleave to an order. This is a modernist dream. In one way or another, we are attached to the idea that if our lives, our organisations, our social theories or our societies, were all 'properly ordered' then all would be well. And we take it that such ordering is possible, at least some of the time. So when we encounter complexity we tend to treat it as distraction.
>
> (Law 1994: 5)

The conditions of contemporary social life that make the cleaving to order so attractive to many represents a serious challenge to schooling, for the state expects the education system to prepare citizens for active participation in a globalised and fast-changing world. One 'space' or discursive practice that purports to offer a little certainty in the context of contemporary schooling is the 'official text' (Apple 1993) that is manifest as policy and curriculum.

The promise of curriculum development

Notwithstanding the often questionable politics behind their development and introduction, new curricula offer a promise of a better educational experience for young people. Sometimes they even offer hope of emancipation and empowerment for students. In their argument against 'fat free schooling' Evans *et al.*

> press pedagogues and policy makers to consider how curriculum and pedagogy would need to be reconfigured to meet individual education and health needs . . . to effect forms of education that deliver empowerment and health.
>
> (Evans *et al.* 2003: 30)

The notion that the curriculum should provide for empowering and emancipatory possibilities for young people is not new, as a (re)reading of Geoff Whitty's (1985) *Sociology and School Knowledge: Curriculum Theory, Research and Politics* will attest. However, the hope of empowerment is not often matched by the happening.

Penney and Harris (Chapter 7) claim that policy (as 'official text') can be a source of either status quo and inequality, or of resistance and challenge to inequity. They suggest that policy 'becomes a force for both promoting and supporting conscious steps towards more socially critical practices and pedagogies in physical education that challenge and extend established "discursive truths" and the thinking and actions they give rise to'. Policy can be translated into official curriculum and in this sense the curriculum embodies these possibilities.

Contemporary HPE curricula in Australia (at least) are, like all curricula, examples of recontextualised knowledge (Bernstein 2000). The recontexualised discourses that are found in the Australian curriculum have their lineage in the 'traditional' fields of knowledge typically found in human movement studies (or sports science or kinesiology) and also in the 'new sociology of education' of the 1970s. Some of the influence of the new sociology of education can be recognised in the emancipatory politics discourse (Giddens 1991). The emancipatory ideals of many of the critical pedagogues has, in some forms at least, been incorporated (perhaps even appropriated) into the new Australia HPE curriculum.

It was Giddens (1991: 210) who described emancipatory politics as 'a generic outlook concerned above all with liberating individuals and groups from constraints which adversely affect their life chances'. As such, emancipatory politics 'makes primary the imperatives of *justice*, *equality* and *participation*' (emphasis in original). When we consider the key principles and values underpinning the Australian HPE curriculum – namely *social justice*, *diversity* and *supportive environments* (Curriculum Corporation 1992: 5) we can see how they resonate with the imperatives of emancipatory politics. Perhaps this is understandable given the education-political context at the time in which the curriculum framework was developed. By the beginning of the 1990s considerable attention had been given to emancipatory discourses within Australian education for over a decade (e.g. Kemmis *et al*. 1983) and they resonated loudly with the Labour (read left-oriented) federal and state governments at the time. Importantly, it is the responsibility of teacher education (ITE) to prepare student teachers to teach this curriculum (Macdonald *et al*. 2000).

However while the imperatives of emancipatory politics are evident in the Australian HPE curriculum framework the same curriculum was also influenced by what Giddens (1991) has termed 'life politics'. While emancipatory politics is primarily concerned with the conditions which liberate the individual to make life choices, life politics assumes a certain level of emancipation and is concerned with the politics of life choices. As such, 'While emancipatory politics is a politics of life chances, life politics is a politics of lifestyle' (Giddens 1991: 214). Giddens offers an important qualification:

It would be too crude to say simply that life politics focuses on what happens once individuals have achieved a certain level of autonomy of action, because other factors are involved; but this provides at least an initial orientation.

(Ibid.: 214)

Bauman (2000: 23) explains that 'we are all engaged nowadays in "life-politics"; we are "reflexive beings" who look closely at every move we take, who are seldom satisfied with the results and always keen to correct them'. Moreover, 'we are perhaps more "critically disposed", much bolder and intransigent in our criticism than our ancestors managed to be in their daily lives, but our critique, so to speak, is "toothless", unable to affect the agenda set for our "life-political" choices'. Kwon and Harris (2002: 13) suggest that the notion of 'life politics' offers insight that enables us to move beyond an emancipatory politics that neglects 'envisioning what comes next after liberation'. As a politics of life choices, life politics is much more complex than making a choice over which brand of jeans or margarine to buy. As Giddens argues:

[L]ife politics concerns political issues which flow from processes of self-actualisation in post-traditional contexts, where globalising influences intrude deeply into the reflexive project of the self, and conversely where processes of self-realisation influence global strategies.

(Giddens 1991: 214)

We are in a difficult space here. Notions of reflexivity, self-actualisation, globalisation and post-modernity are complex concepts and the ways they 'play out' on/in HPE are not immediately obvious.

What is obvious however, is that, as the research on innovation informed us nearly thirty years ago, there is no such thing as a 'teacher-proof' curriculum. The pedagogical process itself is significant here. Lusted's (1986) idea that knowledge is that which is understood and not what is intended is important. Moreover, his notion that 'how one teaches is inseparable from what is taught and the nature of the learner' is also relevant.

We can take the best 'knowledge' available from the 'new sociology of the body' and use it as a basis for our PE curricula. But always the embodied PE teacher must operationalise it. The PE teacher will do pedagogical work on/for the student's body without saying a word and perhaps even in spite of the activities developed to enact the new curriculum. It is complicated stuff. We cannot, no matter how well-intentioned, develop a curriculum that guarantees a positive bodily experience for *all* kids, *all* of the time. Nevertheless, we should continue to work towards developing curricula and pedagogical practices that are intended to produce worthwhile, positive experiences for all young people. We just need to be modest in our claims for the possibilities of our work.

Thoughts on pedagogical work

I am using the term pedagogical work to refer to the work that is done in the process of knowledge production . In a sense this notion is not unlike the way in which Kirk (1992) uses the notion of ideological work in order to avoid some of the difficulties of the term ideology. In my view pedagogical work enables us to avoid some of the confusing thinking that accompanies the ways in which the term pedagogy is used across fields like education, sociology and cultural studies.

While it is usual to think of schools as a key site of learning (knowledge production) and the teacher as a 'flesh and blood' human, pedagogical work is also done by many other 'cultural players' in addition to schools and teachers. Pedagogical work is also done by such diverse media as an instructional video, a lifestyle magazine, a film, a mobile phone text message, a billboard poster, a Nike ad, or even a label on the back of a cereal box. As many of the contributors to this volume have shown, *pedagogical work* in regard to the cult of the body is done within the context of physical culture in general and physical education, health education and school sport more specifically.

Of course we do expect that schooling (and HPE in particular) will do peda-gogical work on the body – after all, that is one of the purposes of the curriculum. However, we certainly don't expect that pedagogical work to be miseducative or oppressive in any way. In considering the ways in which institutional forms of schooling and PETE do pedagogical work on/for the body and health the work of the critical pedagogues has been important.

Pedagogies of the critical persuasion

It was psycho-analyst Alice Miller (1987) who coined the term 'poisonous pedagogies' to refer to the negative parenting practices that were passed down from generation to generation doing damage to successive generations. Over the past twenty years or so there has been considerable analysis of the ways in which certain school-based pedagogical practices actually have poisonous consequences for some young people. Pat Dodds' (1993) analysis of the pedagogical practices that perpetuate the 'ugly isms' typical in many physical education lessons in the USA schooling system provides an early example of the poisonous pedagogies that relate to body knowledge and physical education.

Scholars who have contributed to the identification or naming of poisonous pedagogies within physical education and who have been invested in doing academic work toward social justice most often located their theoretical position under the 'big tent' (Lather 1998) of critical pedagogy. Critical pedagogy scholars have been extremely important in the process of exposing inequities and inequalities related to physical education and health in schools. We know a good deal about how miseducative physical education can be. However, while they have been successful in their critique, by and large, critical pedagogues have been short on offering alternative practices (see O'Sullivan *et al.* 1992). Moreover, the success of critical pedagogies in helping emancipate young people from the tyranny of the cult of the body has been far from successful (see Tinning and Glasby 2002).

As a result of their research into popular culture, schooling and young people, Kenway and Bullen (2001) argue that

> conventionally . . . teachers have a propensity to claim a moral high ground built upon the negative critique of children's culture, popular culture and youth culture. They offer their teaching as a non-oppressive, enlightened, enlightening and empowering alternative to popular pedagogy and the corporate curriculum. But this is not necessarily the way it is understood by students who may experience it as *authoritarian*.
>
> (Kenway and Bullen 2001: 155)

> . . . students do not tend to appreciate teachers who make them feel ashamed about their choices and lifestyles all in the name of helping them . . . [indeed] . . . deconstruction may have an emotional fallout.
>
> (Ibid.: 165)

With similar sentiment on the limits of critique, Crowdes (2000: 25) claims that in many classes in which critical pedagogies are used, students often feel frustrated by 'heavy-handed, and adversarial deconstructions of power imbalance, conflict, and social inequality'. She claims that students 'often report feeling hopeless and cynical. They are often left with their fairly extensive sociological vocabularies and socially aware minds detached from their bodies and agency in matters of conflict resolution and change.' She claims that 'A pedagogic strategy joining *somatic* and *sociological* perspectives intensifies multi-dimensional comprehension of the dynamics of social construction and mindful reconstructions of power and responses to conflict' (p. 27, my emphasis). It seems to me that most of our work is strong in the sociological and rather weak in the somatic.

Bauman (2000) offers another take on the issue of the limitations of critical theory when he suggests that contemporary society has learned to accommodate critique in a way that it remains 'immune to the consequences of that accommodation'. For him, '[t]he kind of modernity which was the target, but also the cognitive frame, of classical critical theory strikes the analyst in retrospect as quite different from the one which frames the lives of present day generations' (Bauman 2000: 25). In other words the emancipatory discourses of the 1970s and 1980s have now been institutionalised (e.g. into the Australian HPE curriculum) and they no longer resonate as important with many young people. Certainly it seems we must offer more than earnest critique if we are to impact on what stands for body knowledge in physical education and health within schools and, I would add, within ITE. From their research, Wright *et al.* (2002) claim that

> if young people are to recognise how truths are constituted it behoves those who seek to educate them to provide the means by which they have choices in the discourses they take up and to understand the effects of their positions on themselves and others.
>
> (Wright *et al.* 2002: 11)

But having choices means more that understanding that you are being duped, oppressed or marginalised. Agency, while vitally important, is always a limited power.

Kimberley Oliver's activist research work in engaging adolescent girls in critical inquiry on the body provides an example of how our earnest attempts to lift the ideological blinkers off our students (in her case adolescent girls) are not always straightforward. Oliver (2001: 161) says that 'despite the pedagogical possibilities of using images from popular culture to engage adolescent girls in critically studying the body, there are also many struggles involved in this type of curriculum work'. Oliver wanted the girls to 'begin to name and recognise some of their unassumed beliefs about the body' (p. 146) and this would seem a useful process. However, in their chapter in this volume Oliver and Lalik 'wonder whether learning critique alone might not leave adolescents with feelings of frustration and helplessness' (p. 22).

In all our interventions as teachers or researchers we have (we are) a body that needs to be considered as we attempt to 'connect the dots'. David Brown's (2002) recognition of the embodied complexity of such issues is important. Brown found PE teachers to be 'living links' acting as a 'cultural conduit' in the process of transmission and maintenance of gender relations in sport and physical education. His research adopts a relational view in which

> patriarchy in the classroom is embedded within the minds *and* bodies of teachers and pupils themselves, sharing a social presence and influencing one another's actions by using the culturally specific gender 'norms' as a point of reference.
>
> (Brown 2002: 2)

In other words, PE teachers' bodies also do pedagogical work *without a word being spoken*. To consider the PE context as a space for defensive work against the 'cult of the body' this 'living link' (to limiting, repressive and oppressive discourses) must be recognised and incorporated into appropriate pedagogical strategies.

Pedagogies and pleasure

If we recognise that popular culture is so significant in doing pedagogical work on the body, surely we need to take seriously the pedagogical forms of that culture and consider its implications for our work in education. According to Kenway and Bullen (2002) it is important to recognise the connection between consumer culture (as a significant element in popular culture) and the non-rational self. They use the term French word *jouissance*, which means 'playful, sensual pleasure', as central to their argument:

> The *jouissance* which children derive from consumer culture is designed to ensure that they unreflexively consume rather than interpret such texts. *Jouissance* is about producing a surge affect, not the reflexive pleasure of

knowing about what is happening as it happens. By its very nature, children's consumer-media culture seeks not to operate at this level of rationality

(Kenway and Bullen 2002: 75)

In response to this understanding Kenway and Bullen argue for developing pedagogies of the popular and the profane. They argue for discovering the 'power of pleasure' and the 'pleasure of power'. This talk of pleasure opens a window into the power of the visceral, corporeal and non-rational. Importantly, in physical education and health much of the pedagogical work done relating to such issues as food, sex and drugs is heavily focused on risk management and consequently emphasises avoidance or abstinence while giving little or no consideration to pleasure (see, for example, Chapter 3). In our pedagogies we continue to privilege the rational and ignore the embodied, sensual and non-rational dimensions of experience.

Kenway and Bullen (2002: 159) also argue for pedagogies that develop or connect with 'life politics'. 'As some schools have discovered, couched in the right way, there is a potentially rich educational agenda associated with life politics and the local and global citizenship activities that go with it'. As I have noted earlier, the Australian HPE is one official text that provides opportunities for such engagement with life politics. However, to date, instances of such engagement are rather rare.

As the distinctions between education, entertainment and advertising diminish, popular culture is increasingly referred to as popular pedagogy, corporate cultural pedagogy and the corporate curriculum. Steinberg and Kincheloe (1997: 3) observed that 'education takes place in a variety of social sites including but not limited to schooling' and that identities are formed and knowledge is produced and legitimated in children's consumer culture. Moreover, corporate pedagogues have become post-modern society's most successful teachers.

In this context, Nicholas Rose (2000: 1398) argues that 'schools have been *supplemented* and *sometimes displaced* by an array of other practices for *shaping identities* and forms of life' (my emphasis). He suggests that advertising, TV soap operas, and lifestyle magazines have become the new regulatory techniques for the shaping of the self, thereby replacing much of the traditional authority of education. This has huge implications for the field of physical education and health. It was only a decade ago that Philip Wexler (1992) observed that schooling is a process of becoming somebody. In other words it was a key site for identity-making for young people. To understand that powerful non-school 'cultural players' also do significant pedagogical work in relation to identity-making, the body and health is to recognise that the quest for the healthy citizen is a tug-of-war in which different vested interests compete for the hearts and minds of young people.

Corporeal pleasure in pedagogy

Earlier I mentioned that pedagogical work was done by the teacher's body by virtue of its materiality. Erica McWilliam (1996: 367) makes the case that ' the body of the teacher needs to be remembered in writing about teaching and learning, because it produces desire in pedagogical events, for good as well as ill'. She contends that it is important to understand the desire to teach and learn as embodied, ' ie., residing in the materiality of students and teachers, not simply in their minds'. Some interesting work relating to these ideas are contained in the edited collection *Taught Bodies* (O'Farrell *et al.* 2000).

McWilliam is interested in ' re-configuring a model of pedagogical instruction that engages quite specifically with materiality of classrooms and bodies' (1996: 373). Since we know that their own bodies are central to the teaching of many physical educators (see, for example, Sparkes 1999), I wonder what this re-configuring might look like in the physical education context. In thinking about the role of the PE teacher's body in enacting out demonstrations (e.g. of skilled movements) McWilliam's (1996) words are informative:

> In performing knowledge acts for the student gaze [for example a demon-stration of a particular movement skill], we ought to be able to acknowledge what Deutscher (1994: 36) calls 'the elating sensation of a physical carnation of one's body as a teacher . . . the overt pleasure produced by the possibility of one's own performance as empowered subject knowledge, the seductive effect of instantaneity between teaching and learning body.
>
> (McWilliam 1996: 310)

What might this desire to perform mean for teacher-receptivity to less teacher centred pedagogies? What messages are conveyed in teacher demonstrations? What messages about the body? What pedagogical work for reproducing the cult of the body is done in such demonstrations? Sparkes' (Chapter 11) account of his heartfelt frustrations when injury prevented him from receiving the 'confirmation of self' he had usually received from physically demonstrating to his PE class is illustrative of both the potentially affirming properties of the student gaze and also of the commonly held belief that teacher demonstrations are an essential part of effective PE teaching. 'No gasps. No confirmation of me. Good PE teachers "do" it. Show don't tell. Shit! Where does that leave me? Time to go' (p. 165). Physicality, manifest as a bodily instantiation of competence, is part of the embodied identity of many (most) PE teachers.

Curriculum, pedagogy and identities

There is a rather complex but significant link between issues of identity, pedagogy and curriculum. Identity (McLaren 1998) and embodiment (Giddens 1991) are central to the post-modern context. However, like much of sociology itself (Turner 1996), curriculum reform has been particularly disembodied. Significantly for HPE teachers the '[b]ody and self are inextricably folded within each other. Rather than a unity of body and self there is a doubling: an *embodied self* (Kenworth Teather 1999: 9). Since, as Elliott (2001: 99) suggests 'the politics of identity is increasingly wrapped around configurations of the body', HPE teachers' engagement with the ideas of a new curriculum will be influenced by their embodied identities.

A significant influence on HPE teacher identities/subjectivities[3] is the central place that physical activity, sport and the body play in their daily lives. Understanding the role played by teachers' embodied identities in the HPE curriculum reform process seems a crucial project. Central to understanding embodiment of the HPE teacher is the way in which they 'come to know' about the body and health. Since most ITE programmes provide for little exposure to, let alone engagement with, alternative discourses of the body and health (see, for example, Wright 2000) to those of the bio-physical sciences, prospective PE teachers' identities are shaped in limited if not uni-dimensional ways. This is a key limitation to creating pedagogical practices that empower young people in terms of bodily knowledge.

Initial teacher education

As in many other Western countries, the preparation of HPE teachers in Australia is not without its critics (e.g. Macdonald *et al*. 2002). The task of preparing teachers to 'deliver' on the 'clever country' national educational agenda that calls for future citizens that are multi-skilled, competent with information technology, literate and numerate in order that they play a productive part in a globalised economy (Luke and Carrington 2001) is daunting. In addition, citizens of our 'clever country' should also be *healthy citizens* who are self-regulating, informed, critically reflective and capable of constructing their own healthy lifestyle and minimising risky behaviours (Tinning and Glasby 2002). What might be the implications of new bodily knowledge in regard to ITE for HPE?

The late Australian educator Garth Boomer once said that ' teachers teach *who* they are'. He was alluding here to the significance of identities in teaching. Since we now know that 'the politics of identity is increasingly wrapped around configurations of the body' (Elliott 2001: 99) and that many HPE teachers' *embodied physicality* is central to their whole orientation to life and teaching, then the relevance of Boomer's comment to teaching in physical education and health becomes increasingly salient.

Foucault informed us that knowledge *makes us its subject*. In other words the process of coming to know something, and the nature of the knowledge itself (see Pronger 1995), has an influence on the type of person we become – on the identities we make. In the process of becoming a HPE teacher what sort of people do student teachers become? The knowledge and ways of thinking that many ITE programmes 'give' student teachers to deal with the problems of working with post-modern young people are predominantly those of science. Indeed many programmes select students into the programme in the first place on the basis of their academic success in science-based school subjects. However, Evans and Davies (Chapter 14) suggest that the

> changes that have occurred in PEH since the 1970s' represent . . . a *paradigmatic shift* in the social basis, logic and coding of PEH knowledge and, concomitantly, of pedagogic modalities and consciousness in schools.

What then, is the appropriate ITE to respond to this paradigmatic shift? It is arguable that our current ITE programmes are not adequately responding to this paradigm shift and accordingly they making the *wrong sort of (teacher) subject* for the task of teaching contemporary HPE curricula to post-modern students.

A brief but relevant aside

Recently an experienced HPE teacher who was head of department at a private girls' school in Brisbane told me that the most frequent issues that she had to deal with as a HPE teacher, were *relationships, peer pressure and sex*. She said issues relating to pregnancy, the Pill, break-ups with boyfriends, negotiating/ mediating peer group disputes etc., were dominant. She suggested that 'HPE teachers are often the interface between kids and their parents in matters relating to sexuality education, and HPE curriculum opens up the space for such issues to be discussed'.

Overall, this teacher considered that the broad focus of her programme of HPE was on developing *life management skills*. This is a rather term vague term but it can be related to the development of knowledge, skills and attitudes consistent with the choice of healthy lifestyle practices . . . practices that contribute to the making of the healthy citizen (see Burrows and Wright's discussion of the Life Education Trust in Chapter 6).

In Chapter 12 Emma Rich *et al.* described how for young anorexic women it is not at all clear who are the relevant (helpful) players: 'should they see a doctor? psychiatrist? the school counsellor?' As the above example reveals, it may be that the school HPE teacher is a beginning player in such matters. The training of the HPE teacher, however, in most cases, would not help them deal with the challenges of such issues. Knowledge of exercise physiology and biomechanics will be of little use here.

A different model

Australian teacher educator Ken Alexander, in providing a rationale for the intro- duction of a new degree programme at Edith Cowan University (ECU) in Western Australia, asked: 'How well suited are existing forms of pre-service professional preparation to meeting the needs of young people in "new times"?' He argues that the new HPE curriculum, with its emphasis on personal development, self- management and decision-making requires a *different teacher education* to that commonly driven by, and conceived within, the discourses of sport and science. In his case his new programme locates its relevant professional knowledge within the fields of youth work, health and physical activity.

The new ITE programme (a double degree BA(Ed)/BSocSc) foregrounds knowledge of *young people* through the study of youth work and counselling. Biophysical and sports science, while included in the programme, is not given privileged status. Behind the new programme at ECU is a desire not only to equip with requisite skills and knowledge, but also to develop certain *types* of HPE teachers – teachers who can understand 'new kids' and the context of 'new times' (Kenway *et al.* 1995). It is envisaged that in the *process* of 'training' these prospective teachers would *become* different types of teachers to their colleagues who develop through programmes that privilege the discourses of sport and science. We are talking here about the development of certain *identities* and a certain orientation to the world.

Given the experiences of the PE head of department mentioned above, and given that the 'reflexive project of the self has disrupted, and revolutionised what is at the heart of the life-world – intimacy, relationships, sexuality, and our notions of the body' (Shapiro 2002: 6), it would seem that this new ITE programme represents something of a paradigm shift that is worth watching. At least that's the hope that Alexander expresses. As to the happening (including pedagogic modalities and consciousness) in the new ITE programme and the teacher subjects it makes, we will have to wait and see.

Research matters

The work of many of the contributors to this volume bear testimony to the analytic power of the theories of Foucault (in particular, see the chapters of Wright; Wright and Burrows; Gard; Garrett; Leahy and Harrison) and Bernstein (see the chapters of Evans and Davies; Penny and Harris) when applied to the field of physical education and health. For Wright (Chapter 2) the theoretical work of Foucault provides a useful starting point in 'taking up the post-structuralist challenge of interrogating the relationship between power and knowledge and between discourse and subjectivity'. Evans and Davies (Chapter 3), however, suggest that while 'the work of Foucault, and other like-minded social theorists, allows us to advance some way in the direction of answering questions' of the post-structuralist challenge, they are drawn to the work of Bernstein as providing a 'more enlightened conceptual scheme'. Chris Shilling (Foreword) has directed our attention to the work of Durkheim which he claims can 'productively be employed to analyse the relationship between the body, education and society' (p. xvi). As Shilling attests, the Bersteinian inspired chapters of Evans and Davies (Chapter 14) and Penny and Harris (Chapter 7) are works heavily influenced by Durkheim.

Working with the ideas of the 'greats', while generative, can also be rather intimidating and most scholars tend to work with(in) rather than extend or develop the theoretical frames of the major social theorists. In this context the work of Evans and Davies' (Chapter 14) is rather rare. Their development of the concept of perfection modes (PFM) to provide better understanding of pedagogical consciousness as *embodied* is a wonderful example of how it is possible (for those with a truly 'deep' understanding of a theory) to refine or develop the ideas of a major theorist (in their case Bernstein) to provide for more sophisticated analyses of education and physical culture.

Thinking sociologically

According to Evans and Davies 'The message is clear, in PE and health we should make research and teaching more not less complex, and "theory", ideas and innovation, not our enemies but friends' (Chapter 1, pp. 11–12). They are correct to claim that good theory can be a catalyst for educational and social change. Their notion of theory being a vehicle for 'thinking otherwise' is rather like the notion of the sociological imagination which Giddens defines as ' . . . *being able to "think ourselves away" from the familiar routines of our daily lives in order to look at them anew*' (Giddens 1991: 18, emphasis in original). Moreover, as Shilling (1993: 22) informs us, the body 'can be conceptualised as occupying a place at the centre of the sociological imagination'.

Importantly, the sociological imagination allows us to 'make the familiar strange' which potentially challenges orthodoxy and provides a check on the possibility of the attraction to certainty. However, as I expressed in my cautionary preface, there is always the danger that we might slip into assuming that if we can just get our thinking straight (by applying the 'right' theorising), if we get our curricula right (the right curriculum development), and if we do our pedagogy right, then the miseducative pedagogical work of the cult of the body will be ameliorated or even eliminated. The shadow of the cleave to order (Law 1994) may be always lurking. In applying the sociological imagination to physical education and health we need to be mindful that ways of theorising do not become forms of a new orthodoxy. Even the major theories have their limitations.

Other connections

In addition to Foucault and Bernstein, there are other generative sources of inspiration for theorising the social body. Law (1994), for example, although heavily influenced by Foucault, argues that we should be seeking a 'modest sociology' that would be less prone to heroic reductionism, always incomplete, aware of the context of its own production, and in which no *a priori* privilege is given to human actors in the process of researching the social. Law (1994: 2) talks of 'relational materialism' in which 'the "social" [is] materially heterogeneous: talk, bodies, texts, machines, architecture, all of these and many more are implicated in and perform the "social"'. What might this mean for understanding the *social* construction of the body? What might it mean for understanding the body *in* nature *and* culture (Kirk 1993)? It seems to me that there are some interesting possibilities for research here. Considering physical culture from the standpoint of relational materialism might include machines and architecture in the analysis. It might see us exploring actor-network theory (Law 1994) as a useful 'tool' for our research.

In moving beyond analysis and towards more empowering body knowledge there is also much to offer from the non-Western discourses of the body. Brian Pronger (2002) in his book *Body Fascism: Salvation in the Technology of Physical Fitness*, conceptualises a 'theory of the body' based on Heidegger's (1938) account of technology *and* Eastern (particularly Zen Buddhist) discourses and practices. Philip Wexler's (1995) 'New Age social theory in education' also connects to non-Western discourses and he considers that 'Any transformatively interested education for a new age will be about the body' (Wexler 1995: 75).

Earlier in this chapter it was noted that our pedagogical strategies were strong in the sociological and rather weak in the somatic. Kristie Fleckenstein (1999: 282) argues for recognition of the somatic. She claims that, while post-structuralist theories 'offer fruitful ways of reconceptualising meaning and identity as fluid processes that are linguistically mediated and constituted', in so doing post-structuralism 'transforms bodies into discourse, corporeality into textuality'. As a way of 'reclaiming corporeality without sacrificing postrstructuralist insights' she argues for the concept of what she calls *somatic mind*:

> The concept of somatic mind – mind and body as a permeable, intertextual territory that is continually made and remade – offers one means of embodying our discourse and our knowledge without totalising either
>
> (Fleckenstein 1999: 281)

For Fleckenstein (ibid.: 287), somatic mind has the potential to blur 'the boundaries of what constitutes flesh and technology, flesh and culture, flesh and other'. There is some resonance here with actor-network theory (Law 1994).

Afterword: the author's body?

Jan Wright (Chapter 2, p. 29) concluded that:

> What the contributors to the book share is a desire to interrogate, to ask questions about the ways in which institutional and cultural processes work to produce particular forms of identity or selves, particularly as these relate to the social construction and control of the body, well-being and health.

Collectively they have provided a sophisticated interrogation. I wonder, however, how the 'particular forms of identity or selves' of each of the authors has played a part in their writing. I am interested in why the authors of this volume write *what* they write. *Why* they seek explanations in particular places (theories) and not others. For example, I wonder why Bourdieu's notion of *habitus* is barely present in the work contained in this volume when it has been used generatively by numerous researchers in our field (e.g. Hunter 2001; Light and Kirk 2000) to pursue similar post-structuralist questions. Answers to these questions (and others of a bio-graphical nature) might provide some insight into the possible embodiments of the authors themselves.

I am suggesting here that what we write (and why we write what we do) is often heavily influenced by our own embodiment. Evans and Davies ('Endnote', Chapter 14 in this volume) ask how pedagogic codes and modalities are acquired and how they come to shape pedagogical consciousness – how they become *embodied*. If we consider that writing a chapter for this book is a pedagogical practice, then how our own embodiments influence what we write, what we select to discuss, analyse or ignore become important questions. In the words of Fleckenstein (1999: 303):

> Identity – cultural and personal – is always subject to the contractions and relaxations of its blood and tissue boundaries, boundaries that evanesce and coalesce in response to and in rhythm with invisible intertextual messages. We exist as somatic minds; we need to write, teach, and live within that realisation.

Hence
  the discursive embodied self
   having written
    then moves on
     changed as it is from the process of writing

Notes

1 With apologies to Ulf Lundgren (1983).
2 Notwithstanding the structuralist lineage of this line and the fact that it might signal a unidimensional 'force' with no possibilities for resistance, I still rather like its evocative power.
3 There is considerable conceptual 'slippage' between the terms identity and subjectivity is some of the literature on the sociology of the body. I would like to use the term subjectivity here (in this paragraph) but that would only reproduce this slippage. Accordingly, I will stick to identity and at least keep some consistency.

References

Apple, M. (1993) *Official Knowledge: Democratic Education in a Conservative Age*, New York: Routledge.

Bauman, Z. (2000) *Liquid Modernity*, Cambridge: Polity Press.

Bauman, Z. (2001) *The Individualized Society*, Cambridge: Polity Press.

Beck, U. (1992) *Risk Society: Towards a New Modernity*, London: Sage.

Bernstein, B. (2000) *Pedagogy, Symbolic Control and Identity: Theory, Research, Critique*, revised edition, London: Rowman & Littlefield.

Bourdieu, P. (1991) *Language and Symbolic Power*, Oxford: Polity Press.

Brown, D. (2002) 'Living links and gender resources in teaching PE: the social construction of masculinity in teaching physical education', paper presented at the Association for Physical Education in Higher Education (AIESEP) conference, LaCoruna, Spain, 2002.

Crowdes, M. (2000) 'Embodying sociological imagination: pedagogical support for linking bodies to minds', *Teaching Sociology* 28: 28–40.

Curriculum Corporation (1992) *National Statement on Health, Australian Education Council Curriculum and Assessment Committee.*

Dodds, P. (1993) 'Removing the ugly 'isms' in your gym: thoughts for teachers on equity', in J. Evans (ed.) *Equality, Education and Physical Education*, London: Falmer Press.

Elliott, A. (2001) *Concepts of the Self*, Oxford: Polity Press.

Evans J. and Davies, B. (1986) 'Sociology, schooling and physical education', in J. Evans (ed.) *Physical Education, Sport and Schooling: Studies in the Sociology of Physical Education*, London: Falmer Press.

Evans, J., Evans, R., Evans, C. and Evans, J.E. (2003) 'Fat free schooling: the discursive production of ill-health', *International Studies in the Sociology of Education* 12(2): 191–215.

Fleckenstein, K. (1999) 'Writing bodies: somatic mind in composition studies', *College English* 61(3): 281–306.

Giddens, A. (1991) *Modernity and Self-Identity. Self and Society in the Late Modern Age*, Cambridge: Polity Press.

Giddens, A. (1994) *Beyond Left and Right: The Future of Radical Politics*, Cambridge: Polity Press.

Heidegger, M. (1938) *The Age of the World Picture. The Question Concerning Technology and Other Essays*, New York: Garland.

Hunter, L. (2001) 'The bodies we work with: students' bodies as a site for learning', paper presented at the ACHPER state conference, Brisbane.

Kelly, P., Hickey, C. and Tinning, R. (2000) 'Producing knowledge about physical education pedagogy: problematising the activities of expertise', *Quest* 52(3): 284–96.

Kemmis, S., Cole, P. and Suggett, D. (1983) *Orientations to Curriculum and Transition: Towards the Socially-critical School*, Melbourne: Victorian Institute of Secondary Education.

Kenway, J. (1998) *Education in the Age of Uncertainty: An Eagle's Eye View*, Geelong: Deakin University.

Kenway, J. and Bullen, E. (2001) *Consuming Children: Education – Entertainment – Advertising*, Buckingham: Open University Press.

Kenway, J., Bigum, C. and Fitzclarence, L. (1995) 'New education in new times', *Journal of Education Policy* 9(4): 317–33.

Kenworth Teather, E. (1999) 'Introduction: geographies of personal discovery', in E. Kenworth Teather (ed.) *Embodied Geographies: Spaces, Bodies and Rites of Passage*, London: Routledge.

Kirk, D. (1992) 'Physical education, discourse, and ideology: bringing the hidden curriculum into view' *Quest* 44: 35–56.

Kirk, D. (1993) *The Body, Schooling and Culture*, Geelong: Deakin University.

Kirk, D. (1999) 'Physical culture, physical education and relational analysis', *Sport, Education and Society* 4(1): 63–75.

Klein, N. (2000) *No Logo*, London: Flamingo.

Kwon, S.Y. and Harris, J. (2002) 'Working out your life: the discourse of lifestyle', paper presented at the International Sociological Association, Brisbane, July 2002.

Lather, P. (1998) 'Critical pedagogy and its complicities: a praxis of stuck places', *Educational Theory* 48(4): 487–97.

Law, J. (1994) *Organizing Modernity*, Oxford: Blackwell.

Light, R. and Kirk, D. (2000) 'High school rugby, the body and the reproduction of hegemonic masculinity', *Sport, Education and Society* 5(2): 163–77.

Luke, A. and Carrington, V. (2001) 'Globalisation, literacy, curriculum practice. Langauge and literacy in action', in R. Fisher, M. Lewis and G. Brooks (eds) *Language and Literacy in Action*, London: Routledge/Falmer.

Lundgren, U. (1983) *Curriculum Theory, Between Hope and Happening: Text and Context in Curriculum*, Geelong: Deakin University.

Lusted, D. (1986) 'Why pedagogy?', *Screen* 27(5): 2–14.

Macdonald, D., Glasby, T. and Carlson, T. (2000) 'The health and physical education statement and profile Queensland style', *ACHPER Healthy Lifestyles Journal* 47(1): 5–8.

Macdonald, D., Hunter, L., Carlson, T. and Penney, D. (2002) 'Teacher knowledge and the disjunction between school curricula and teacher education', *Asia-Pacific Journal of Teacher Education* 30(3): 259–75.

McLaren, P. (1998) 'Revolutionary pedagogy in post-revolutionary times: rethinking the political economy of critical education', *Educational Theory* 48(4): 431–62.

McWilliam, E. (1996) 'Touchy subjects: a risky inquiry into pedagogical pleasure', *British Educational Research Journal* 22(3): 305–17.

Miller, A. (1987) *For Your Own Good: Hidden Cruelty in Child-rearing and the Roots of Violence*, London:Virago.

O'Farrell, C., Meadmore, D., McWilliam, E. and Symes, C. (eds) (2000) *Taught Bodies*, New York: Peter Lang.

Oliver, K. (2001) 'Images of the body from popular culture: engaging adolescent girls in critical inquiry', *Sport, Education and Society* 6(2): 143–64.

O'Sullivan, M., Siedentop, D. and Locke, L. (1992) 'Toward collegiality: competing viewpoints among teacher educators', *Quest* 22: 266–80.

Petersen, A. and Lupton, D. (1996) *The New Public Health: Health and Self in the Age of Risk*, Sydney: Allen and Unwin.

Pronger, B. (1995) 'Rendering the body: the implicit lessons of gross anatomy', *Quest* 47: 427–46.

Pronger, B. (2002) *Body Fascism: Salvation in the Technology of Physical Fitness*, Toronto: University of Toronto Press.

Rose, N. (2000) 'Community, citizenship, and the third way', *American Behavioural Scientist* 43(9): 1395–411.

Shapiro, S. (2002) 'The life-world, body movements and new forms of emancipatory politics', in S. Shapiro and S. Shapiro (eds) *Body Movments: Pedagogy, Politics and Social Change*, Cresskill, NJ: Hampton Press.

Shilling, C. (1993) 'The body, class and social inequities: equality, education and physical education', in J. Evans (ed.) *Equality, Education and Physical Education*, London: Falmer Press.

Sparkes, A. (1997) 'Reflections on the socially constructed physical self. The physical self: from motivation to well-being', in K. Fox (ed.) *The Physical Self: From Motivation to Well-Being*, Champaign, IL: Human Kinetics.

Sparkes, A. (1999) 'Understanding physical education teachers: a focus on the lived body. Learning and teaching in physical education', in C. Hardy and M. Mawer (eds) *Learning and Teaching in Physical Education*, London: Falmer Press.

Steinberg, S. and Kincheloe, J. (eds) (1997) *Kinderculture: The Corporate Construction of Childhood*, Boulder: Westview Press.

Tinning, R. and Glasby, T. (2002) 'Pedagogical work and the 'cult of the body': considering the role of HPE in the context of the "new public health"', *Sport, Education and Society* 7(2):109–19.

Wexler, P. (1992) *Becoming Somebody: Toward a Social Psychology of School*, London: Falmer Press.

Wexler, P. (1995) 'After postmodernism: a new age social theory in education', in R. Smith and P. Wexler (eds) *After Postmodernism: Education, Politics and Identity*, London: Falmer Press.

Whitty, G. (1985) *Sociology and School Knowledge: Curriculum Theory, Research and Politics*, London: Methuen.

Wright, J. (2000) 'Bodies, meanings and movement: a comparison of the language of a physical education lesson and a Feldenkrais movement class', *Sport, Education and Society* 5(1): 35–51.

Wright, J., O'Flynn, G. and Macdonald, D. (2002) 'Physical activity in the lives of young women and men: embodied identities', paper presented to the Australian Association for Research in Education Annual Conference, Brisbane 2002.

Index

Sport, Education and Society

EDITOR
John Evans
Loughborough University, UK

Sport, Education and Society is an international journal which provides a focal
point for the publication of research on pedagogy, policy and the wide range of
associated social, cultural, political and ethical issues in physical activity and sport.
The journal concentrates both on the forms, contents and contexts of physical
education and sport found in schools, colleges and other sites of formal education.
The journal also focuses on pedagogies of play, callisthenics, gymnastics and sport
found in familial environments, various sport clubs, the leisure industry, as well as
private fitness and health studios, dance schools, gymnastic clubs and rehabilitation
centres.

Sport, Education and Society encourages contributions not only from sports
scientists and educationalists working in the field of pedagogy but also from
professionals with interests in theoretical and empirical issues relating to pedagogy,
policy and the curriculum in physical activity and sport.

This journal is also available online.
Please connect to www.tandf.co.uk/online.html for further information.

To request a sample copy please visit: **www.tandf.co.uk/journals**

SUBSCRIPTION RATES

2004 – Volume 9 (Increased to 3 issues per year)
Print ISSN 1357-3322
Online ISSN 1470-126X
Institutional rate: US$345; £209
(includes free online access)
Personal rate: US$130; £80 (print only)

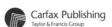
Carfax Publishing
Taylor & Francis Group

ORDER FORM   cses

PLEASE COMPLETE IN BLOCK CAPITALS AND RETURN TO THE ADDRESS BELOW

Please invoice me at the ☐ **institutional rate** ☐ **personal rate**

Name _____

Address _____

_____

_____

Email _____

Please contact Customer Services at either:

Taylor & Francis Ltd, Rankine Road, Basingstoke, Hants RG24 8PR, UK
Tel: +44 (0)1256 813002   **Fax:** +44 (0)1256 330245   **Email:** enquiry@tandf.co.uk   **Website:** www.tandf.co.uk

Taylor & Francis Inc, 325 Chestnut Street, 8th Floor, Philadelphia, PA 19106, USA
Tel: +1 215 6258900 **Fax:** +1 215 6258914   **Email:** info@taylorandfrancis.com   **Website:** www.taylorandfrancis.com